First Responder: Skills in Action

NATIONAL SAFETY COUNCIL

Boston   Burr Ridge, IL   Dubuque, IA   New York   San Francisco   St. Louis
Bangkok   Bogotá   Caracas   Kuala Lumpur   Lisbon   London   Madrid   Mexico City
Milan   Montreal   New Delhi   Santiago   Seoul   Singapore   Sydney   Taipei   Toronto

Other titles available from the National Safety Council

National Safety Council: *First Aid: Taking Action*

National Safety Council: *Standard First Aid, CPR, and AED*, 2e

National Safety Council: *First Aid*, 2e

National Safety Council: *CPR and AED*, 2e

National Safety Council: *Bloodborne and Airborne Pathogens*

National Safety Council: *Pediatric First Aid, CPR, and AED*, 2e

National Safety Council: *Basic Life Support: Healthcare and Professional Rescuers*

About the National Safety Council

Founded in 1913, the National Safety Council (NSC) is a nonprofit membership organization devoted to making our world safer. Its mission is to educate and influence people to prevent accidental injury and death. For more than 90 years, the National Safety Council has been the leader in protecting life and promoting health in the workplace. The Council has helped make great improvements in safety with an expanded focus on safety on the roads and in the home and community. Working through its 48, members, and in partnership with public agencies, private groups, and other associations, the Council serves as an impartial information gathering and distribution organization. The NSC disseminates safety, health, and environmental materials through a network of regional offices, chapters, and training centers.

The NSC's First Aid and CPR/AED courses have grown to meet the changing needs of emergency responders at all levels of expertise. Upon completing this course, you will join millions of emergency responders trained to protect life and promote health.

Author Acknowledgements

Many National Safety Council staff and affiliates have contributed to the production of this book and we would like to acknowledge the following people for their assistance:

Paul Satterlee, MD, Medical Director, for reviewing and providing oversight of the content;

Tom Lochhaas, Editorial Services, for providing technical writing services;

Donna M. Siegfried, Executive Director, Emergency Care, for providing vision and support;

Barbara Caracci, Director of Emergency Care Programs and Training, for providing oversight of content and interfacing with McGraw-Hill staff on all areas of development and production;

Donna Fredenhagen, Product Manager, for providing marketing support;

Kathy Safranek, Project Administrator, for providing day-to-day assistance.

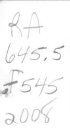

Higher Education

FIRST RESPONDER: SKILLS IN ACTION

Published by McGraw-Hill, a business unit of The McGraw-Hill Companies, Inc., 1221 Avenue of the Americas, New York, NY 10020. Copyright © 2008 by the National Safety Council. All rights reserved. No part of this publication may be reproduced or distributed in any form or by any means, or stored in a database or retrieval system, without the prior written consent of the National Safety Council, including, but not limited to, in any network or other electronic storage or transmission, or broadcast for distance learning.

✪ This book is printed on recycled, acid-free paper containing 10% postconsumer waste.

1 2 3 4 5 6 7 8 9 0 QPV/QPV 0 9 8 7

ISBN 978–0–07–352196–1
MHID 0–07–352196–5

Publisher, Career Education: *David T. Culverwell*
Senior Sponsoring Editor: *Claire Merrick*
Developmental Editor: *Michelle Zeal*
Outside Developmental Services: *Julie Scardiglia*
Senior Marketing Manager: *Lisa Nicks*
Senior Project Manager: *Sheila M. Frank*
Senior Production Supervisor: *Laura Fuller*
Senior Coordinator of Freelance Design: *Michelle D. Whitaker*
Cover/Interior Designer: *Studio Montage*
 (USE) Cover Image: *(c) National Safety Council/Rick Brady, photographer*
Lead Photo Research Coordinator: *Carrie K. Burger*
Photo Researcher: *Pam Carley*
Compositor: *Electronic Publishing Services Inc., NYC*
Typeface: *11.5/13 Minion*
Printer: *Quebecor World Versailles, KY*

ISSN 1932-5576

Photo Credits: Figure 6.1: © AP Photo/The Examiner, Jay Westcott; **Figure 11.11:** © Mediscan; **Figure 11.12:** © SIU/Visuals Unlimited; **Figure 13.1:** © Tierbild Okapia/Photo Researchers, Inc.; **Figures 13.2, 13.3:** © Dr. P. Marazzi/Photo Researchers, Inc.; **Figure 13.4:** © Custom Medical Stock Photo; **Figure 13.13:** Courtesy Trauma.org; **Figures 13.20, 13.21:** © Dr. P. Marazzi/Photo Researchers, Inc.; **Figure 13.22:** © Image courtesy Bradley R. Davis; **Figure 13.24:** © Dr. P. Marazzi/Photo Researchers, Inc.; **Figure 13.27, Figure 14.5:** © Mediscan; **CO 16:** © Rick Wilking/Reuters/Corbis; **Figure 17.8:** © Mediscan; **Figure 18.11:** © Brent Larson/fStop/Getty Images; **Figure 18.12:** © Joyce Naltchayan/AFP/Getty Images; **Figure 18.13:** © Vincent Laforet/Pool/Reuters/Corbis; **CO 19:** © David McNew/Getty Images; all other photographs © National Safety Council/Rick Brady, photographer.

NATIONAL SAFETY COUNCIL MISSION STATEMENT
The mission of the National Safety Council is to educate and influence people to prevent accidental injury and death.

DISCLAIMER
Although the information and recommendations contained in this publication have been
compiled from sources believed to be reliable, the National Safety Council makes no guarantee as to, and assumes no responsibility for, the correctness, sufficiency, or completeness of such information or recommendations. Other or additional safety measures may be required under particular circumstances.

www.mhhe.com

Detailed Table of Contents

Chapter 19

The National Incident Management

System and Mass-Casualty Incidents . . 306

Appendix A:

Answers to "Do You Understand?"

Index of Skills

Preface

Congratulations on your decision to become a First Responder!

As a First Responder, you will be an important part of the Emergency Medical Services (EMS) system, providing crucial emergency care for people who are injured or suddenly ill. This text and the accompanying supplements are designed to provide you with the knowledge and skills so that you can give immediate, on-scene care to ill and injured individuals. The text and other materials cover all the information in the U.S. Department of Transportation (DOT) First Responder National Standard Curriculum, as well as additional information typically included in First Responder training. This course is based on the latest Guidelines for CPR and Emergency Cardiac Care.

The National Safety Council developed *First Responder: Skills in Action* as a combination text and workbook to provide you with all the information and step-by-step skills you need to fill an essential role as part of an emergency healthcare team. A list format is used throughout the text, as appropriate, to present information in an easily grasped format. Additionally, the text focuses on information essential for First Responder practice rather than providing extensive tangential information.

In using this book, begin by reading the Chapter Preview to get a glimpse of the chapter topics. From there, read the "You Respond To. . ." case study, which provides a typical emergency scenario that a First Responder may encounter in the field. By the end of the chapter, you will know what to do in this emergency.

As you move through each chapter, you'll notice that information is organized so that you can learn and review essential information in a manner emphasizing patient care priorities. Features such as "Need to Know," "Need to Recognize," and "Need to Do" help you focus on the essential information you need to treat patients effectively in the field. The Skills provide step-by-step directions and images so that you can give patients quality emergency care.

Also included throughout the text are the four consistent steps of the standard First Responder patient assessment. The four primary actions for standard First Responder patient care are also emphasized, along with additional emergency care steps to take depending on the particular injury or illness.

Throughout each chapter, you will have multiple opportunities to test your knowledge. "Do You Understand?" workbook sections appear in key places within each chapter to help you check your understanding as you read, and multiple-choice review questions are included at the end of each chapter to ensure you have mastered key chapter content. Answers to both are provided in the Appendix.

First Responders come from all walks of life. Whether you are providing care in an industrial, community, rural, or other setting, or employed as a firefighter, police officer, lifeguard, or in another role, this book and its accompanying supplements will help you provide effective emergency patient care—while helping to keep you safe.

Key Features

- **Chapter Preview.** This listing of topics at the opening of the chapter provides learners with a bulleted list of the major chapter topics.

- **You Respond To ...** Each chapter opens with a typical emergency situation to which First Responders may be called. The scenario pertains to information discussed in the chapter and helps set expectations for how learners can apply their knowledge by the end of the chapter.

- **Introduction.** The introduction provides readers with a brief overview of the core chapter content.

- **Icons.** For what First Responders **Need to Know, Need to Recognize,** and **Need to Do.**

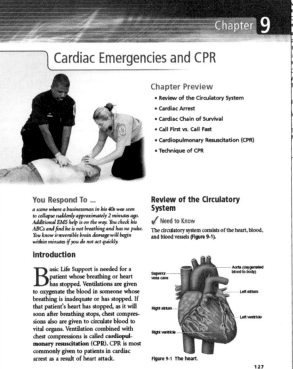

Information in most chapters is organized in a consistent pattern to help readers learn and review key information and emergency care priorities. "Need to Know" sections present information that learners should understand to be able to provide effective patient care. "Need to Recognize" sections focus on patient assessment as the basis of all emergency care, including the signs and symptoms of injuries and illness First Responders are likely to encounter in emergency care. "Need to Do" sections provide the steps for actions to take in each emergency situation.

- **Standard First Responder Assessment.** The four assessment steps taken with every emergency patient are included along with the assessments for specific injuries and illnesses to reinforce the consistent approach used in all emergencies.

- **Standard First Responder Patient Care.** The four primary actions taken by First Responders caring for any patient are highlighted along with additional steps to take depending on the particular injury or illness.

---

224   First Responder: Skills in Action

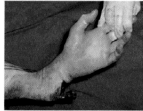

Figure 14-5 Open fracture.

☑ **Muscle Injuries.** Common muscle injuries include strains, contusions, and cramps. These injuries are usually less serious than fractures and joint injuries. Muscle injuries are typically caused by overexertion, careless or sudden uncoordinated movements, or poor body mechanics, such as lifting a weight with the back bent or twisted.

In some cases, the type of injury may be obvious, while in many cases you will recognize only that a musculoskeletal injury is present but will not know what kind. The emergency care for most patients with musculoskeletal injuries is the same regardless of the type.

🔍 Do You Understand?

1. Large forces are more likely to result in _____ or _____ (types of musculoskeletal injuries).

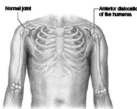

Figure 14-6 A deformity may occur with a dislocation.

2. An elderly patient suffering trauma is more likely than a younger patient to suffer a fracture because of _____.

3. What may result from a dislocation that can cause a serious or even life-threatening condition? _____

Assessment of Musculoskeletal Injuries

✓ Need to Know

Remember to perform the initial assessment of any patient and care for any life-threatening conditions before performing a physical examination. Musculoskeletal injuries are usually not life threatening, except in cases of severe bleeding, but may nonetheless be serious and result in pain and disability.

☑ Ask a responsive patient what happened and what he or she felt when the injury occurred.

☑ If large forces were involved in the injury, consider the potential also for a spinal injury. Particularly if the patient is unresponsive, do not move him or her unnecessarily to assess a musculoskeletal injury.

■■ Need to Recognize

Perform the standard assessment:

1. Size up the scene before beginning emergency medical care.
2. Complete the initial assessment.
3. Perform a physical examination as appropriate.
4. Complete ongoing assessments.

In addition:

♦ Expose the injury site (control bleeding as needed).

♦ Recognize that the amount of pain or swelling is not a good indicator of the seriousness of the injury.

♦ Assess for circulation, sensation, and movement (CSM) below the injury site:
— Check for a pulse below the injury (radial pulse in the wrist or pedal pulse in the foot) and for skin color and temperature.
— Check for sensation by touching the patient's fingers or toes to determine whether the patient can feel your touch or feels a tingling sensation or numbness.
— Check movement by asking the patient to wiggle the fingers or toes, unless doing so causes pain.

♦ A lack of circulation or possible nerve damage indicated by abnormal sensation or movement indicates a need for immediate medical treatment.

Signs and symptoms of musculoskeletal injuries (Figure 14-7):

♦ Deformity of the area or angulation of the extremity (compare to the other extremity)
♦ Pain and tenderness
♦ A feeling or sound of bone ends grating together (crepitus)
♦ Swelling
♦ Skin discoloration: Bruising or a pale or light blue skin color (an ashen color in dark-skinned individuals), along with cool skin, may indicate a lack of blood flow below the injured area.
♦ Bone ends exposed in an open wound
♦ Joint locked into position
♦ Abnormal sensation (numbness, tingling)
♦ Inability to move the area
♦ Difference in temperature from the opposite extremity

Emergency Care of Musculoskeletal Injuries

✓ Need to Know

Any movement of a musculoskeletal injury can cause further injury, pain, and swelling. With a fracture or dislocation, movement of the extremity could cause the bone to move, further injuring soft tissues such as blood vessels and nerves. Movement also generally increases blood flow, which may increase internal bleeding and swelling.

Injuries to Muscles and Bones   225

Manually stabilizing or splinting the injured area is therefore a key part of emergency care.

▶ Need to Do

Perform standard patient care:

1. Ensure EMS has been activated.
2. Take body substance isolation precautions.
3. Maintain the patient's airway and provide artificial ventilation if needed.
4. Comfort, calm, and reassure the patient while awaiting additional EMS resources.

In addition:

♦ After any life threats have been controlled, allow the patient to remain in a position of comfort.
♦ Cover open wounds with a sterile dressing.
♦ Put a cold pack on an area of painful, swollen, deformed extremity to reduce swelling and pain, except on an open fracture.
♦ Do not try to replace bones protruding from a wound.
♦ Stabilize an injured extremity manually, or have the patient manually support the area.
— Support above and below an injury.
— Pad the area to prevent pressure and discomfort.
— When in doubt, manually stabilize the injury.
♦ Follow local protocol to administer oxygen if it is available and you are so trained.
♦ If appropriate, splint the extremity.

🔍 Do You Understand?

1. What three things should you assess distal to a musculoskeletal injury?

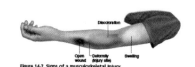

Figure 14-7 Signs of a musculoskeletal injury.

- **Skills.** Key First Responder actions are presented visually in easy-to-follow step-by-step procedures.

- **Do You Understand?** These workbook sections appear in key places within chapters to help learners confirm their understanding of preceding topics and retain information. Correct answers and explanations are located in the Appendix.

- **Tables.** Informative tables provide readers with detailed information to help them understand the topics presented, including the latest injury statistics from the National Safety Council.

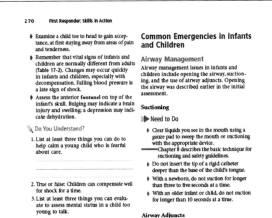

270   First Responder: Skills in Action

- Examine a child toe to head to gain acceptance, at first staying away from areas of pain and tenderness.
- Remember that vital signs of infants and children are normally different from adults (Table 17-2). Changes may occur quickly in infants and children, especially with decompensation. Falling blood pressure is a late sign of shock.
- Assess the anterior fontanel on top of the infant's skull. Bulging may indicate a brain injury and swelling; a depression may indicate dehydration.

Do You Understand?

1. List at least three things you can do to help calm a young child who is fearful about care.

2. True or false: Children can compensate well for shock for a time.
3. List at least three things you can evaluate to assess mental status in a child too young to talk.

n your initial assessment, you find that an unresponsive toddler is breathing lowly and has a pulse of 40 along with igns of poor perfusion. What should ou do?

Common Emergencies in Infants and Children

Airway Management

Airway management issues in infants and children include opening the airway, suctioning, and the use of airway adjuncts. Opening the airway was described earlier in the initial assessment.

Suctioning

▶ Need to Do

- Clear liquids you see in the mouth using a gauze pad to sweep the mouth or suctioning with the appropriate device.
  Chapter 8 describes the basic technique for suctioning and safety guidelines.
- Do not insert the tip of a rigid catheter deeper than the base of the child's tongue.
- With a newborn, do not suction for longer than three to five seconds at a time.
- With an older infant or child, do not suction for longer than 10 seconds at a time.

Airway Adjuncts

▶ Need to Do

Use an oral airway to maintain the airway open in an unresponsive child without a gag reflex. Remove the airway if the child gags, coughs, or otherwise responds to an attempt to insert it.

- Use the oral airway to maintain an open airway but not for initial ventilations.

ble 17-2

rmal Vital Signs

nt	Infant	Child	Adult
mal Respiratory Rate at Rest	20-30	18-30	12-20
mal Pulse Rate at Rest	80-150	70-130	60-100
mal Blood Pressure (systolic/diastolic)	84-106/56-70	98-124/50-80	118-140/60-90

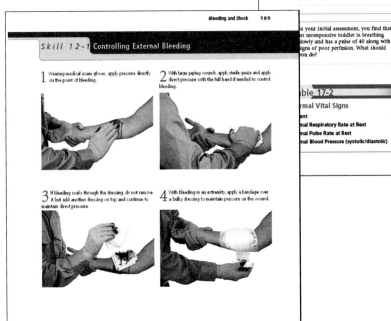

Bleeding and Shock   189

Skill 12-1 Controlling External Bleeding

1 Wearing medical exam gloves, apply pressure directly on the point of bleeding.

2 With large gaping wounds, apply sterile gauze and apply direct pressure with the full hand if needed to control bleeding.

3 If bleeding soaks through the dressing, do not remove it but add another dressing on top and continue to maintain direct pressure.

4 With bleeding in an extremity, apply a bandage over a bulky dressing to maintain pressure on the wound.

- **Conclusion.** At the end of the chapter, this feature summarizes the First Responder's role relative to the chapter topic, noting the primary actions that a First Responder must undertake.

- **Key Terms** used in the chapter are listed at the end of the chapter to help ensure learners know appropriate medical and other emergency terminology helpful for providing care and communicating with other EMS professionals. Page numbers are provided for the defining explanation of these terms to make review convenient when needed.

- **Review Questions** in multiple-choice format included at the end of each chapter help learners review chapter content and continue to reinforce knowledge and skills. Answers are provided in the Appendix.

Ventilation Devices and Oxygen | 25

Key Terms

airways (p. 111)
bag mask (p. 116)
bulb syringe (p. 110)
flow meter (p. 121)
nasal airway (p. 116)
nasal cannula (p. 122)
nasopharyngeal airway (NPA) (p. 116)
nonrebreathing mask (p. 122)
oral airway (p. 114)
oropharyngeal airway (OPA) (p. 114)
oxygen delivery device (p. 121)
oxygen reservoir (p. 120)
pressure regulator (p. 121)
suction (p. 110)
supplemental oxygen (p. 121)

Review Questions

1. In an infant, you should not suction more than how many seconds at a time?
   a. 2
   b. 5
   c. 10
   d. 15

   To determine the maximum depth of the suction tip's insertion, measure from the
   a. eyebrow to the corner of the mouth.
   b. outside corner of the eye to the earlobe.
   c. nostril to the earlobe.
   d. earlobe to the corner of the mouth.

   If a patient vomits,
   a. sweep out solids and fluid with your finger before suctioning.
   b. sweep out solids and fluid with your finger after suctioning.
   c. sweep out solids and fluid with your finger during suctioning.
   d. do not use your finger to sweep the mouth; use suction only.

4. To choose the correct size oral airway, measure from the
   a. eyebrow to the corner of the mouth.
   b. outside corner of the eye to the earlobe.
   c. nostril to the earlobe.
   d. earlobe to the corner of the mouth.

5. Use a nasal airway rather than an oral airway in a patient who
   a. is wearing dentures.
   b. needs oxygen.
   c. is responsive.
   d. may have a spinal injury.

6. The bag of a bag mask for use on an infant is
   a. about 1/3 the volume of an adult bag.
   b. about 1/2 the volume of an adult bag.
   c. the same volume as a child bag.
   d. the same volume as an adult bag.

7. The best way to connect oxygen tubing to a bag mask is
   a. to an oxygen reservoir bag.
   b. to the bag you squeeze.
   c. to a portal in the mask.
   d. Oxygen tubing cannot be attached to a bag mask.

8. Give ventilations by squeezing the bag over
   a. 1 second.   c. 3 seconds.
   b. 2 seconds.   d. 4 seconds.

9. Oxygen may be delivered to a patient through
   a. any resuscitation mask.
   b. a resuscitation mask with a special port.
   c. only a nonrebreathing mask.
   d. any face shield.

10. Which oxygen delivery device is best to use for ventilating an unresponsive nonbreathing patient?
    a. Nasal cannula
    b. Resuscitation mask
    c. Nonrebreathing mask with reservoir bag
    d. Bag mask with reservoir bag

The Well-Being of the First Responder | 29

Following a natural disaster, rescue efforts are generally coordinated through a governmental agency. As always, make personal safety your top priority. Work with the disaster response team, and do not deviate from the rescue plan (Chapter 18).

Natural disasters often pose more hazards than one might think. Many injuries and deaths after natural disasters result from hazards such as electricity, hazardous materials, and fast water rather than directly from the disaster. Minimize your risk by carefully surveying the scene, avoiding obvious hazards, and using caution when operating rescue equipment. For example, gasoline-operated rescue equipment such as chain saws, generators, and sump pumps should never be used in confined spaces.

Unsafe Buildings and Structures

Buildings and other structures may be unsafe because of a fire, explosion, natural disaster, or deterioration. Many different problems may be present, such as:

- An injured victim may be confined or trapped.
- The atmosphere may contain a hazardous gas.
- Communication with a victim may be impossible.

As always, personal safety is the primary concern. The exact or probable location of the victim should be established and a rescue plan devised. Never enter an unsafe building alone. Leave this type of rescue to personnel with proper training and equipment.

Wreckage

Wreckage from an automobile, aircraft, or machinery is hazardous. Hazards include sharp pieces of metal, glass, fuel, and moving parts. In addition, the wreckage may be unstable. Attempt rescue of a victim from wreckage only if you have the proper equipment and training and only after the wreckage has been adequately stabilized. Specific rescue techniques are described in Chapter 18.

Do You Understand?

1. True or false: In an emergency scene where fumes may be present, you may run in and remove the patient if you hold your breath.

2. True or false: A First Responder's responsibilities at a hazardous scene include protecting bystanders.

3. At the scene of a vehicle crash, your responsibilities include:
   a. Removing the victim as quickly as possible from the vehicle
   b. Removing any power lines that have fallen onto the vehicle
   c. Using warning devices to warn oncoming traffic
   d. Disarming the vehicle's airbag

Conclusion

Your well-being as a First Responder depends on understanding and coping with the stress of emergencies, protecting yourself from infectious disease, and staying safe in hazardous scenes. Always remember that safety is your highest priority in any emergency.

Key Terms

acquired immunodeficiency syndrome (AIDS) (p. 19)
airborne transmission (p. 20)
bloodborne transmission (p. 20)
body substance isolation (BSI) (p. 21)

critical incident (p. 18)
Critical Incident Stress Debriefing (CISD) (p. 18)
critical incident stress management (CISM) (p. 18)
debriefing (p. 18)
decontamination (p. 22)
defusing (p. 18)

Publisher's Acknowledgements

David M. Andrade, BS, Paramedic, EMS Instructor
Lt. of Training, Stratford EMS, Central High School
Bridgeport, CT

Neal Arrington
Palmetto Safety Services
Goose Creek, SC

Mendee Bayless-Tarnowski, BS, NREMT-P
Hennepin County Medical Center
Minneapolis, MN

Paul A. Bishop
Monroe Community College, Public Safety
Training Center
Rochester, NY

Bryan E. Bledsoe, DO, FACEP
Midlothian, Texas

Keith W. Bowman, NREMT-B
Wilmington, DE

Dr. Nicholas J. DiCicco
Camden Community College
Blackwood, NJ

H. Stephen Erb, CIC
Rochester, NY Fire Academy
Rochester, NY

Sandra K. Eustice
Chippewa Valley Technical College
Eau Claire, WI

Jeffrey S. Force, BA, NREMT-P
Pikes Peak Community College
Colorado Springs, CO

Dan Garner
Education Affiliates
Medix School
Smyrna, GA

Jay D. Johns III, NREMT-P, BS, Ed.
EMS Educator-EMT-P Department
Southwestern Illinois College, Memorial Hospital
Belleville, IL

Bob Lynch, EMT-P/IC
Tennessee Technological University
Cookeville, TN

Anthony E.Marzano, CEM, EMT-B
Will County Emergency Management Agency
Joliet, IL

Stephen J. Nardozzi
Westchester Community College
Department of Prehospital EMS
Valhalla, NY

John Pelazza, Paramedic, EMS Coordinator
Bridgeport Hospital
Bridgeport, CT

Del Preuss
Minnesota State Community and Technical
College
Moorhead, MN

Robb S. Rehberg, PhD, ATC, NREMT
Director of Emergency Services
Coordinator, Office of Emergency Management
Montclair State University
Upper Montclair, NJ

Dr. Harold F. Risk
St. Cloud State University
St. Cloud, MN

Dave Sarazin, M.Ed., NREMT-P
Lake Superior College ERTC
Duluth, MN

Craig Spector, President
CPR Heart Starters, Inc.
Warrington, PA

Jeremy Tiermini, MSS, ATC
Finger Lakes Community College
Canandaigua, NY

Marilyn B. Vojta, M.A., EMSI
Darien EMS
Darien, CT

Advance Comments From the Field

The text had good study materials built into it. Good incorporation of new AHA BLS guidelines and good self-review questions.

Jeffrey S. Force, BA, NREMT-P
Pikes Peak Community College
Colorado Springs, CO

I REALLY like the outline style. It is organized and logical, and seems easy for a First Responder to follow. I prefer minimal elaboration from the text because it allows me to supplement and reinforce the information with lecture in class. This format provides students with "need-to-know" information while requiring them to gain the practical knowledge and "whys" from the instructor.

Mendee Bayless-Tarnowski, BS,
NREMT-P
Hennepin County Medical Center
Minneapolis, MN

I was very impressed with the layout—the content was very good and easy for everyone to understand. I was especially impressed with the key words and their page references for easy access. The review questions were well done.

Keith W. Bowman, NREMT-B
Wilmington, DE

I am thrilled with the streamlined appproach you have taken. Your text is straight to the point. The levels of discussion are consistent throughout the chapter, making the content very easy for a student with no medical training to comprehend. It seems that it would be very easy to instruct with and add instructor touches in the classroom.

The "Do You Understand?" sections are a major strength. An instructor can cover the material and immediately review it with students to assure that there was an adequate exchange of information.

Bob Lynch, EMT-P/IC
Tennessee Technological University
Cookeville, TN

I was very impressed with the manuscript and thought it was well written and well planned. The preliminaries come first and then the more detailed parts come afterwards. I actually do teach in this order. I think the order is well planned.

I like the way each chapter opens with a scenario and then closes with a summary and review questions. I also like the chapter preview, which gives the reader a look at what's coming up in the chapter, as well as the "Need to Know" and "Need to Recognize" sections. I also like the use of lots of bulleted points instead of paragraphs. I think it will make the text easy to understand. The material and content is very well done and appropriate for this level of course.

David M. Andrae, BX, Paramedic,
EMS Instructor
Lt. of Training, Stratford EMS,
Central High School
Bridgeport, CT

I found it very easy to follow and the important material was clearly defined by the headings before each segment. I like the brief "Need to Know" segment at the beginning of each topic.

You have done an excellent job of making sure that the topic is easy to follow and that the information is concise and to the point. The content was very accurate, and written at a level that was easy to understand for First Responders.

John Pelazza, Paramedic,
EMS Coordinator
Bridgeport Hospital
Bridgeport, CT

The quality of the writing is excellent. It really provides the right information in an appropriate manner. I really like the depth of information.

I would use every chapter, focusing primarily on the chapters involving hand-on emergency skills. The overall content of the material is excellent. I have yet to see a chapter that I didn't like better than the current text I am using!

Jeremy Tiermini, MSS, ATC
Finger Lakes Community College
Canandaigua, NY

First Responder: Skills in Action

NATIONAL SAFETY COUNCIL

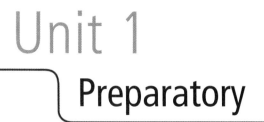
Unit 1
Preparatory

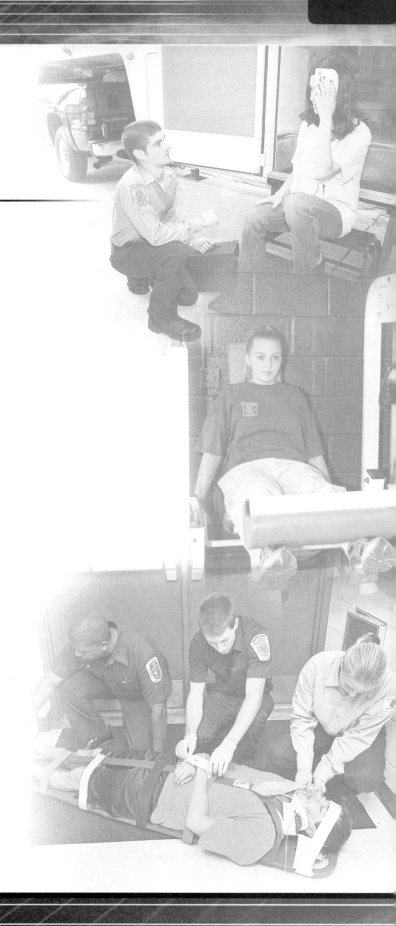

Chapter 1

Introduction to the EMS System

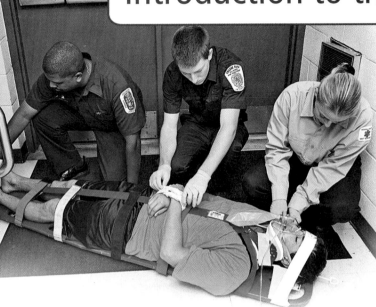

Chapter Preview

- Emergencies
- The Emergency Medical Services System
- Accessing EMS
- Roles and Responsibilities of First Responders
- Medical Oversight

You Respond To ...

a nearby construction scene when radioed by a foreman. A construction worker has fallen from a low ladder. He has a sharp pain in one leg but says he can move the leg and does not think it is broken. No one has called 911 yet, and the worker and foreman look to you for a decision about what to do.

Introduction

Congratulations on your decision to become a First Responder! First Responders are an essential part of the **Emergency Medical Services (EMS) system,** which provides needed emergency care for people who are injured or suddenly ill.

- **First Responders** are often the first *trained* persons to reach an ill or injured patient.

- A First Responder is an individual, paid or volunteer, routinely summoned to provide care in an emergency.

- First Responders, unlike lay persons, have a professional duty to respond to the scene of a medical emergency and to provide emergency medical care to the ill or injured.

- First Responders, unlike lay persons, usually have ready access to first aid supplies and equipment for providing care until more advanced medical care is available.

In some occupations, such as law enforcement and fire fighting, First Responders are required to respond to and assist at the scene of a medical emergency. First Responders may also work in many other occupations and roles that, on occasion, involve assisting at the scene of a medical emergency. Examples include:

- Industrial safety officers
- Prison guards
- Lifeguards
- Daycare attendants
- Athletic trainers
- Ski patrol members
- Civil defense personnel
- Disaster team members

Regardless of your occupation, when called, you have a duty to quickly and safely respond to the scene of the medical emergency, provide necessary emergency medical care, activate the EMS system, assist EMS personnel, and document the actions you took.

Emergencies

A medical emergency is any situation in which a person suddenly needs medical care. Typically the person is injured in an accident or experiences sudden illness.* The emergency may be life-threatening, which means the person may die if he or she does not receive treatment very soon. In the United States every year:

- ☑ Almost 40 million visits are made to emergency departments because of injuries
- ☑ 2 million people are hospitalized because of injuries
- ☑ 140,000 die from injuries
- ☑ 180,000 die from heart attacks
- ☑ 162,000 die from strokes

Tables 1-1 and 1-2, respectively, list the most common causes of injuries for which patients go to a hospital emergency department and the

*The term **sudden illness** is generally used to describe medical conditions that occur suddenly and require emergency care until the patient can be seen by a medical professional. This term will be used throughout this text. "Sudden" illness is generally different from other illness situations in which the sick person is already under the care of a healthcare professional or has time to see a healthcare professional for a nonemergency condition. In some cases a person with a nonemergency chronic illness, such as diabetes or asthma, may suddenly experience an emergency situation as a result of that illness. That emergency, such as a person with asthma having an attack and not being able to breathe, is then called sudden illness.

Table 1-1

Injuries Annually Treated in Hospital Emergency Departments

Falls	7,989,000
Motor vehicle crashes	4,582,000
Struck by or against object	4,209,000
Cut or pierced by object	2,544,000
Overexertion and strenuous movements	1,686,000
Assault	1,608,000
Bites and stings (other than dog bites)	998,000
Poisoning (includes drug overdose)	750,000
Burns	516,000
Attempted suicide	438,000

Source: National Safety Council, Injury Facts 2005.

Table 1-2

Annual Deaths Due to Selected Injuries

Motor vehicle crashes	45,549
Suicide	31,655
Poisoning (includes drug overdose)	17,550
Falls	16,257
Assault by firearm	11,829
Choking	4,934
Drowning	3,447
Smoke, fire, flames	3,159
Mechanical forces	2,871
Assault by sharp objects	2,074
Bicycle crashes	767
Cold exposure	646
Water transport/boating accidents	617
Other breathing threats	583
Electrocution	454
Heat exposure	350
Burns	102
Venomous animals and plants	76

Source: National Safety Council, Injury Facts 2005.

annual deaths resulting from the most common types of injuries. These statistics, however, show only how common injuries are. If you compare the numbers of those who die from injuries with the numbers of those given emergency medical treatment for injuries, it is readily seen that millions of people every year are saved from death, disability, or pain and suffering by Emergency Medical Services. First Responders have a large role in the success of this system.

- ☑ As **Figure 1-1** shows, motor vehicle crashes account for most accidental injury deaths, followed by injuries in the home, public places, and work. Injuries and sudden illness may strike at any time in any place.

- ☑ When an emergency occurs outside a hospital or other healthcare facility, First Responders usually have a role in providing care until the patient can receive advanced medical help through the EMS system.

The Emergency Medical Services System

✓ Need to Know

As a First Responder, you are part of the **Emergency Medical Services (EMS) system,** a complex healthcare system designed to pro-

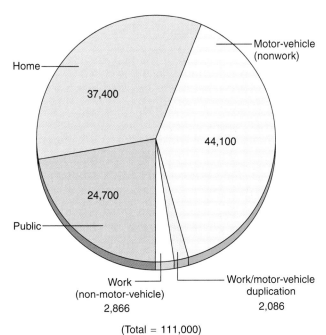

Figure 1-1 Unintentional injury deaths by class, United States, 2004. (National Safety Council, Injury Facts 2005.)

vide immediate, on-scene care to ill and injured patients.

Until the 1970s, the quality of emergency care outside of hospitals was poor. Ambulance attendants were trained only to retrieve ill or injured patients and rush them as rapidly as possible to the hospital to receive emergency care. The Emergency Medical Services Act of 1973 established a nationwide system of emergency healthcare. The EMS system as it exists today has evolved over the years to a highly sophisticated network of services for providing emergency care as quickly and effectively as possible. Anywhere in the United States, a single telephone call for help initiates an often complex set of actions and responses to rush medical care to the patient rather than just rushing the patient to the hospital.

Accessing EMS

The EMS system is activated when someone calls for help, usually with a telephone call to 911 or another local emergency number. Most communities have a centralized 911 system: the call to 911 for any type of emergency reaches a **dispatcher** who then sends the needed resources to the scene.

In the basic 911 system, callers need to identify their name, location, and the number they are calling from in addition to information about the injured or ill person or other emergency. Many communities now have an **enhanced 911** system that automatically provides the dispatcher with the caller's phone number and location when a land telephone line is being used. This information can be lifesaving if the call is interrupted or comes from a young child or patient who cannot identify their location.

Even with the enhanced 911 system, however, callers should not assume the dispatcher knows their location. The caller may need to specify the exact location—such as to say you are with a patient in the backyard—to prevent the loss of precious time while EMTs knock at the front door. With calls from cellular telephones the dispatcher cannot know the caller's location.

The process of the EMS response begins when someone recognizes that an emergency has occurred and proceeds through a number of steps to the point where the patient is receiving in-hospital care.

EMS Response to Emergencies

A typical EMS response to a medical emergency involves a series of steps (**Figure 1-2**):

1. **Medical emergency occurs**—The emergency begins when a person is injured or suddenly becomes ill. This can occur anywhere and at anytime.

2. **Recognition of the emergency and activation of EMS**—Often the injured or ill person cannot call for help. The emergency may be discovered by someone nearby such as a family member or fellow worker, who calls for help and activates the EMS system. The call is usually received by a centralized EMS dispatcher. This person is highly skilled in obtaining information and determining what emergency equipment will likely be required. The EMS dispatcher will dispatch the appropriate EMS unit.

3. **First aid by a citizen responder**—A person who is nearby or who discovers the injury or illness may provide first aid if he or she has been trained. The prompt initiation of first aid or cardiopulmonary resuscitation (CPR) by bystanders often means the difference between life and death for the patient. The dispatcher may also give the lay person instructions for care to give the patient until help arrives. This should be maintained until the first component of the EMS system arrives.

4. **First Responder arrival**—The first EMS personnel to arrive at the scene of a medical emergency are usually First Responders.* First Responders may be police officers, fire fighters, industrial safety officers, or similar persons often close to the scene and who have a professional duty to respond. The First Responder often assumes care of the patient from citizen responders and gathers information concerning the patient. Citizen responders do not frequently deal with injured or ill persons and may experience fear or apprehension. Your caring and professional attitude can help allay the citizen responder's fears as well as the patient's. Often assisted by the

*Note: First Responders are generally part of the EMS system and may be sent to the emergency scene by the dispatcher after a citizen has activated EMS. In other situations, a First Responder may already be on the scene, such as a lifeguard who is present and recognizes the emergency. In this case, the First Responder is the one who initiates the call to the dispatcher to activate EMS. This text will generally use the phrase "Ensure that EMS has been activated" to cover all situations.

citizen responder, you provide emergency care until arrival of the **Emergency Medical Technicians (EMTs)**.

5. **Arrival of additional EMS resources**—Often, Emergency Medical Technicians (EMTs) or **Paramedics** arrive next and assume care of the patient.

6. **Emergency medical care at the scene**—EMTs continue any emergency care measures begun by First Responders and initiate any additional care that may be required for which they are trained.

7. **Transportation to the receiving facility**—Following appropriate on-scene stabilization and care, the patient is transported to a hospital emergency department or other specialized facility appropriate for caring for the patient's problem. During transport, EMTs may make contact with the emergency department or other facility, advising them of the patient's condition. Additional care is provided during transport. Receiving facilities include:
    *   Emergency departments
    *   Specialty facilities
        *   Trauma centers
        *   Burn centers
        *   Pediatric centers
        *   Perinatal centers

    In addition, a poison center may be contacted for additional information or treatment guidance.

8. **Transfer to an in-hospital care system**—Upon arrival at the hospital emergency department or other facility, the staff there assumes care of the patient. This emergency care team often consists of trained emergency nurses, emergency physicians, and other healthcare professionals. After stabilization, the patient receives any additional care needed from other healthcare professionals, including physicians, social workers, physical therapists, and many others. The goal of definitive care is to return the patient to his or her previous state of health.

    *   Your instructor will inform you of any ways in which your local EMS system varies from this general approach, along with any specific state or local statutes or regulations affecting your EMS system.

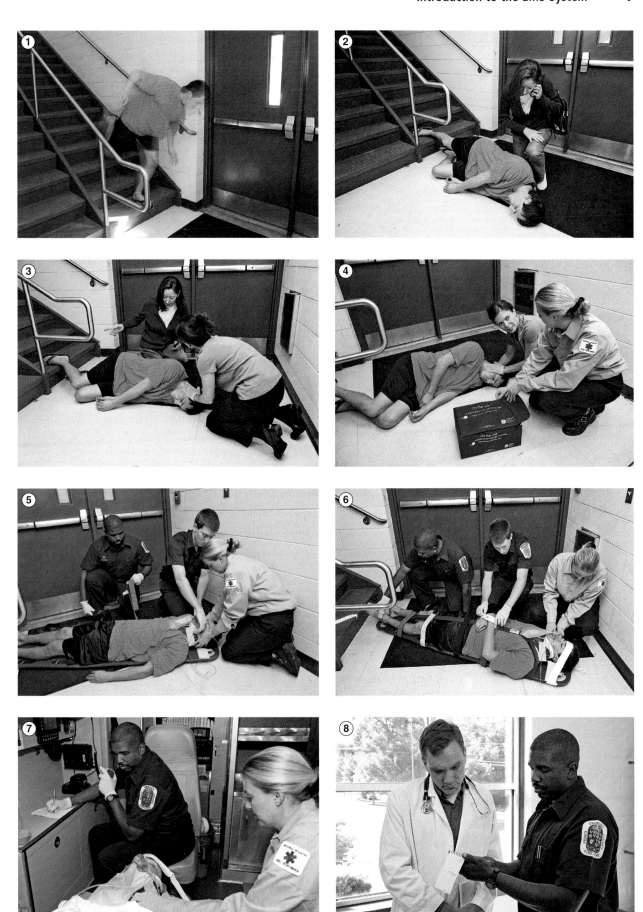

Figure 1-2 Steps in the EMS response to a medical emergency.

First Responders in Emergencies

✓ Need to Know

The first phase of the emergency response begins even before the emergency occurs, involving the preparation of equipment and personnel.

- ☑ The emergency equipment used by First Responders must be clean, complete, and readily available for use.
- ☑ This requires frequent checks of both equipment and supplies:
  - ◦ All equipment must be safe and in good working order.
  - ◦ Dated supplies must be checked and replaced before expiration dates.
  - ◦ Oxygen cylinders must be kept full.
  - ◦ Dressings, bandages, and other equipment must be replaced as soon as they are used.

Another important preparation for the emergency response is **preplanning**. Preplanning involves preparing a response plan in anticipation of different emergencies:

- ☑ Many industrial plants have prearranged plans for emergency response. These plans identify key personnel, locations of supplies, a mechanism for notifying EMS, and evacuation routes for removing patients.
- ☑ Many fire departments and EMS systems preplan responses to areas with a likelihood of an emergency occurring, such as sports stadiums, theatres, public buildings, and industrial plants. The preplan involves inspection of the site and identification of any potential hazards present at the scene.

An equally important component of preparation is the training of First Responders, beginning with this course and continuing thereafter. You must continually strive to keep your skills and knowledge up to date. Infrequently used skills should be practiced. Continuing education is also essential.

You may be notified of a medical emergency in different ways:

- ☑ If you are a member of a police department, volunteer fire department, or rescue squad, you may receive the call via telephone, pager, or radio.
- ☑ Disaster team members, industrial safety officers, and civil defense personnel may receive the call for emergency assistance similarly.

- ☑ In other situations, lifeguards, ski patrol members, and athletic trainers are often already at or near the scene when an emergency occurs.

As soon as you receive the call, you should gather the necessary medical equipment and go to the scene. If the scene is some distance away, you will respond in the appropriate vehicle.

- ☑ Fire, police, and rescue personnel usually have vehicles equipped with the necessary warning equipment such as emergency lights and sirens. First Responders in an emergency vehicle should adhere to local laws and guidelines regarding use of the emergency warning equipment.
- ☑ If you must respond to the scene of a medical emergency in a private vehicle, you should obey all traffic laws and signs; never drive a private vehicle as if it were an emergency vehicle. Many crashes have occurred when well-meaning people were hurrying to a crash scene or hospital. An emergency response is dangerous even in an equipped emergency vehicle and much more so in a private one without warning equipment.

Components of an EMS System

Every EMS system has 10 classic components:

- ☑ **Regulation and policy:** guidelines for training, equipment, treatment standards, and protocols for EMS personnel
- ☑ **Resource management:** physical resources such as vehicles, equipment, facilities, and other resources
- ☑ **Human resources and training:** the recruitment and training of people who work or volunteer within the EMS system
- ☑ **Transportation:** ambulances and air transport
- ☑ **Facilities:** hospital emergency departments and specialized facilities in the area
- ☑ **Communications:** emergency calls to dispatcher and communication system among EMS personnel
- ☑ **Public information and education:** injury and illness prevention programs as well as first aid and CPR courses and programs
- ☑ **Medical oversight:** direction of the EMS system by a physician

☑ **Trauma systems:** a network of healthcare professionals who provide care for serious trauma patients

☑ **Evaluation:** a program of quality assurance to ensure the EMS system meets the community's needs most effectively

EMS Personnel

The Emergency Medical Services system includes a number of different professionals with different levels of training and responsibilities (Box 1-1).

Do You Understand?

1. The enhanced 911 system automatically provides the dispatcher with the caller's telephone number and _____ when using a land telephone line.
2. What does a First Responder usually do after arriving at an emergency scene where a citizen responder is already giving a patient first aid? _____
3. Who typically transports the patient to a hospital emergency department? _____

BOX 1-1

EMS PROFESSIONALS

Dispatcher

A 911 call for help is usually received by an EMS dispatcher, also called an emergency medical dispatcher (EMD) or dispatch. The dispatcher may be located in a centralized law enforcement agency, fire station, or other site. This person is trained in obtaining information and determining what emergency personnel and equipment will likely be needed. The EMS dispatcher then sends the appropriate EMS unit to the scene.

First Responder

Usually the first person to arrive at the scene of a medical emergency is a First Responder, sometimes called an emergency medical responder. The First Responder often takes over care of the victim from those giving first aid. The First Responder also gathers any information concerning the victim, controls the scene, and prepares for the arrival of an ambulance. The First Responder, assisted if needed by bystanders, provides emergency care until more advanced emergency care professionals arrive. This care includes **Basic Life Support,** basic care for the patient's airway, breathing, and circulation.

Emergency Medical Technician (EMT)

EMTs usually arrive in an ambulance equipped for Basic or Advanced Life Support.

They take over the medical care of the victim, give necessary medical care at the scene, and transport the victim for definitive medical care. EMTs with different levels of training perform different medical treatments. The EMT-Basic (EMT-B) has the minimum level of EMT training and can give emergency patient care at a higher level than a First Responder. The EMT-Intermediate (EMT-I) has more advanced training and skills and may give some medications as well as use some **Advanced Life Support** techniques. The EMT-Paramedic has the highest level of EMT training and may perform advanced techniques such as endotracheal intubation, medication administration, electrocardiography (ECG), and other skills.

Medical Director

The medical director is a physician within the EMS system who oversees the care given by First Responders and EMTs. The medical director establishes protocols for medical care to be given to victims at the scene. The medical director, or another physician designated as the medical control physician, is available for consultation by radio or telephone to EMS personnel giving care.

4. Name two ways you can keep your skills and knowledge up to date after your First Responder course.

_____

_____

Roles and Responsibilities of First Responders

 Need to Do

First Responders' roles and responsibilities fall into four categories: general responsibilities, patient care responsibilities, responsibilities at the scene, and personal responsibilities and characteristics.

General Responsibilities

1. Respond in a safe and rapid manner to the scene of the medical emergency.

2. Maintain your personal safety. This is always a top priority. When facing a life-threatening emergency, it is easy to accidentally overlook hazards at the scene. If you become injured, however, you too will become a patient and will not be able to help the person who needs your care. In addition, personal safety involves using personal protective equipment and taking other steps to prevent the possibility of infectious disease transmission (Chapter 2).

3. If the nature of the emergency requires specialized personnel or equipment, contact the EMS system to request additional resources to be sent to the scene.

4. Gain access to the patient. Tell the patient and family members or bystanders present that you are a trained EMS emergency worker. Again, make sure the scene is safe for both you and the patient. If the scene is not safe, you may have to move the patient carefully to a safe area. Only move a patient when absolutely necessary.

5. When safety for both you and your patient has been assured, begin actual emergency care for the patient. After safety, the patient's needs are the highest priority.

6. Document the emergency and your actions to meet local recordkeeping requirements.

Patient Care Responsibilities

Patient care follows a systematic procedure described in following chapters and emphasized throughout this text.

1. Determine whether there are any immediate threats to the patient's life **(Figure 1-3)**. This involves ensuring the patient's airway is open, the patient is breathing adequately, the patient has a pulse and adequate circulation, and the patient's spine is protected from movement. Give any care needed for life-threatening problems based on your patient **assessment.**

2. Activate the EMS system if it has not been activated.

3. Further assess the patient, if appropriate, to detect other medical problems or life threats, and provide care as needed. Ask others present on the scene what happened.

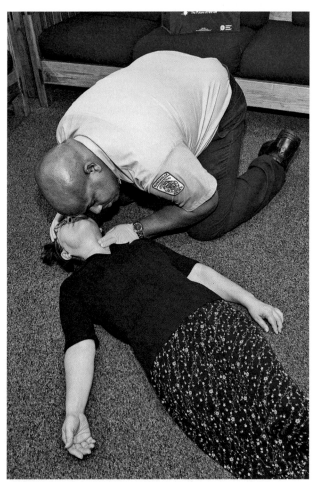

Figure 1-3 Assess first for threats to the patient's airway, breathing, and circulation.

4. Provide any indicated emergency care and remain with the patient until more highly trained personnel arrive at the scene.

5. Assist other EMS personnel with patient care as needed. In some communities and situations, you may be needed to accompany the patient in the ambulance.

6. Maintain the patient's privacy and confidentiality (Chapter 3).

Responsibilities at the Scene

In addition to direct patient care, First Responders may have other responsibilities at the scene:

1. Size up the scene to identify any safety issues, to determine how many patients need help, and to determine what other resources are needed.

2. In some situations, it may be necessary to take actions at the scene to access the patient. Remember the priority for safety, however. If fire, downed electrical lines, fast water, ice, heights, or other dangers prevent you from reaching the patient, you should summon EMS so that personnel specially trained in rescue can be dispatched.

3. Maintain safety of others at the scene, in addition to yourself and the patient. This may include the patient's family members, bystanders, passing motorists, etc. Dangers at the scene may include traffic, fire, and spilled hazardous materials.

4. Assist other emergency personnel as required or requested. Relay any information you have gathered regarding the patient and the emergency. Describe what happened, how the patient was found, the results of your patient assessment, and any care you have rendered. You may also need to assist with other patients at the scene.

5. Cooperate with other public safety workers such as law enforcement, fire personnel, and other EMS providers.

6. Other responsibilities at the scene may include:

- Assisting in directing traffic flow
- Summoning other appropriate help such as the fire department, police, rescue group, power company, and so on
- Controlling, directing, or asking bystanders for help

- Other supplemental responsibilities as dictated by your job or specific EMS system, such as shutting down equipment or notifying other personnel

Personal Responsibilities and Characteristics

Your First Responder training does not end with the completion of this course. You must continually strive to keep your skills and knowledge up to date. This may be accomplished through continuing education programs, reading, and refresher training. In addition, it is important to maintain a current knowledge of local, state, and national issues affecting EMS.

As a First Responder, you should manifest these personal characteristics:

1. Maintain a caring and professional attitude. Ill and injured patients and their family members, as well as bystanders, are sometimes difficult to work with. You must be compassionate and understand their concerns and fears. Never make insensitive, rude, or potentially embarrassing remarks that may be overheard by the patient, family members, or others at the scene.

2. Respect all patients, family members, and bystanders. Do not discriminate in the care you provide or how you behave based on any differences in the person's appearance, religion, age, gender, sociocultural background, or behavior.

3. Maintain composure. Learn to control your feelings. Understand that a patient's or family member's anger or other strong emotions often result from their fears and concerns.

4. Maintain a professional appearance. A neat and clean appearance accompanied by professional behavior helps ease a patient's concerns. An untidy First Responder may cause the patient additional stress.

5. Maintain personal fitness and health. As a First Responder, you may at any time be called upon to lift or move a patient or perform another physically demanding task. Therefore, it is important to be in good physical condition. Daily exercise, attention to diet, and a healthy lifestyle are important aspects of the job. Your good health will also help you cope with the physical and psychological stresses of giving emergency care.

Do You Understand?

1. True or false: Your top priority in any emergency is maintaining your personal safety.

2. What do you do if you discover special equipment or skills are needed at the emergency scene?_____

3. Your *first* responsibility in patient care is to

   a. fully assess the patient.

   b. talk to others at the scene to find out what happened.

   c. accompany the patient in the ambulance.

   d. determine whether there are immediate threats to the patient's life.

Medical Oversight

✓ Need to Know

Medical oversight in an EMS system refers to the responsibility of a physician, usually called the **medical director** or medical control, who oversees out-of-hospital emergency medical care. Medical oversight includes direct and indirect medical control. The medical director leads the medical emergency response team and has responsibility for making decisions about how emergency care is delivered.

Direct Medical Control

☑ The medical director is personally involved in patient care provided by EMS personnel through instructing **prehospital care** providers. This medical control is sometimes referred to *online control*.

☑ The medical director or another physician designated as medical control at the communications base station stays in contact with emergency care providers through radio or cellular telephone communications and sometimes may be physically present to oversee emergency operations **(Figure 1-4)**.

☑ Through direct control, the medical director or medical control can authorize a specific patient treatment not covered by standard protocols for patient care.

Indirect Medical Control

☑ Indirect medical control refers to offline or prospective direction provided by the medical

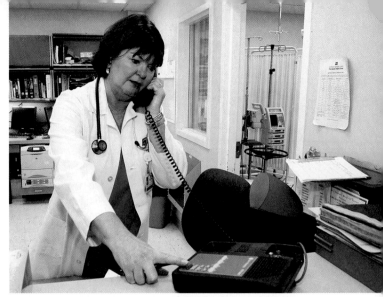

Figure 1-4 The medical director often maintains online communication with EMS personnel in the field.

director. The medical director is responsible for developing protocols, or standing orders, that dictate how EMS providers are to provide patient care in different situations without having to speak directly to the base station for authorization.

☑ Indirect medical control also includes the design of the specific EMS system; standards of training for EMS providers, usually including First Responders; and quality assurance programs.

In most states, First Responders, like other EMS care providers, function under the guidance and control of the EMS system's medical director.

☑ State laws vary somewhat, but generally a First Responder is considered a designated agent of the medical director and provides care as an extension of that physician's authority.

☑ Your instructor will explain your exact relationship with the medical director within your system as well as specific state laws and regulations regarding your role in providing emergency care.

Conclusion

As a First Responder, you will function within the Emergency Medical Services (EMS) system, along with other EMS personnel, to provide care to injured or ill patients in emergencies. Your roles and responsibilities help ensure that in an emergency, the patient receives good initial care until others with higher levels of medical training arrive at the scene and take over. In this way First Responders help save lives.

Key Terms

Advanced Life Support (p. 9)

assessment (p. 10)

Basic Life Support (p. 9)

citizen responder (p. 6)

direct medical control (p. 12)

dispatcher (p. 5)

Emergency Medical Technician (EMT) (p. 6)

Emergency Medical Services (EMS) system (p. 3, 5)

enhanced 911 (p. 5)

First Responder (p. 3)

indirect medical control (p. 12)

medical director (p. 12)

medical oversight (p. 12)

Paramedic (p. 6)

prehospital care (p. 12)

preplanning (p. 8)

sudden illness (p. 4)

Review Questions

1. EMS can be activated by
   a. EMTs.
   b. citizens.
   c. emergency department physicians.
   d. dispatchers.

2. Replace used bandages and other supplies
   a. at the end of your shift.
   b. at the beginning of your shift.
   c. as soon as possible.
   d. before leaving the emergency scene.

3. Which of the following has the highest level of training?
   a. Paramedic
   b. EMT-B
   c. First Responder
   d. EMT-I

4. How long should you remain at the scene when treating a patient?
   a. Until the patient says you may go
   b. Until you have done everything you can do
   c. Until more highly trained personnel arrive and take over
   d. Until you have completed all final written reports

5. In addition to providing patient care, First Responders often
   a. act as law enforcement personnel to investigate the scene.
   b. transport patients to the hospital if they do not require an ambulance.
   c. grant interviews to local media.
   d. assist in directing traffic.

6. Indirect medical control by the medical director often includes
   a. setting standards for First Responder training.
   b. funding lobbying efforts for local legislation.
   c. coming to the emergency scene to supervise operations.
   d. communicating with responders by radio.

The Well-Being of the First Responder

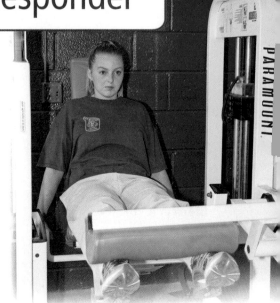

Chapter Preview

• Emotional Aspects of Emergency Medical Care

• Preventing Disease Transmission

• Scene Safety

You Respond To . . .

a scene where two vehicles have crashed in an intersection. One driver has gotten out of his vehicle and has moved away, but the other is slumped over the wheel, apparently unresponsive. Bystanders are crowding around. You see a pool of gasoline that has leaked from the vehicle's ruptured gas tank.

Introduction

Staying physically and psychologically safe and healthy as a First Responder involves a number of factors. Because emergency situations frequently are stressful, First Responders need to understand stressful incidents, particularly death, and how to manage **stress.** Providing emergency care to patients also carries a risk of infectious disease, but First Responders can minimize this risk through appropriate precautions and the use of personal protective equipment. Finally, because emergency scenes often involve many hazards for First

Responders, as well as patients and bystanders, it is crucial to follow basic guidelines for scene safety.

Emotional Aspects of Emergency Medical Care

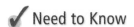 Need to Know

Providing emergency care is stressful. Many situations cause strong emotional reactions—it is only human that we feel stress when confronting serious trauma, injured children, death, and other incidents. Patients and family members too experience severe stress. Stress itself cannot be eliminated, but First Responders can learn how to cope with stress, reduce the effects of stress, and seek help when needed after a critical incident.

Stress

Stress is the result of any experience that causes psychological strain or an imbalance. Stress is a mental and emotional state that also has many physical effects on the body. We all feel stress almost everyday, and most people learn to cope with minor stress, but emergency care frequently involves more severe stress that can impact one's psychological and physical functioning.

Stressful Situations

For many people, any type of injury or illness is stressful. Some First Responders who give emergency care on a regular basis may become used to "routine" injuries and illness situations, while for others the day-to-day job produces much stress. Knowing that the patient's pain and suffering are temporary and that most patients recover fully helps minimize the stress of less severe emergency situations. But many emergency situations are more stressful, often affecting caregivers emotionally. These are particularly stressful situations:

- ☑ Multiple-casualty incidents
- ☑ Injured or ill infants or children
- ☑ Death of a patient
- ☑ Traumatic amputations
- ☑ Violent behavior
- ☑ Abuse of an infant, child, elder, or spouse
- ☑ Death or injury of a coworker or other public safety personnel

▶ Need to Recognize

As emergency personnel feel the stress of these situations, so too do patients and their family members, as well as bystanders at the scene. Stress may lead to different emotional reactions in different people, including:

- ♦ Anger
- ♦ Pain
- ♦ Fear
- ♦ Anxiety or panic
- ♦ Guilt
- ♦ Depression
- ♦ Confusion or delusion

Realize that a patient, family member, or bystander experiencing strong emotions is reacting to the stress caused by the emergency. Do not react personally to their emotions or behavior. Be empathetic and try to help patients cope with their stress while giving emergency care. Chapter 11 includes additional information on working with patients experiencing behavioral emergencies.

Death and Dying

▶▶ Need to Do

Medical emergencies sometimes involve the death or dying of a patient, always a stressful situation for everyone affected. Although people respond in individual ways to the death or dying of another, or to their knowledge of their own death coming, these responses generally fall into a pattern of grieving. Most people pass through identifiable stages of grief that help them cope with the death or dying. Not everyone passes through all five stages in the same order or even through all stages. Recognizing a patient's or family member's stage of grieving, however, will help you know how to respond to the person.

Denial

A patient who is severely injured or dying, and family members, may psychologically refuse to accept the reality of the situation. This defense mechanism helps lower stress because the person does not have to deal with the reality of death. This is sometimes called a "not me" reaction because people in this stage refuse to believe this is happening to them.

Anger

The initial response after realizing that the injury, death, or dying is real, is often anger. "Why me?" the patient or family member may wonder. This anger may be directed at you or others at the scene. It is important not to respond personally to anger directed at you or become defensive, but to listen to the patient or family member and be empathetic about what they are feeling.

First Responders may also respond with anger in emergencies involving severe stress. This is often a normal reaction. Talk with coworkers and others to help work through these feelings rather than allowing them to be directed at others.

Bargaining

With this defense mechanism, the grieving person tries to put off the reality of the injury or dying by bargaining. "Let me live a little longer and I'll never do this again," the person may think. The person is struggling to keep hope alive. A patient or family member may look to you to support their hope. In this case, do not offer false hope or reassurance, but assure the person that everyone is doing everything possible. Be sensitive and understanding of their emotional reaction.

Depression

Depression frequently occurs when the patient or family member realizes the inevitability or reality of death or disability. The patient or family member may be overwhelmed with sadness, despair, or mourning. The person may cry or become silent and withdrawn. Again, this is a normal response. Be supportive and continue to help meet the person's needs while respecting his or her emotional state.

First Responders may also experience depression after a stressful emergency situation. This normal reaction usually passes in a day or two; if not, do not hesitate to seek professional help to cope with the continuing stress caused by the emergency.

Acceptance

In this stage, the patient or family member accepts the death or disability. The person's emotional state may now be calm or may continue to be angry or sad. Often, family members need more support in this stage than the patient. Acceptance may be the final stage in the grieving process, or the person may again experience one or more of the earlier stages.

Dealing with Dying Patients and Family Members

▶ Need to Do

While giving care to dying patients, provide emotional support also to the patient and family members. Respect their needs and feelings, and help them maintain their dignity. Allow them to share and communicate their feelings.

- Help maintain the privacy of the patient and family members.

- Allow family members to express their fear, rage, anger, or despair. Be tolerant and do not respond defensively if anger is directed at you.

- Listen empathetically to both the patient and family members.

- Use a gentle tone of voice and a reassuring touch, if appropriate.

- Do not give false reassurance, but let them know that everything that can be done to help will be done.

- Comfort the family.

- Give the patient and family members as much control as possible over the situation.

Stress Management

✓ Need to Know

First Responders, like everyone else, may experience many stresses in their lives related to their job, relationships, financial responsibilities, and other dimensions of living. Added to this is the frequent job stress caused by emergencies. Most stress cannot be prevented, but understanding the factors involved and recognizing the signs and symptoms of unhealthy stress when it occurs are important first steps in learning to manage your stress in a productive rather than destructive manner.

Everyone feels stress at one time or another, but in some ways the stress of being a First Responder is different from most other people's stress. People generally talk over stressful situations with friends and family members; this is a coping strategy that reduces stress. Because of the unique experiences of working in emergency scenes, First Responders and other emergency personnel often feel their family members and friends do not understand what they are feeling because they have not had the same experiences. They may not seem to understand what you are going through in your work, and this may cause you frustration when you want to share your experiences and feelings. Being on call often adds still more stress for both you and family members.

The difficulty First Responders often have communicating with family and friends about their work sometimes leads to sharing more with coworkers and other emergency personnel than with family members. This can cause family members to feel they are being kept at some distance or being ignored, causing additional stress and misunderstanding. It is important to recognize this pattern when it develops so that you can keep it from interfering with your personal life. Most important are good communication and listening to others as well as making the effort to share with them.

Signs and Symptoms of Stress

◼ Need to Recognize

Again, stress is a normal part of everyday life. But when stress becomes severe and is not being adequately managed, it begins to have disruptive effects on an individual's life and health. Following are warning signs that stress has gotten out of control:

- Irritability to family members, friends, and coworkers

- Inability to concentrate
- Difficulty sleeping or having frequent nightmares
- Anxiety
- Indecisiveness
- Guilt
- Loss of appetite
- Loss of interest in sexual activities
- Feeling isolated
- Loss of interest in work

Managing Stress

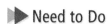 Need to Do

You can reduce the stress you feel and its effects on you with lifestyle changes, changing how you balance different aspects of your life, work changes, and professional help if needed.

Lifestyle Changes

Stress not only disrupts one's life but may also lead to "job burnout." Adapting a healthy lifestyle including a good diet and regular exercise helps reduce stress while promoting a longer, richer life. Following are accepted guidelines for a low-stress, healthy lifestyle:

- If you smoke or use tobacco, investigate smoking cessation programs that can help you stop.
- Eat a healthy diet based on a variety of nutrient-dense foods within the basic food groups, choosing foods with limited amounts of saturated and trans fats, cholesterol, added sugars, and salt.
- Reduce your consumption of beverages containing caffeine.
- Avoid or reduce consumption of alcoholic beverages. Although some people may drink in an effort to reduce stress, in the long term, alcohol use increases stress.
- Control body weight by avoiding overeating.
- Engage in regular physical activity and reduce sedentary activities to promote health and psychological well-being as well as maintain a healthy body weight. Try to engage in approximately 60 minutes of moderate- to vigorous-intensity activity on most days of the week.

- If you find it difficult to relax, learn relaxation techniques such as meditation and visual imagery techniques.

Balancing Your Life

All too often people are consumed by their work. This can be a particular cause of stress for First Responders. You may need to deliberately and conscientiously work to include, in your daily and weekly schedule, more time with family or friends, sports or recreational activities, and times for relaxing.

Work Changes

Sometimes much of your stress results from your work schedule, especially if it prevents you from spending time with family members or engaging in activities you enjoy that also help lower stress. If so, do not hesitate to request a different work shift that would better meet your needs for time with others. If the nature of the work, rather than the schedule, is a cause of unmanageable stress, you may also need to request a rotation to a less stressful assignment.

Professional Help

The changes and techniques discussed may be enough to reduce stress to a manageable level. In some instances, however, you may find that you cannot solve the problem alone or with the help of family members. There is no shame in seeking help from those professionally trained in reducing stress and handling other emotional problems. Your employer may have a program for such assistance or can refer you to a mental health professional or social worker as appropriate. You can also speak to a member of the clergy or your personal physician. Often the cost of professional help is covered by health insurance.

Critical Incident Stress

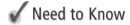 Need to Know

The preceding sections focus on many types of personal or job-related stress. In addition, specific programs have been developed to help First Responders and other emergency personnel with the often severe stress that results from one emergency situation, or a series of emergency situations, called critical incident stress.

Critical incident stress is a normal stress response to abnormal circumstances. The following are **critical incidents** that often may result in severe stress experienced by First Responders:

- ☑ Death or serious injury of a coworker in the line of duty
- ☑ Multiple-casualty incident
- ☑ Suicide by an emergency services worker
- ☑ Serious injury or death of a child
- ☑ Involvement in an emergency generating excessive media interest
- ☑ An emergency involving violence
- ☑ Providing patient care to someone you know
- ☑ Any disaster
- ☑ Any emergency that has an unusual impact on emergency workers

Programs of **critical incident stress management (CISM)** are available in most public safety departments or EMS systems for those who experience uncontrollable stress resulting from any of these situations or from an accumulation of events. Talk with your employer to learn more about this program in your system.

Critical Incident Stress Management

CISM programs involve comprehensive services from a team of counselors, mental health professionals, and others trained in helping emergency personnel cope with the stress of critical incidents and the job in general. Services usually include:

- ☑ Pre-incident stress education
- ☑ On-scene peer support
- ☑ One-on-one support
- ☑ Disaster support services
- ☑ Critical Incident Stress Debriefing (CISD)
- ☑ Follow-up services
- ☑ Support programs for spouse and family members
- ☑ Community outreach programs
- ☑ Other health and welfare programs such as wellness programs

Critical Incident Stress Debriefing (CISD) is a special program to help emergency personnel cope with the severe stress of an emergency situation. The program usually involves a team of peer counselors and mental health professionals. The goal of CISD is to accelerate the normal recovery process after experiencing a critical incident. CISD techniques

include defusings and debriefings. Participation in CISD programs is voluntary and confidential and is recommended for all First Responders significantly affected by a critical incident.

A **defusing** is a short session that is typically less formal and less structured than a debriefing. The session occurs a few hours after the critical incident and usually lasts only 30 to 45 minutes. The defusing allows personnel to vent and begin to resolve their feelings. This session may eliminate the need for a formal debriefing or may enhance the formal debriefing if one is needed.

A **debriefing** is a team meeting generally held within 24 to 72 hours after a major incident. Counselors encourage an open discussion among those involved in the incident about their feelings, fears, and reactions. Like a defusing, a debriefing is voluntary and is not an investigation or interrogation of emergency personnel. Everything spoken in the session is private and confidential. The CISD leaders and mental health personnel present in the debriefing evaluate the needs of emergency personnel involved and offer suggestions to help manage their feelings and overcome their stress.

✎ Do You Understand?

1. Family members who have just learned that an individual is dying are likely to *first* experience _____.

2. True or false: When speaking with family members of a dying patient, it is best to not acknowledge the coming death but to give reassurances that all will be well.

3. Who is likely to experience stress in their lives?
   - a. Everyone
   - b. People with chronic depression
   - c. People with chronic anxiety
   - d. People with chronic illness

4. List at least four lifestyle changes you can make to reduce your stress.

_____ _____

_____ _____

Preventing Disease Transmission

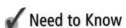 **Need to Know**

When caring for a patient in any emergency situation, there is some risk of transmission of infectious disease. That risk is very low, however, and taking steps to prevent disease transmission greatly reduces that risk. It is best to assume any patient being treated may have an infectious disease and to take the appropriate steps to protect yourself. In addition, assess the individual situation for the risks and act accordingly. For example, in a situation involving the likelihood of significant blood splashing, eye protection may be needed, whereas in most other situations it is unnecessary to wear goggles or eye shields.

Serious Infectious Diseases

Serious infectious diseases include those caused by bloodborne and airborne **pathogens.** Bloodborne pathogens are those transmitted from one person to another through contact with the infected person's blood. Bacteria or viruses that cause such diseases are also present in some other body fluids, such as semen, vaginal secretions, and bloody saliva or vomit. Other body fluids such as nasal secretions, sweat, tears, and urine do not normally transmit pathogens. Three serious bloodborne infections are HIV, hepatitis B, and hepatitis C. Tuberculosis is a serious airborne infection.

HIV

Acquired immunodeficiency syndrome (AIDS) is caused by the **human immunodeficiency virus (HIV).** People with AIDS are more susceptible to opportunistic infections, which invade the body as the disease progresses. The disease is eventually fatal. The greatest risk involves exposure to the almost 1 million HIV-positive people in the United States, a fourth of whom are unaware of their infection. The only reliable way to determine if a person has HIV is through a blood test. HIV is transmitted through an infected person's body fluids, including:

- ☑ Blood
- ☑ Semen
- ☑ Vaginal secretions
- ☑ Breast milk
- ☑ Other body fluids if blood is present

Although HIV can sometimes be detected in saliva, tears, urine, and other body fluids, exposure to these fluids from an infected person does not result in transmission of the virus. Casual contact with those infected with HIV also does not result in transmission of the virus.

No **vaccine** is currently available for HIV, and there is no cure for AIDS. Therefore, preventive measures are very important, as described in following sections.

Hepatitis B

Hepatitis B, also called serum hepatitis, is caused by the hepatitis B virus (HBV). HBV is transmitted by blood and materials contaminated with blood or body fluids. HBV infections are a major cause of liver damage, cirrhosis, and liver cancer. Because of routine hepatitis B vaccinations, the number of new infections per year has declined, but the CDC reports that HBV still infects about 80,000 people in the United States yearly, and there are about 1.25 million chronic carriers. About 5,000 people die every year of liver problems associated with HBV infection.

The most common mode of transmission of HBV is direct contact with infectious blood. Exposure to HBV on contaminated environmental surfaces is another common mode of transmission. At room temperature, the virus may survive for several days in dried body fluids on surfaces such as tables and faucets. HBV is easily transmitted because it can live longer outside the body and because very little blood is needed to cause infection. HBV can also be spread by sharing such personal items as a razor or toothbrush or by drug paraphernalia such as needles and syringes. HBV is not transmitted in food or water, in fecal matter, through the air, or through casual contact.

A vaccine is available for HBV, and First Responders are recommended to receive this along with other recommended immunizations. Those who are not vaccinated can prevent infection by protections against exposure to blood.

Hepatitis C

Hepatitis C is a liver disease caused by the hepatitis C virus (HCV). This virus lives in the blood of people with the disease and is spread via the blood. The CDC reports that an estimated 2.7 million people in the United States have chronic HCV infection, and about 25,000 new infections occur each year. Many people who carry HCV have some liver damage but do not feel sick from it. In others, cirrhosis of the liver may develop, resulting in eventual liver failure. Blood tests can be done to determine if a person has HCV. The CDC recommends HCV testing for healthcare workers and others who have been exposed to HCV-positive blood.

There currently is no vaccine available for HCV and no cure. Therefore, preventive measures are especially important.

Tuberculosis

Tuberculosis (TB) is transmitted through the air, typically when an infected person coughs or sneezes. TB made a comeback in the 1980s and 1990s and, although now again declining, about 16,000 cases are reported each year. Some forms of the tuberculosis bacteria have become resistant to treatment. Healthcare workers generally use precautions when caring for people known or suspected to have TB, but rarely does a First Responder need to take special precautions against airborne disease. Use of a face mask with a one-way valve protects a rescuer giving rescue breathing to a nonbreathing patient.

How Infectious Diseases Are Transmitted

The transmission of infectious disease occurs through a process involving four stages:

1. **The process begins with a person (or animal) carrying an infection.**

2. **The infectious pathogen (disease-causing bacteria, virus, fungus, or parasite) leaves the infected person's body.** For example:
   - The person may bleed from a cut, and in that blood is the pathogen.
   - The person may sneeze out little droplets carrying the pathogen.

3. **The infectious pathogen reaches another person and enters his or her body.** This can happen in a number of ways:
   - The person may come into contact with the infected person's blood, other body fluid, or infectious material in a way that the pathogen enters his or her body through mucous membranes or nonintact skin (**bloodborne transmission**).
   - The person may inhale the pathogen in tiny droplets in the air (**airborne transmission**).
   - The person may be bitten by an insect, such as a tick or mosquito, carrying the pathogen (**vector transmission** of bloodborne pathogen).

Transmission of a pathogen from one person to another is said to occur through direct or indirect contact:

- **Direct contact** occurs with contact with an infected person or fluids or substances from that person.
- **Indirect contact** occurs with contact with contaminated objects, food or drink, droplets in the air, or vectors such as insects.

4. **The second person develops the infection.** Just having the pathogen enter the body does not automatically mean a person will become ill. He or she may have been vaccinated against the disease, which means the body will kill the pathogen before it can cause disease. A person's natural immune system may also be able to kill some pathogens and thereby prevent illness. Or the person may become infected. The process then starts over.

OSHA Regulations

✔ Need to Know

Because bloodborne diseases are very serious, the United States Occupational Safety and Health Administration (OSHA) has created safety standards for those who are likely in their work to encounter the body fluids of others, including many First Responders (www.osha.gov). The **Occupational Exposure to Bloodborne Pathogens Standard** (the Standard) was designed to eliminate or minimize employees' exposure to human blood and other potentially infectious materials (OPIM), such as other body tissues and cell cultures. The Standard applies to all employees who, as part of their job, may reasonably expect to be exposed to blood and OPIM that may contain pathogens. The Standard applies to employees who may be at risk, even if their job does not generally involve giving emergency care or working near or with bloodborne pathogens.

If required by your job, you may take a separate training course for preventing bloodborne and airborne diseases. In the course you will learn more detail about the principles of disease prevention described here. Your instructor will tell you more about the local, state, and federal regulations that apply to you.

Preventing Disease Transmission

▶▶ Need to Do

The prevention of infectious disease is based on guidelines to prevent contact with a patient's blood or other body fluids and substances. These guidelines are often called **body substance isolation (BSI),** universal precautions, or standard precautions **(Box 2-1).** The guidelines involve handwashing and personal hygiene practices, the cleaning and disinfection of equipment used in patient care, and the use of personal protective equipment such as barrier devices and medical exam gloves. In addition, follow your local

system's requirements for the use and cleaning of equipment and the disposal of used gloves and other disposable care equipment and supplies.

Handwashing

Handwashing is a simple but very important step for preventing the transmission of bloodborne pathogens. Follow these general guidelines for handwashing;

- ▶ Wash any exposed skin, ideally with antibacterial or antimicrobial soap, as soon after an exposure as possible.
- ▶ While washing, be gentle with any scabs or sores.

BOX 2-1

INFECTION CONTROL TERMINOLOGY

Because of changes in infection control terminology over the last two decades, there has been some confusion about the exact meanings and applications of the terms *universal precautions, body substance isolation,* and *standard precautions.*

Universal precautions is the term the CDC originally promoted in 1987 for actions to protect providers of first aid and healthcare from exposure to bloodborne pathogens. Universal precautions apply to all people's blood, semen, vaginal secretions, and other body fluids containing visible blood or to any objects potentially contaminated with any of these. In its 1991 Bloodborne Pathogens Standard, OSHA required the use of universal precautions, which it defined as: "an approach to infection control. According to the concept of Universal Precautions, all human blood and certain human body fluids are treated as if known to be infectious for HIV, HBV, and other bloodborne pathogens." Many healthcare and first aid providers continue to use the term *universal precautions* in part because it exists within federal, and many state, laws.

At the same time, many healthcare institutions were following principles of body substance isolation (BSI), an infection-control concept that originated in efforts to control all infections (not just bloodborne pathogens) occurring within healthcare facilities. BSI precautions assume that *any* body fluid or moist body tissue is potentially infectious.

In 1996, the CDC published new guidelines called **standard precautions** intended primarily for infectious disease control within healthcare facilities. Standard precautions combine the major features of universal precautions and BSI precautions. Although some providers feel that standard precautions have replaced universal precautions, the CDC states: "Standard precautions were developed for use in hospitals and may not necessarily be indicated in other settings where universal precautions are used, such as child care settings and schools."

Because standard precautions are more rigorous than universal precautions, this text will use the term *standard precautions.* Recognize, however, that in many first aid situations, universal precautions are appropriate.

Occupational Safety and Health Administration (OSHA).
Division of Healthcare Quality Protection (DHQP) through The Centers for Disease Control and Prevention.

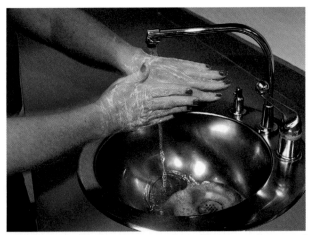

Figure 2-1 Handwashing is an effective means of helping prevent disease transmission.

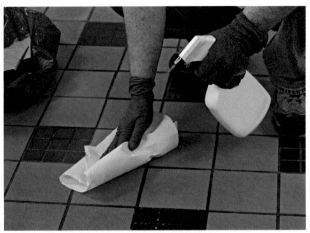

Figure 2-2 Disinfect an area after a spill of blood or potentially infectious material.

- Wash all surfaces thoroughly, including the backs of hands, wrists, between the fingers, and under fingernails **(Figure 2-1)**.
- Wash hands immediately after removing medical exam gloves or other personal protective equipment.

For handwashing after caring for a patient, you can use facilities such as restrooms, janitor closets, and laboratory sinks, as long as soap is available, but do not use sinks in areas where food is prepared. Remember to scrub thoroughly using soap—merely wetting the hands will not prevent infection.

Antiseptic towelettes and antibacterial or antimicrobial handwashing liquid can be used when soap and running water are not available. When used for the initial cleaning after being exposed to a patient's blood or body fluids, however, a thorough scrubbing with soap and water is still needed as soon as possible.

Equipment Disinfection

After providing emergency care involving a patient's body fluids, you may need to decontaminate or sterilize the area or equipment. **Decontamination** is the use of physical or chemical means to remove, inactivate, or destroy bloodborne pathogens on a surface or item so that it is no longer infectious. To **sterilize** something means to use a chemical or physical procedure to destroy all microbial life on the item. The following are general guidelines for decontamination and sterilization. Use the specific protocols required by your EMS system and employer.

- All reusable sharps, such as knives, scissors, and scalpels, must be cleaned and sterilized after being used.

- Decontaminate equipment and working surfaces, bench tops, and floors with an approved **disinfectant** such as a 10% bleach solution **(Figure 2-2)**.
- Disinfect personal items such as jewelry and nail brushes after handwashing.
- Use utensils, such as tongs or a dustpan, to clean up broken glass and other contaminated materials for disposal in a biohazard container.

Personal Habits

During and after care for a patient when you may be exposed to bloodborne pathogens, prevent the entry of pathogens into your mouth or eyes by keeping your hands away from your face. In general, follow these guidelines:

- Do not smoke.
- Do not put on lip balm, hand lotion, or cosmetics.
- Do not eat or drink.
- Do not handle your contact lenses.
- Do not use a sink used for food preparation for any other cleanup.

Personal Protective Equipment

Personal protective equipment (PPE) consists of barriers such as medical exam gloves and resuscitation masks used when caring for a patient in an emergency **(Figure 2-3)**. In some settings, you may also have access to other forms of PPE, such as jumpsuits or aprons, face shields or face masks, eye shields or goggles, and caps and booties that you wear to protect yourself from exposure to blood and OPIM.

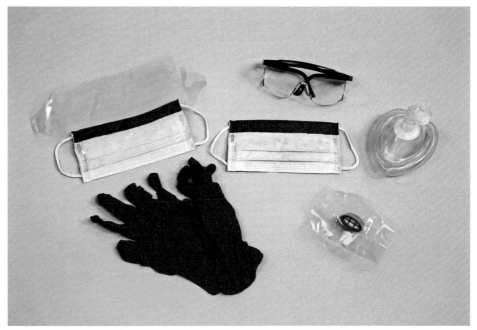

Figure 2-3 Personal protective equipment.

Gloves

Medical exam gloves are a type of barrier that, like other barriers, separate you from potentially infectious materials. When possible, wear gloves whenever providing care, not just when blood or other body fluids are obviously present. Follow these guidelines:

- *Check that your gloves are intact.* If a hole or tear is present, replace the glove immediately with a new one.

- *Do not use petroleum-based hand lotions.* These lotions may cause latex gloves to disintegrate.

- *Remove contaminated gloves carefully.* Do not touch any part of the contaminated outside surface of the gloves as you remove them **(Skill 2-1).**

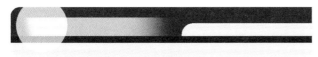

GLOVE LATEX ALLERGY

People who frequently wear latex medical exam gloves have a potential risk of uncovering a latex allergy. This reaction may include a skin rash or even cause breathing difficulty. If you experience signs of an allergy when wearing gloves, ask your employer for latex-free or hypoallergenic gloves made of nitrile or vinyl.

- *Dispose of gloves properly.* After touching any material that may be infected by bloodborne pathogens, dispose of your gloves in a container safe for biohazardous waste.

- *Always change gloves between patients.* Also, wash your hands before and after each patient contact.

- *Wear heavier utility gloves when cleaning a spill or when disinfecting equipment.*

Masks

Resuscitation masks and other types of barriers should be used for personal protection when giving a patient rescue breathing or CPR. These are described fully in Chapter 7.

Surgical (cloth) masks may be used to protect one's mouth and nose in situations in which blood may splash. In some situations, it may be advisable to put a surgical mask on a cooperative patient who is coughing. If there is reason to suspect the patient may have an airborne infection such as tuberculosis, you may wear a high-efficiency particulate air (HEPA) respirator if available. Follow local protocols for using masks.

Eye Protection

Because bloodborne pathogens can enter the body through the mucous membranes of the eyes, eye protection is needed in situations involving the possibility of being splashed by blood. Protective

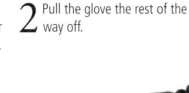

Skill 2-1   Removing Contaminated Gloves

1 With one hand, grasp your other medical exam glove at the wrist or palm and pull it away from your hand.

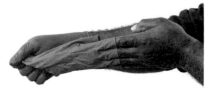

2 Pull the glove the rest of the way off.

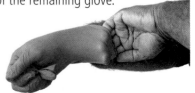

3 Holding the removed glove balled up in the palm of your gloved hand, insert two fingers under the cuff of the remaining glove.

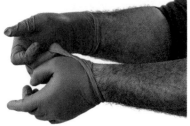

4 Remove the glove by stretching it up and away from the hand and turning it inside out as you pull it off.

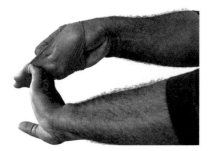

5 Dispose of gloves in a biohazard container, and wash your hands.

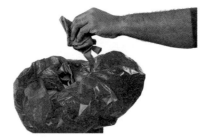

equipment includes eye shields, safety glasses and goggles, and side splash shields that may be applied to prescription glasses.

Protective Clothing

In situations with the likelihood of large blood splashes, protective clothing may be needed, such as a gown or jumpsuit. Follow your local protocols. Remember that if your uniform is soiled by a patient's blood or other body fluids, change it as soon as possible and handle the soiled clothing appropriately because it may transmit infection.

Improvising Personal Protection Equipment

In unexpected circumstances, you may not have medical exam gloves or other PPE with you when potentially exposed to bloodborne pathogens in an emergency. Be creative in using items at hand

to avoid contact with potentially infectious material. Using a plastic bag, a sheet, or a towel, or even removing an article of clothing to use as a barrier, is better than being unprotected. Dispose of or decontaminate any articles you use as barriers as you would any contaminated item.

Standard Precautions

Standard precautions, formerly called universal precautions, are body substance isolation guidelines to be used in all patient treatment situations. These precautions consider all blood and OPIM to be contaminated. In most emergency situations, you cannot readily identify precisely a body fluid present to evaluate whether it may be infectious. Therefore, OSHA recommends using standard precautions with *every* body fluid. Following standard precautions means using PPE and following all the safety guidelines previously described.

If an Exposure Occurs

Even when you follow all safety guidelines and standard precautions, when giving care in an emergency, an unexpected exposure can occur. If so, you need to take immediate action:

- If blood or OPIM splashes in your eyes or other mucous membranes, flush the area with running water for 20 minutes if possible.
- Immediately wash any exposed area well with soap, using an antibacterial or antimicrobial soap if possible.
- Treat any scabs and sores gently when cleaning your skin.
- Report the exposure to your supervisor as soon as possible.
- Save any potentially contaminated object for testing purposes.
- Seek medical care as soon as possible.

OSHA requires employers to inform you how to make an incident report if you are exposed. After receiving your report, your employer must take additional steps to assist you in receiving any needed tests and medical treatment.

Recommended Immunizations and Tests

First Responders are generally recommended to be immunized against hepatitis B as well as tetanus, a common infection that may enter the body through any broken skin. First Responders should ensure they have had a tetanus booster within the last 10 years. Annual TB skin tests may also be recommended; your instructor will tell you about these and other immunizations available in your community.

Do You Understand?

1. Which of the following is *not* a bloodborne infectious disease?
   a. HIV
   b. Tuberculosis
   c. Hepatitis B
   d. Hepatitis C

2. Who is covered by the OSHA Bloodborne Pathogens Standard?

   _____

3. True or false: You should wash your hands after providing patient care if you wore medical exam gloves and removed them correctly.

4. If a patient's blood splashes in your eyes, you should flush them out with running water for _____ minutes.

Scene Safety

Need to Recognize

Many emergency scenes have hazards. Learn to expect the unexpected, and be aware that, at any time, even a seemingly safe emergency scene can turn dangerous. Even when the scene appears safe, approach slowly and carefully and assess the scene for potential hazards. **If at any time the scene appears unsafe, retreat to a safe distance, ensure that dispatch has been notified, and await the arrival of personnel trained to deal with hazardous situations.** This principle cannot be overemphasized. *Never* enter a hazardous scene unless you have the necessary training and equipment to do so safely! Well-meaning rescuers have often become victims themselves because they forgot to be on the lookout for obvious and not-so-obvious scene hazards.

Look for any hazards, such as the following:

- Smoke, flames
- Spilled gasoline or chemicals, fumes, hazardous materials placards
- Downed electrical wires
- Risk of explosion, building collapse
- Roadside dangers, high-speed traffic
- Deep or fast-moving water, ice
- Potential for violence from someone present at the scene

General Principles for Scene Safety

Need to Do

1. Personal protection is the first goal: Ensure it is safe for you to approach the patient. If the scene is unsafe, consider whether you can make it safe. If not, do not enter.

2. Assess the scene also for risks to the patient. The patient may need protection from factors such as extreme temperatures. In some situations, if hazards are present that threaten the patient but it is safe for you to approach briefly, you may have to move the patient (see Chapter 5).

3. Protect bystanders from hazards at the scene by not allowing them to enter the scene and by asking those already present to move away immediately. Never allow other First Responders, bystanders, or family members to enter an apparently unsafe scene.

Specific Scene Dangers

The following sections describe important safety principles at different emergency scenes.

Hazardous Materials Incidents

Hazardous materials are common in our society and pose a special hazard for emergency personnel. When you approach an emergency scene, pay attention for possible clues of a hazardous material. Persons who transport or store significant amounts of most hazardous materials are required to post placards identifying the presence of the hazardous material **(Figure 2-4)**. These placards include a visual warning as well as a number identifying the specific hazardous material. The placard's number is identified in the *Emergency Response Guidebook* published by the U.S. Department of Transportation (DOT) (http://hazmat.dot.gov/pubs/erg/gydebook.htm). If you suspect a hazardous material is present, check the scene from a safe distance upwind, using binoculars. If no placard is present but a hazardous material is suspected, try to obtain additional information before approaching the scene. Because some vehicles carrying certain hazardous materials may not be required to post placards, you should always be cautious.

If hazardous materials may be present, do not enter the scene. Retreat to a safe distance and call for help following your local protocol. Most fire departments have specially trained hazmat teams for managing these incidents. While awaiting the hazmat team, prevent bystanders and other First Responders from entering the scene. Only when notified that hazardous materials have been contained and the scene is safe should you enter to provide patient care.

Hazardous materials may also be present in the home, such as natural gas, gasoline, kerosene, pesticides, and many other substances. Because many hazardous materials do not have an odor, never assume that a scene is safe because you do not smell an odor. Some hazardous materials, such as natural gas, are explosion hazards. If there is any chance of gas or fumes being present, be careful not to provide an ignition source. Even turning on a light switch or using a telephone or radio may generate a spark that sets off an explosion. When you call for help, stay well clear of the scene with your telephone or radio.

Chapter 18, EMS Operations, discusses hazardous materials incidents in more detail.

Motor Vehicle Crashes

Traffic is probably the most frequent danger faced by emergency personnel, including First Responders. Many emergency personnel have been injured or killed attempting to help patients injured in traffic accidents. If the accident scene appears unsafe due to dangerous traffic, wait for the arrival of EMS personnel, law enforcement officers, or additional help.

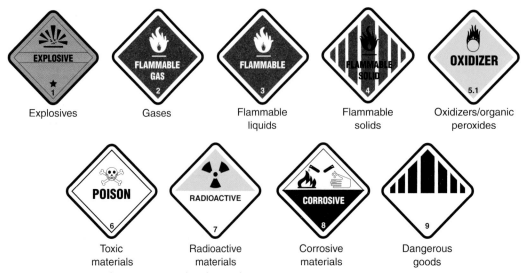

Explosives	Gases	Flammable liquids	Flammable solids	Oxidizers/organic peroxides

Toxic materials	Radioactive materials	Corrosive materials	Dangerous goods

Figure 2-4 Hazardous materials placards.

When arriving at an accident scene, always attempt to park your vehicle so that it does not block traffic. Give other First Responders and emergency vehicles proper access to the scene. The only reasons to park in the roadway or block traffic are to:

- Protect the injured person
- Protect any rescuers, including yourself
- Warn oncoming traffic when their vision of the scene may be blocked

If possible, warning devices such as reflectors, flares, or lights should be placed along the roadway.

Vehicle crash scenes can be extremely dangerous for rescuers because of the risks of passing vehicles, downed electrical wires, fire or explosion, vehicle instability, and so on. Rescuers have also been injured by accidentally setting off an automatic airbag when attempting to reach a victim pinned inside. For all these reasons, it is crucial to ensure the scene is safe before approaching the vehicle. Do not try to stabilize the vehicle unless you have special training. Never try to remove a patient trapped inside a vehicle, but wait for those with appropriate training. You may be able to provide some care through an open window or the back seat.

Hostility, Violence, and Crime Scenes

Occasionally a victim or family member shows hostility when you approach or offer help. Rage or hostility may be due to the injury or illness or to emotional factors. Many emergency victims are afraid of losing control, and fear may turn into anger. Drug or alcohol abuse may also cause hostile behavior. If a person seems hostile, first try to quietly explain who you are and that you are there to help. Often, after the patient realizes that you are not a threat but are there to help, the hostility will dissipate. But if the person refuses your care or threatens you, retreat from the scene and call for help from law enforcement personnel. Never try to restrain, argue with, or force care on a victim. Chapter 11 discusses how to deal with behavioral emergencies such as violent people.

Hostile family members can also be a problem, usually because of their fears. Listen to what they have to say and act accordingly. If at any time your personal safety appears threatened, retreat to a safe distance and wait for law enforcement officers and other EMS personnel.

Hostile crowds are a unique threat that can develop when you least expect it. As a rule, one cannot reason with a hostile crowd. If you find a hostile crowd when you arrive, wait at a safe distance until law enforcement and EMS personnel arrive. Approach the scene only when declared safe by police officers. Never approach a hostile crowd.

Suicide occurs at an alarming rate in this country. If you respond to a suicide scene, enter only after determining that the scene is safe. If it is not, wait for responding emergency personnel or law enforcement officers. Never enter a suicide scene alone. If a suicide has occurred and the person is obviously dead, do not touch anything. Protect the scene for responding law enforcement personnel. If the scene is safe and the person is still alive, begin emergency care. Do not touch any items such as a weapon, medication bottle, suicide note, or other items. Concentrate on care of the patient and leave the rest to law enforcement personnel.

In any situation in which a crime may have been committed, take care not to disturb anything in the scene except as needed to provide patient care. It is important to maintain a chain of evidence, if possible, by not touching or moving items on the scene. However, patient care remains the higher priority.

Fire Scenes

Fire scenes require special precautions:

- Never enter a burning or smoky building unless you have special training and are functioning within your role in a fire department. Firefighters are highly trained and use special equipment that protects against fire and smoke.
- Do not let others enter or approach a fire scene.
- Make sure a fire unit is responding, and then try to gather information for responding units, such as the possible number of victims, the cause of the fire, the presence of any explosives or chemicals, and other relevant facts. Relay this information immediately to emergency officials. Never attempt to enter a building that is on fire or contains smoke.
- Always touch doors before opening them. Never open a door that is hot to touch.
- Never use an elevator if there may be fire in the building.
- Never approach a vehicle in flames.

Electricity

Downed electrical lines are a major hazard to both the patient and emergency personnel. Always look for downed wires at an accident scene, and follow these guidelines if you see downed wires:

- Never attempt to move downed wires.
- Notify the power company immediately.
- If the downed wires are across a vehicle, do not touch the vehicle or allow anyone else to do so. Tell anyone in the vehicle to remain still and not exit the vehicle. Never attempt to remove a patient from a vehicle with downed wires across it no matter how seriously injured the patient may be.
- If wires are down across chain link fences, metal structures, or bodies of water or similar hazards, do not touch the fence, structure, or water. Instead, await the arrival of the power company.
- If there is any doubt about downed wires, *do not approach the scene.*

Water and Ice

Deep water and ice involve several hazards.

- Never enter the water unless you have been properly trained and only as a last resort.
- If you are called to assist a person who is in deep water, try to get a flotation device or rope to the patient. Many items commonly found around water will float, such as personal flotation devices, spare tires, plastic jugs, ice chests, gas cans, and so on.
- If a rope is available, try to throw one end of it to the victim and then tow the victim to shallow water where you can render aid.
- If spinal injury is suspected, do not attempt to move the patient from the water until the spine has been adequately immobilized. Instead, float the patient to the side and render care there. If the patient requires lifesaving care that cannot be given in the water, such as CPR, you may have to remove the patient from the water.

Other aquatic environments are equally hazardous. Fast water often occurs following natural disasters such as floods and hurricanes. Never enter fast water but wait until personnel trained in fast-water rescue arrive. A fast-water rescue requires careful planning, proper equipment, and adequate resources.

Ice involves the risks of both drowning and hypothermia. Cold-water immersion is serious and can quickly doom even the best of swimmers. Ice rescue should be left for specially trained personnel who have the necessary safety equipment. Never attempt an ice rescue alone.

Natural Disasters

Natural disasters include tornados, hurricanes, earthquakes, forest and range fires, and others.

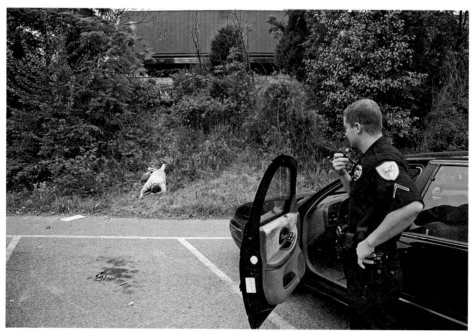

Figure 2-5 When a scene appears unsafe, or is a potential crime scene, ensure that dispatch has been notified.

Following a natural disaster, rescue efforts are generally coordinated through a governmental agency. As always, make personal safety your top priority. Work with the disaster response team, and do not deviate from the rescue plan (Chapter 18).

Natural disasters often pose more hazards than one might think. Many injuries and deaths after natural disasters result from hazards such as electricity, hazardous materials, and fast water rather than directly from the disaster. Minimize your risk by carefully surveying the scene, avoiding obvious hazards, and using caution when operating rescue equipment. For example, gasoline-operated rescue equipment such as chain saws, generators, and sump pumps should never be used in confined spaces.

Unsafe Buildings and Structures

Buildings and other structures may be unsafe because of a fire, explosion, natural disaster, or deterioration. Many different problems may be present, such as:

- An injured victim may be confined or trapped.
- The atmosphere may contain a hazardous gas.
- Communication with a victim may be impossible.

As always, personal safety is the primary concern. The exact or probable location of the victim should be established and a rescue plan devised. Never enter an unsafe building alone. Leave this type of rescue to personnel with proper training and equipment.

Wreckage

Wreckage from an automobile, aircraft, or machinery is hazardous. Hazards include sharp pieces of metal, glass, fuel, and moving parts. In addition, the wreckage may be unstable. Attempt rescue of a victim from wreckage only if you have the proper equipment and training and only after the wreckage has been adequately stabilized. Specific rescue techniques are described in Chapter 18.

Do You Understand?

1. True or false: In an emergency scene where fumes may be present, you may run in and remove the patient if you hold your breath.

2. True or false: A First Responder's responsibilities at a hazardous scene include protecting bystanders.

3. At the scene of a vehicle crash, your responsibilities include:
   a. Removing the victim as quickly as possible from the vehicle
   b. Removing any power lines that have fallen onto the vehicle
   c. Using warning devices to warn oncoming traffic
   d. Disarming the vehicle's airbag

Conclusion

Your well-being as a First Responder depends on understanding and coping with the stress of emergencies, protecting yourself from infectious disease, and staying safe in hazardous scenes. Always remember that safety is your highest priority in any emergency.

Key Terms

acquired immunodeficiency syndrome (AIDS) (p. 19)

airborne transmission (p. 20)

bloodborne transmission (p. 20)

body substance isolation (BSI) (p. 21)

critical incident (p. 18)

Critical Incident Stress Debriefing (CISD) (p. 18)

critical incident stress management (CISM) (p. 18)

debriefing (p. 18)

decontamination (p. 22)

defusing (p. 18)

direct contact (p. 20)

disinfectant (p. 22)

hepatitis (p. 19)

human immunodeficiency virus (HIV) (p. 19)

indirect contact (p. 20)

Occupational Exposure to Bloodborne Pathogens Standard (p. 20)

pathogen (p. 19)

personal protective equipment (PPE) (p. 22)

standard precautions (p. 21)

sterilize (p. 22)

stress (p. 14)

tuberculosis (TB) (p. 20)

universal precautions (p. 21)

vaccine (p. 19)

vector transmission (p. 20)

Review Questions

1. Bargaining, a reaction of a dying patient, involves
   a. offering payment for extra care.
   b. discussing one's last will and testament with relatives.
   c. trying to put off the reality of the coming death.
   d. anger at caregivers and EMS personnel.

2. To help family members cope with a dying patient
   a. give them as much control as possible over the situation.
   b. stay away from them as much as possible.
   c. keep them busy with "make-work" tasks to avoid thinking about the situation.
   d. report their reactions to social services agencies.

3. Critical incident stress management programs for First Responders are usually run by
   a. fire chiefs and law enforcement managers.
   b. counselors and mental health professionals.
   c. First Responder course instructors.
   d. other First Responders.

4. In most patients, bloodborne diseases can also be transmitted by the patient's
   a. tears.
   b. semen.
   c. saliva.
   d. urine.

5. The OSHA Bloodborne Pathogen Standard mandates precautions applying to blood and
   a. the respiration of patients with TB.
   b. foodborne illnesses.
   c. toxic chemicals.
   d. all other potentially infectious materials.

6. Equipment used in providing patient care may be disinfected using
   a. iodine.
   b. rubbing alcohol.
   c. bleach solution.
   d. sterile saline.

7. Which substance should not come into contact with latex medical exam gloves?
   a. Petroleum-based hand lotions
   b. Water
   c. Any body fluid from the patient
   d. Waterless antiseptic towelettes

8. OSHA recommends following standard precautions with
   a. blood and semen.
   b. blood, urine, and semen.
   c. blood, vomit, and semen.
   d. any body fluid.

9. If a hazardous material is spilled at an emergency scene,
   a. call it in and then remove a contaminated patient from the scene.
   b. call it in and stay away and let trained personnel manage the scene.
   c. first remove the patient and hose him or her off as quickly as possible.
   d. hose down the entire scene first.

10. How should you attempt to manage a hostile crowd at the scene?
    a. Try to reason with them.
    b. Leave immediately in your vehicle.
    c. Wait at a safe distance for law enforcement and EMS personnel.
    d. Restrain anyone who may potentially become violent.

Legal and Ethical Issues

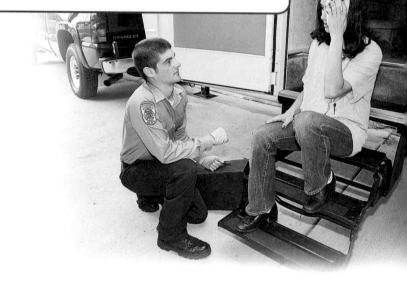

Chapter Preview

- Regulations
- Scope of Practice
- Standard of Care
- Ethical Responsibilities
- Consent
- Abandonment
- Negligence
- Confidentiality
- Special Situations

You Respond To ...

a scene where an injured man is lying on the sidewalk. He is responsive but his words are heavily slurred, and he seems confused and disoriented. You notice his pupils are dilated. One leg is bleeding heavily, soaking the fabric of his pants. You ask if you can help him and stop the bleeding, but he waves you away and mumbles, "I'm okay —it's not bad."

Introduction

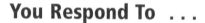oth lay people and trained rescuers often worry about being sued by a victim or patient given care. Lawsuits against First Responders who provide emergency care at the scene of an accident are rare, however, and are usually unsuccessful when the First Responder understands and adheres to basic legal principles related to emergency care. This chapter addresses the general legal principles of emergency care. Because states vary somewhat in their laws,

your instructor will update you about laws in your area that apply to you.

Regulations

✓ Need to Know

Federal, state, and often local laws and regulations govern the practice of emergency medicine and stipulate the requirements for registering or becoming certified as a First Responder. Such laws also state what you can and cannot do as a First Responder under the medical oversight of the medical director, as described in Chapter 1.

Scope of Practice

Scope of practice refers to the level of care that can be provided by a healthcare professional with a specified level of training. Individuals cannot practice outside or beyond their level of training. The scope of care for First Responders is defined at the national level by the United States Department of Transportation's *First Responder: National Standard Curriculum*, on which this text and your training are based. Some state laws may modify certain aspects of the First Responder scope of care, as your instructor will explain as needed. Scope of care is further defined within a particular EMS system through the process of medical oversight. This process includes protocols and standing orders developed by the medical director, as well as direct oversight. These factors collectively define what you can and should do as a First Responder when delivering emergency care.

Standard of Care

Standard of care is closely related to scope of practice but refers to *how* you provide care as well as *what* specific care you give. The standard of care refers to the minimal quality of care First Responders are trained to provide. In legal terms, you are expected to give the same care as a reasonable, prudent First Responder with similar training would give a patient in similar circumstances.

The national standards of care for First Responders are based on training guidelines in the *National Standard Curriculum* as well as accepted medical authorities, including the EMS medical director. Essentially, what you are taught in your First Responder training comprises the standards of care applicable to you. As long as you give care as you have been taught, you are meeting the standard of care and cannot be held legally liable for a negative patient outcome.

As explained in the later section on negligence, if you neglect to follow the standard of care—to act as you have been trained—and the patient suffers as a result of your negligence, then you may be legally liable for your actions.

Ethical Responsibilities

 Need to Do

While laws and regulations narrowly define scope and standards of care along with specific legal requirements, ethical principles are generally broader. As a healthcare provider and First Responder, you accept the ethical responsibility to provide the best patient care possible. This involves the following responsibilities:

1. Make the physical and emotional needs of the patient your highest priority when providing care.

2. Practice your caregiving skills until you are certain you have mastered all skills.

3. Regularly attend continuing education and refresher programs to learn new information

and skills and to ensure continued mastery of your present skills.

4. After each patient care episode, review your performances to see if you can improve your response time, give better care to improve patient outcomes, or communicate more effectively.

5. Be honest in your reporting and documentation.

 Do You Understand?

1. True or false: Standards of care require you to perform any patient care that an EMT would provide in the same circumstances.

2. True or false: You may be legally liable for acting outside your scope of practice.

3. When providing patient care, your ethical responsibilities make what your highest priority?

Consent

 Need to Know

All people have a fundamental right to decide what can or cannot be done to their body—including what medical or emergency care they will accept. Therefore, before you can provide care for a patient, you must obtain the victim's **consent** whenever the victim (or victim's guardian) is competent to give consent **(Figure 3-1).** The victim gives consent based on the information you provide. A competent adult has the right to refuse care.

Competence

When seeking the victim's consent to give emergency care, first determine whether the victim is competent to consent. **Competent** means the person is able to understand what is happening and the implications of his or her decision about receiving or refusing emergency care. A victim may not be competent because of intoxication, the influence of a drug, or altered mental status caused by a severe injury.

In cases of children or mentally incompetent adults, consent must be given by a parent or legal guardian. The legal age at which a person is no longer considered a minor varies among states, and in some states, emancipated minors under the usual legal age have a court order giving them many adult rights, including the right to consent.

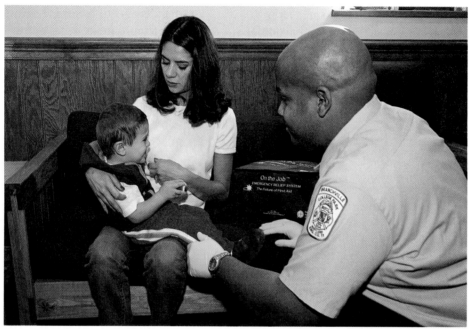

Figure 3-1 You must have consent before providing patient care.

In an emergency, when the parents or guardians of a child or mentally incompetent adult cannot be reached quickly to give permission, care should be given on the assumption that their consent would be given if possible (implied consent).

Expressed Consent

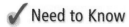 Need to Do

Expressed consent means the patient explicitly grants permission for you to give care, usually with a verbal agreement or a nod. Expressed consent must be obtained from every responsive, mentally competent adult before giving emergency care. To obtain consent you must:

1. Identify yourself to the patient.
2. State your level of training.
3. Explain what you think may be wrong.
4. Describe the care you plan to give and its benefits.
5. Explain any risks related to the care.

Implied Consent

✔ Need to Know

When a patient is unresponsive, confused, or seriously injured, he or she may not be able to grant consent. In these cases, the law assumes that the patient would, if able, grant consent for life-saving care. This

is termed **implied consent.** Implied consent also applies to children and mentally incompetent adults who obviously need emergency care when their parents or guardians cannot be reached to give consent.

Refusal of Consent

▶ Need to Do

Some victims, even those who desperately need it, will refuse the care you offer. Competent adult victims have the right to refuse medical care, and you must honor their wishes. The refusal may be verbal or indicated by shaking the head or pulling away from you. Ideally, the refusal should be verbal so that the person's competence can be evaluated. The person should be informed of and fully understand all the risks and consequences associated with refusing emergency medical care. Once treatment begins, the patient still has the right to withdraw from emergency medical care at any time. Follow these guidelines when a victim refuses to give consent for care:

- When in doubt, err in favor of providing care.
- Do not argue with the victim or question the victim's personal beliefs.
- Do not try to give care. Touching a victim who refuses care may make you guilty of battery (discussed in the next section).
- Allow responding EMS units to arrive and evaluate the situation. You should not make an independent decision regarding the refusal of care.

REFUSAL OF MEDICAL COVERAGE

I hereby voluntarily acknowledge and state that I have been advised regarding the state of my present physical condition. I have been advised of the risks/complications of my condition and the dangers of refusing medical treatment. I understand the risks, complications and/or dangers of refusing medical treatment as explained by Red County Rescue Service personnel. With full knowledge of the possible consequences of my refusal of care, I hereby voluntarily refuse medical care and transportation by Red County Rescue Service. Furthermore, I, for myself, my heirs, executors, administrators and assigns forever release and fully discharge Red County Rescue Service, its officers, employers, medical consultants, hospitals, borrowed servants or agents from any and all liability or claims of whatever nature arising out of Red County Rescue Service's efforts to provide me with medical care and/or transportation and my consequent refusal, and I, therefore, agree to hold them completely and totally harmless and without fault unconditionally. *I have read and fully understand all of the above.*

☐ Medical Control Contact   Talked to:_____

☐ Patient refused specific treatment (explain in narrative) _____

Date____/____/____   Signature **X**_____   Date____/____/____   Witness **X**_____

Figure 3-2 Refusal of care form.

- If possible, have the victim sign a refusal form or at least try to have a witness hear the victim's refusal. Many EMS systems provide First Responders with a Refusal of Care form for this situation **(Figure 3-2)**.

- While awaiting arrival of additional EMS resources, you should:

  1. Try again to persuade the victim to accept care.

  2. Determine whether the victim is competent to make a rational, informed decision and is not under the influence of alcohol or other drugs or responding to the effects of illness or injury.

  3. Inform the victim again why care is needed and what may happen if care is refused.

  4. Consult medical oversight as directed by your local protocol.

  5. Consider calling for the assistance of law enforcement.

  6. Report your assessment findings and any emergency medical care you have provided.

Assault and Battery

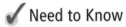
Need to Know

Assault is the crime of threatening, either verbally or physically, to touch another person without consent. **Battery,** touching another person without consent, is a crime. If you provide emergency care to a competent victim who refuses your care, you may be found guilty of assault or battery, and the victim may also file a lawsuit against you.

Advance Directives

An **advance directive,** such as a **living will,** is a legal document in which a person states his or her wishes not to receive specified types of medical care. The document is developed and signed while the person is competent to make decisions regarding future situations when the person may be unable to express his or her wishes. A **durable power of attorney** for healthcare is a type of advance directive by which a person gives another person the legal right and responsibility to make care decisions, including the right to refuse certain types of care. A common type of advance directive is a **Do Not Resuscitate (DNR) order,** in which the person, in advance of a situation, refuses to accept resuscitative efforts in case of cardiac arrest **(Figure 3-3)**. Often, such orders are made by people with a terminal illness or a medical condition that reduces the likelihood of full recovery from arrest. Advance directives generally must be signed and witnessed, and some states require a physician's signature as well.

If an advance directive is brought to your attention when you are about to provide care to a victim, follow your local protocol based on your state's laws. Remember that DNR orders refer only to resuscitative care for victims whose heart has stopped—it does not refer to other kinds of treatment. If there is any doubt, or if a written directive is not present, give care as usual. In the case of an unresponsive adult, other adults, including family members, cannot refuse care for the victim without a formal advance directive. If family members ask you to provide care, even when a DNR order is present, it is usually best to give care until you turn over patient care to responding EMS professionals.

HENNEPIN COUNTY
RESUSCITATION GUIDELINES

Check all boxes that apply Category	Recommended action	Medical response will provide	Medical response not provided
[ ] CPR	Call 911	Full treatment as appropriate	
[X] DNR (No CPR)	Call 911 Except for cardiac arrest	Active treatment up to the point of cardiac arrest	If in cardiac arrest: No intubation No ventilatory assistance No chest compressions No defibrillation
[ ] Hospice or comfort care	Call M.D. or R.N May call ambulance for routine transport May call 911 for urgent needs	Comfort and hygiene care	If in cardiac arrest: No intubation No ventilatory assistance No chest compressions No defibrillation

Patient/Client Name John Doe

I understand this document identifies the level of care to be rendered in situations where death may be imminent. I make this request knowingly and I am aware of the alternatives. I expressly release, on behalf of myself and my family, all persons who shall in the future attend to my medical care of any and all liablility whatsoever for acting in accordance with this request of mine. Furthermore, I direct these guidelines be enforced even though I may develop a diminished mental capacity at some future time. I am aware that I can revoke these guidelines at any time by simply expressing my request verbally or in writing to my caretaking, family, physician, or designated heath care provider.

John Doe 5/31/06
Patient/Client or Authorized Signature "Relationship" Date

I have witnessed the above signature:

Larry Johnson
Witness Signature

Scott ... MD 1234 Hospital Drive 5/31/06
Physician's Signature Address Phone # Date

THE ABOVE 3 SIGNATURES AND 2 DATES ARE REQUIRED FOR THIS FORM TO BE VALID AND ITS INTENT CARRIED OUT

PATIENT COPY - BLUE CHART COPY - PINK PHYSICIAN COPY - YELLOW

Figure 3-3 A typical advance directive.

Abandonment

While it is important to obtain consent from a patient before beginning treatment, it is also critical to ensure that a patient will continue to receive care once treatment is initiated. Once you have initiated emergency care for a patient, you have a legal obligation to continue that care until another person with equal or higher training arrives and takes over the patient's care. Generally, your obligation to render care ends when EMTs take over. If you fail to continue care before they do, you could be sued for **abandonment,** a form of negligence. Even only assessing the patient is considered care: If you assess a patient and release that patient before EMTs arrive and the patient later dies or suffers, you are still guilty of abandonment. Leaving a victim who refuses care, without waiting for EMTs to arrive and assess the victim, may also constitute abandonment.

A special case of abandonment may occur if you believe a person is dead and do not attempt resuscitation. Unless if the patient is obviously dead and resuscitation is obviously impossible, you must attempt resuscitation. The conditions in which death can be assumed include decapitation, rigor mortis (the stiffening of the body that occurs hours after death), or tissue decomposition (occurs after a day or more).

Remember that if you are unsure what to do in any situation, call medical control for advice.

Negligence

Negligence is failing to care for a patient following the accepted standard of care. Negligence includes both not giving care and giving improper or poor-quality care. In either case, if the patient suffers further injury or disability, you may be sued for negligence. Legally, four conditions must be present for negligence to have occurred:

1. **There must be a duty to act.** When acting in your role as a First Responder, you usually have a legal obligation to give emergency medical care, although state laws vary in terms of how this duty is defined. In some locales,

duty may be defined differently for volunteer First Responders and First Responders in paid positions. In addition, some laws differentiate between care given during work hours and care given during time off. In almost all cases, however, once you offer a victim care and begin to provide treatment, you have a **duty to act** and to meet the standard of care for First Responders.

2. **The duty to act is breached.** This happens if you fail to give care or to meet the standard of care, whether willfully (gross negligence) or unintentionally.

3. **The patient suffers injury or damage.** The damages a patient may sue for include not only physical injury and disability but also emotional and psychological damage, such as pain and suffering.

4. **The patient's injury or damage resulted from your actions or inactions.** You can be sued for harm or damage that resulted from your actions or inactions, called "proximate cause." While you cannot be sued for the initial injury that occurred before you began care (e.g., a spinal fracture related to a head injury), you can be sued for any injury that results from your actions (e.g., paralysis resulting from improperly moving a patient with a spinal injury).

Good Samaritan Laws

Negligence can be charged only when you have a duty to act. In some situations, however, you may be providing emergency care voluntarily rather than in your role as a First Responder. In most states you are not legally obligated during your off hours to stop at the scene of an accident, for example, to provide emergency care; your instructor will tell you about the laws in your state and your obligations under them. To protect persons with emergency care training who voluntarily provide emergency care, most states have **Good Samaritan laws.** Such laws generally protect First Responders who act in good faith and within the scope of their training. These laws vary from state to state, and your instructor will inform you of the legal protections in your state.

Confidentiality

As a First Responder, you will often learn things about patients that are generally considered private. When gathering the patient's history from the patient or family members, you may learn about previous medical problems, physical problems, medication use, and other personal information. Your assessment findings and the emergency care you provide are also confidential information. You have an ethical responsibility to respect the patient's right to privacy and should never talk about this information with others, including family members and coworkers.

In addition, the patient's right to privacy and confidentiality of all information is legally protected by the **Health Insurance Portability and Accountability Act (HIPAA),** which applies to all providers of healthcare. This law generally specifies that you must not disclose any information about a patient, including his or her identity—even through casual conversation—except when that information is needed by others providing treatment. Violations may lead to civil or criminal penalties.

The HIPAA regulations are complex and detailed, particularly in reference to the management of written records. Always follow the specific policies of your EMS system.

As a general rule, do not talk about specific patients at all with others not involved in the patient's care. When in doubt, consider everything you know about a patient to be confidential.

This principle of confidentiality does not apply to communication with other EMS or healthcare personnel involved in the patient's care who may need this information. In some cases, you may also need to provide information to law enforcement personnel at the scene. Otherwise, never release any confidential information about the patient without a written release form signed by the patient.

A release is not required when providing information in reports required by law, such as when reporting abuse or a gunshot wound, or when subpoenaed by a court to testify.

Do You Understand?

1. When do you have implied consent to treat a patient?

_____

2. True or false: If a competent adult patient refuses consent, you should leave the scene immediately.

3. You may be guilty of _____ if you fail to meet the standard of care when treating a patient.

Special Situations

Legal considerations are involved in certain other situations, such as those involving medical identifications, crime scenes, reportable events, and documentation.

Medical Identification Insignia

▶ Need to Do

Medical identification insignia include necklaces, bracelets, and cards worn or carried by patients who have certain medical conditions such as allergies, diabetes, epilepsy, and heart conditions **(Figure 3-4)**. Not looking for such an insignia in your patient assessment may be negligence.

Crime Scenes

If you are providing emergency care at a scene where a crime may have been committed, take precautions to preserve evidence that may be important later:

- Make sure the scene is safe before entering to provide patient care.
- Ensure that law enforcement personnel have been notified and are responding.
- Do not disturb any item at the scene unless emergency medical care requires it. Remember that emergency medical care of the patient is your top priority.
- Observe and document anything unusual at the scene.
- If possible, when removing a patient's clothing to expose an injury, do not cut through holes in clothing from gunshot or stabbing wounds.
- When law enforcement personnel have responded, follow their directions. If they request that you not touch anything, explain what is necessary to provide essential patient care.

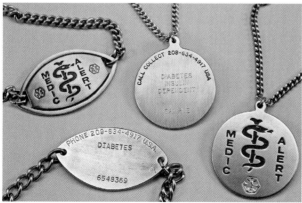

Figure 3-4 Examples of medical information insignia.

Reportable Events

First Responders are obligated under federal and state laws to report certain situations to the appropriate authorities. Your instructor will inform you what events must be reported in your area and how to file reports. Typically, these situations include:

- Child, elder, and spouse abuse or domestic violence
- Certain crimes, such as gunshot and knife wounds, suspicious burns, rape and sexual assault
- Vehicle crashes
- Certain infectious diseases
- Exposure to a patient's body fluids

Documentation

✓ Need to Know

Documenting patient assessment findings and care is nearly as important as the care itself. Your verbal report and written record help other EMS professionals assess and treat the patient. A patient's condition often changes by the time he or she reaches the hospital. Therefore, your documentation of the patient's condition when seen by you immediately after the emergency provides much information for EMTs and emergency department staff.

In addition, your record is a legal document. Should you be called to court for any reason, the written record helps support what you saw, heard, and did at the scene. Complete the record as soon as possible after the emergency while the facts are fresh in your memory. State and local EMS requirements for documentation vary, and many EMS systems have printed forms used by First Responders **(Figure 3-5)**. Your course instructor will tell you about the forms used in your system.

✎ Do You Understand?

1. List at least four precautions to take when giving emergency care at a crime scene.

   _____ _____

   _____ _____

2. True or false: You may be obligated to report child abuse to the authorities.

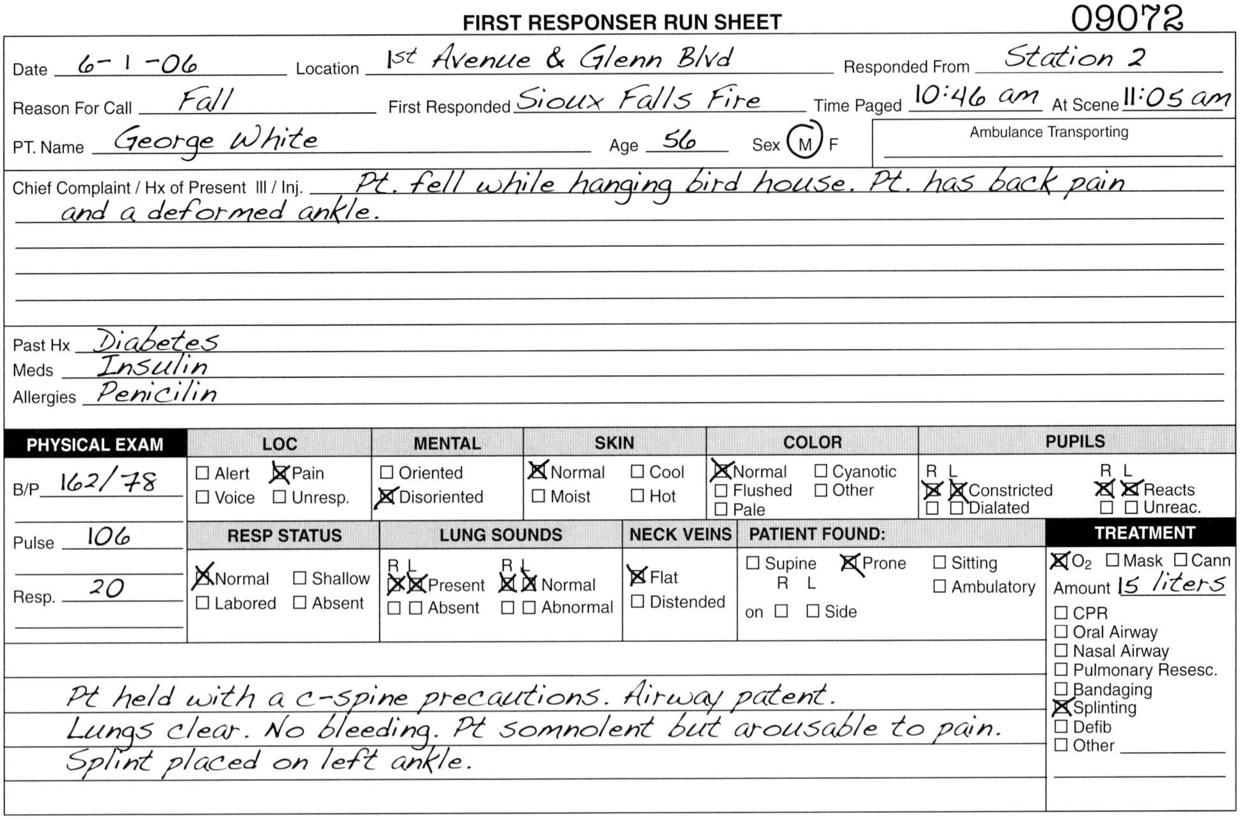

FIRST RESPONSER RUN SHEET   09072

Date _6-1-06_ Location _1st Avenue & Glenn Blvd_	Responded From _Station 2_
Reason For Call _Fall_ First Responded _Sioux Falls Fire_	Time Paged _10:46 am_ At Scene _11:05 am_
PT. Name _George White_ Age _56_ Sex (M) F	Ambulance Transporting

Chief Complaint / Hx of Present Ill / Inj. ___Pt. fell while hanging bird house. Pt. has back pain___
___and a deformed ankle.___

Past Hx _Diabetes_
Meds _Insulin_
Allergies _Penicilin_

PHYSICAL EXAM	LOC	MENTAL	SKIN	COLOR	PUPILS
B/P _162/78_	☐ Alert ☒ Pain ☐ Voice ☐ Unresp.	☐ Oriented ☒ Disoriented	☒ Normal ☐ Cool ☐ Moist ☐ Hot	☒ Normal ☐ Cyanotic ☐ Flushed ☐ Other ☐ Pale	R L ☒ ☒ Constricted ☐ ☐ Dialated R L ☒ ☒ Reacts ☐ ☐ Unreac.

Pulse _106_	RESP STATUS	LUNG SOUNDS	NECK VEINS	PATIENT FOUND:	TREATMENT
Resp. _20_	☒ Normal ☐ Shallow ☐ Labored ☐ Absent	R L ☒ ☒ Present R L ☐ ☐ Absent ☒ ☒ Normal ☐ ☐ Abnormal	☒ Flat ☐ Distended	☐ Supine ☒ Prone R L on ☐ ☐ Side ☐ Sitting ☐ Ambulatory	☒ O₂ ☐ Mask ☐ Cann Amount _15 liters_ ☐ CPR ☐ Oral Airway ☐ Nasal Airway ☐ Pulmonary Resesc. ☐ Bandaging ☒ Splinting ☐ Defib ☐ Other _____

Pt held with a c-spine precautions. Airway patent.
Lungs clear. No bleeding. Pt somnolent but arousable to pain.
Splint placed on left ankle.

Figure 3-5 A typical report form used by First Responders.

Conclusion

In addition to your general ethical responsibility for giving patients the best care possible, you have legal obligations for giving correct care and acting properly in an emergency. When dutifully following the general principles related to emergency care, you will not have to be concerned with being sued if a patient has a negative outcome.

Key Terms

abandonment (p. 36)

advance directive (p. 35)

assault (p. 35)

battery (p. 35)

competent (p. 33)

consent (p. 33)

Do Not Resuscitate (DNR) order (p. 35)

durable power of attorney (p. 35)

duty to act (p. 36)

expressed consent (p. 34)

Good Samaritan laws (p. 37)

Health Insurance Portability and Accountability Act (HIPAA) (p. 37)

implied consent (p. 34)

living will (p. 35)

negligence (p. 36)

scope of practice (p. 32)

standard of care (p. 33)

Review Questions

1. Scope of practice is defined in part by
   a. how First Responders behave in other parts of the country.
   b. protocols developed by the medical director.
   c. observing the care given by Paramedics.
   d. international research associations.

2. Which of the following is *not* a reason why an adult patient may be considered incompetent to refuse care?
   a. Intoxication
   b. Unresponsiveness
   c. Religious beliefs about medical treatment
   d. Altered mental status caused by injury

3. The crime of assault occurs if
   a. you touch a patient without consent.
   b. you give care different from your training.
   c. you verbally threaten a patient.
   d. your care causes the patient to experience pain.

4. In which situation can you *not* be found guilty of negligence?
   a. Harm or damage resulted from your faulty action.
   b. Harm or damage resulted from your inaction
   c. Pain but no physical disability resulted from your faulty actions
   d. Disability resulted from the injury despite the care you gave

5. With whom should you never discuss a patient's injury?
   a. Your spouse
   b. Your supervisor
   c. Law enforcement personnel at the scene
   d. Healthcare personnel not present at the scene

6. What may result if you fail to look for medical insignia during your assessment of a patient?
   a. Negligence
   b. Abandonment
   c. Breach of confidentiality
   d. Transmission of infectious disease

7. You should document the patient care you provided in an emergency
   a. before going off duty at the end of your shift.
   b. any time before going on your next call.
   c. as soon as possible after the emergency.
   d. during your weekly report.

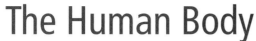

Chapter 4

The Human Body

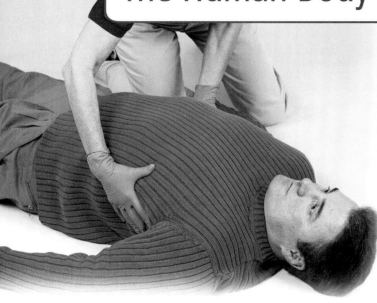

Chapter Preview

• Body Regions and Directions

• Body Systems

• Respiratory System

• Circulatory System

• Musculoskeletal System

• Nervous System

• The Skin

• Other Body Systems

You Respond To . . .

a scene where an older woman lies on the floor unresponsive. Her breathing is very slow, and her skin is pale and cool. You see no signs of injury. You take her pulse and find that her heart rate is slower than normal.

Introduction

The human body is composed of many different organs and tissues working together to sustain life and allow for activity. A minor injury or illness may damage only a specific body part or function, but a serious injury or sudden illness can threaten body functions necessary for life. Understanding the human body can help you recognize the effects of injuries and illnesses and help you give more effective emergency care.

Body Regions and Directions

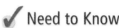 Need to Know

To prevent confusion when describing different areas of the body, such as to report the location of a patient's injury or signs and symptoms, special terms are used by healthcare providers for body regions. Directional and positional terms typically are used to describe the relationship of body structures or the patient's position.

Body Regions and Cavities

The following are key terms referring to body regions (**Figure 4-1**):

☑ The term **extremities** refers to both the arms and legs. Many emergency care principles are the same for all the extremities, so this term is often used rather than saying "arms and legs."

☑ The term **thorax** refers to the chest area enclosed by the ribs (including the back of the body). The **thoracic cavity** is the area inside the chest where the heart and lungs are located.

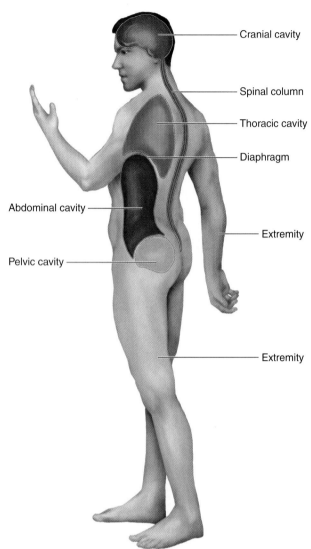

Figure 4-1 Major regions and cavities of the body.

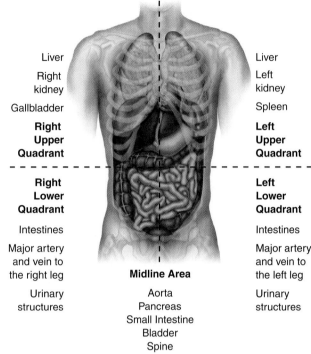

Figure 4-2 Abdominal quadrants.

☑ The term **abdomen** refers to the area immediately below the thoracic cavity. In the **abdominal cavity** are located the stomach, intestines, and other organs. Between the thoracic cavity and the abdominal cavity is the **diaphragm,** a muscle that moves with breathing.

☑ The term **pelvis** refers to the area below the abdomen and specifically to the pelvic bones between the hip and the lower spine. In the **pelvic cavity** are located the bladder and other organs.

☑ The term spine, or **spinal column,** refers to the bones of the neck and back, as well as to the nerves, or **spinal cord,** that run through the vertebrae.

Because many important organs are situated within the abdomen, **abdominal quadrants** are used to describe specific injuries or signs and symptoms. **Figure 4-2** shows the four quadrants of the abdomen and the underlying organs. The upper and lower quadrants are divided by a line passing through the umbilicus. These descriptions, like all directional terms referring to the body, are based on the **anatomical position,** with the patient face forward and palms facing forward.

Directional Terms

All positional and directional terms are based on the anatomical position shown in **Figure 4-3**. The following are key directional and positional terms used to describe injuries and signs and symptoms:

☑ **right, left** refer to the *patient's* right and left, divided by a **midline** down the center of the body

☑ **lateral, medial** away from the midline of the body, toward the midline of the body

☑ **anterior, posterior** the front or back of the body

☑ **proximal, distal** closer or farther away from the trunk of the body (used to describe the relative position of two structures; e.g., the knee is proximal to the ankle, the wrist is distal to the forearm)

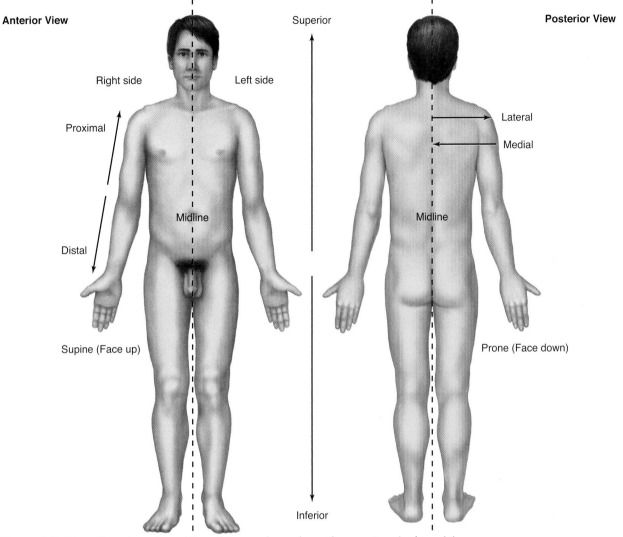

Figure 4-3 Directional and positional terms based on the anatomical position.

☑ **superior, inferior** toward the head, toward the feet (used to describe the relative position of two structures; e.g., the mouth is superior to the chin, the nostrils are inferior to the eyes)

☑ **prone, supine** lying facedown, lying faceup

Body Systems

An **organ** is a body structure that accomplishes one or more specific functions. In most cases, several organs work together to achieve a larger function. For example, the heart, arteries, veins, and capillaries work together to circulate blood to all parts of the body. The organs that work together to perform a major body function are called a **body system.**

Although we can talk about each system as if it is separate from other body systems, in fact, body systems are closely interrelated and work together to perform many functions. For example:

☑ Blood carries oxygen from the lungs (respiratory system) to the body cells, all of which need a continual supply of oxygen to stay alive. Nerve sensors (nervous system) detect the amount of oxygen and carbon dioxide in the blood and speed up or slow down the heart beat (cardiovascular system) and breathing to change the oxygen level.

☑ If body temperature drops, muscles in the extremities (musculoskeletal system) start shivering to produce heat, which is then carried by the blood (cardiovascular system) to vital organs.

Understanding the close relationships of body systems will help you understand what is happening in the body in injuries and illness so that you can provide emergency care most effectively.

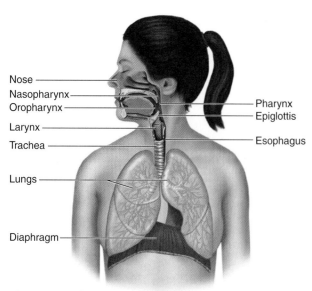

Nose
Nasopharynx
Oropharynx
Larynx
Trachea
Lungs
Diaphragm

Pharynx
Epiglottis
Esophagus

Figure 4-4 The respiratory system.

Respiratory System

✓ Need to Know

The main functions of the **respiratory system** are to bring air into the lungs, allow oxygen from the air to enter the blood, and remove carbon dioxide from the blood into the air breathed out (exhaled). This process is called respiration.

The primary organs of the respiratory system are the structures of the airway and the lungs (**Figure 4-4**):

- ☑ The **airway** is the path air takes from the nose and mouth to the lungs.
- ☑ Air entering the nose or mouth passes through the **pharynx** (throat) to the **trachea,** the tube carrying air through the neck.
- ☑ The trachea branches into the left and right **bronchi** (singular: bronchus), the passageways into the lungs.
- ☑ These tubes branch into smaller passages in the lungs and eventually end in the **alveoli,** the tiny air sacs where oxygen and carbon dioxide pass into and out of small blood vessels called capillaries.

The pharynx also leads to the **esophagus,** the tube that carries food to the stomach, so another structure, called the epiglottis, is very important for breathing:

- ☑ The **epiglottis** is a tissue flap that prevents solids and liquids from entering the trachea and blocking the airway or reaching the lungs.
- ☑ The epiglottis directs food and drink to pass instead to the esophagus and stomach.

Breathing depends on muscular movements under the control of the nervous system:

- ☑ When the diaphragm (the large muscle below the lungs) contracts and moves down, the thoracic cavity and lungs expand, pulling air into the lungs.
- ☑ In the lungs, oxygen enters the blood and carbon dioxide leaves the blood.
- ☑ When the diaphragm relaxes and moves up, the thoracic cavity contracts, and air carrying the carbon dioxide flows back out of the lungs.

Emergency Care Related to the Respiratory System

■ Need to Recognize

Respiration, one of the most vital functions in the body, can be affected by many different injuries and illnesses.

- ◆ An **airway obstruction** is a physical blockage of the airway that prevents the flow of air, such as **choking** on a piece of food lodged in the pharynx. In an unresponsive person lying supine, the tongue may block the opening into the pharynx.
- ◆ Chest injuries may also affect respiration. A broken rib may puncture a lung, making breathing ineffective. A penetrating injury into the lungs caused by a sharp object may alter the lung pressures needed for inhaling, thereby keeping the lungs from filling with air.
- ◆ Breathing is controlled by the brain, so other factors that affect the nervous system may also cause respiratory emergencies. A poisoning or drug overdose, for example, may severely depress nervous system functions, slowing breathing to the point where the body is not getting enough oxygen.
- ◆ Asthma is a common illness, especially in children, in which airway tissues swell and make it hard for the person to breathe in.

In infants and children, anatomical structures are smaller and the airway is more easily obstructed than in adults. Infants' and children's tongues take up proportionally more space in the mouth and may obstruct the airway more easily. In addition, the trachea is more flexible. The primary cause of cardiac arrest in infants and children is an uncorrected respiratory problem.

Circulatory System

✔ Need to Know

The **circulatory system** consists of the heart, blood, and blood vessels throughout the body (**Figure 4-5**). The primary functions of the circulatory system are to:

☑ Transport oxygen and nutrients in the blood to all parts of the body.

☑ Remove carbon dioxide and other wastes.

The heart has four chambers, the left and right **atria,** the upper receiving chambers of the heart, and the left and right **ventricles,** the lower pumping chambers.

☑ The ventricles pump the blood through two loops or cycles in the body:

1. The right ventricle pumps blood to the lungs to pick up oxygen and release carbon dioxide. The blood returns to the left atrium, from which it moves through a one-way valve to the left ventricle.

2. The left ventricle pumps the oxygenated blood into all areas of the body to release oxygen for use by body cells and pick up carbon dioxide for removal. The blood returns to the right atrium, from which it moves through a one-way valve to the right ventricle to be pumped again to the lungs.

☑ The heart is composed of muscle (**myocardium**) that contracts to create the pumping action. **Contractions** are controlled by electrical signals under nervous system control.

☑ The blood flows from the heart to body areas through the **arteries (Figure 4-6).** With the heart beat, pulsing **blood pressure** changes occur in the arteries that can be felt in certain body locations as the **pulse.**

The most commonly measured pulses are in the carotid, femoral, radial, and brachial arteries:

☑ The carotid arteries are the major arteries of the neck, where the pulse can be palpated on either side.

☑ The femoral artery is the major artery of the thigh, where the pulse can be palpated in the crease between the abdomen and thigh.

☑ The radial artery is the major artery of the lower arm, where the pulse can be palpated on the palm side of the wrist.

☑ The brachial artery is a primary artery of the upper arm, where the pulse can be palpated on the inside of the arm between the elbow and the shoulder.

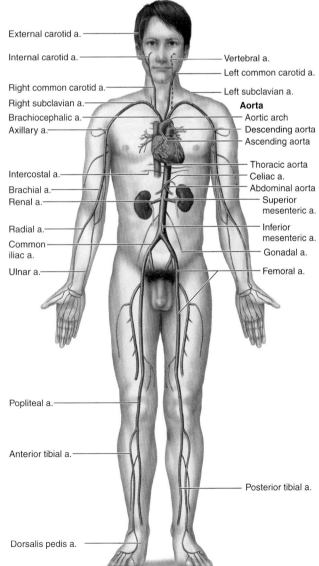

Figure 4-6 Major arteries of the body.

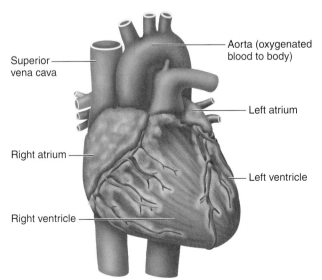

Figure 4-5 The heart.

Arteries progressively branch into smaller vessels that eventually reach **capillaries,** small blood vessels with thin walls where oxygen and carbon dioxide are exchanged with body cells. From the capillaries, the blood drains back to the heart through the **veins.** Blood flows more evenly through veins, which do not have a pulse. Arteries are generally deeper in the body than veins and are therefore more protected and less likely to be damaged by injuries.

The heart rate, which can be measured as the pulse, is affected by many factors:

☑ The average resting heart rate in adult males is 64 to 72 beats per minute, and in adult females, 72 to 80 beats per minute.

☑ The heart rate of infants and children is higher.

☑ With exercise, fever, or emotional excitement, the heart rate increases to meet the body's greater need for oxygen.

Emergency Care Related to the Cardiovascular System

◼ Need to Recognize

Cells begin to die in vital organs such as the brain after only a few minutes without oxygen. The delivery of oxygen to body cells can be diminished by any injury or illness that affects the heart, blood, or blood vessels.

⧫ Bleeding may be so severe that not enough blood is left in circulation to provide the body with enough oxygen.

⧫ Arterial bleeding is most severe because the blood may spurt out under pressure, leading within minutes to the life-threatening condition of shock. **Shock** occurs when vital body organs are not receiving enough oxygen.

⧫ Bleeding from veins is generally slower but can still be serious or life-threatening if it continues.

⧫ Capillary bleeding is usually minor and stops by itself as the blood clots.

Stroke is another type of blood vessel problem involving arteries in the brain. A blood clot or bleeding in the brain may reduce circulation to a part of the brain, causing mental and physical impairments.

Problems involving the heart also affect tissue oxygenation:

⧫ If the heart muscle does not receive enough oxygenated blood because of blocked cardiac arteries, part of the cardiac muscle may die, commonly called a heart attack or **acute myocardial infarction.** Heart muscle can tolerate interrup-

tion of the blood supply for only very short periods. The heart may stop (**cardiac arrest**).

⧫ **Dysrhythmia** (also called arrhythmia), an irregular heartbeat, is another type of heart problem that may reduce the heart's pumping ability.

⧫ **Fibrillation** is a serious dysrhythmia, common after a heart attack, in which the heart muscle flutters rather than pumping blood.

Musculoskeletal System

✓ Need to Know

The **musculoskeletal system** combines the skeletal system **(Figures 4-7 and 4-8)** and the muscular system along with the structures that join them (ligaments and tendons). The musculoskeletal system's primary functions are the following:

☑ The skeletal system provides shape and support for the body as a whole.

☑ The muscles act on the bones, allowing for movement.

☑ Groups of bones protect vital internal organs: The ribs protect the heart and lungs, the

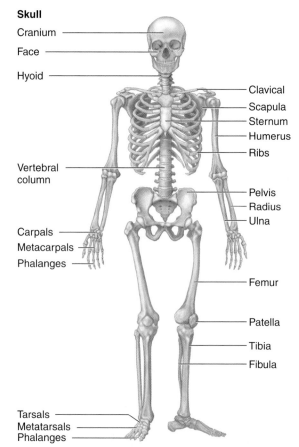

Figure 4-7 The skeletal system.

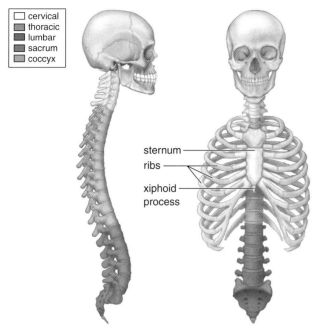

cervical
thoracic
lumbar
sacrum
coccyx

sternum
ribs
xiphoid
process

Figure 4-8 The spine and rib cage.

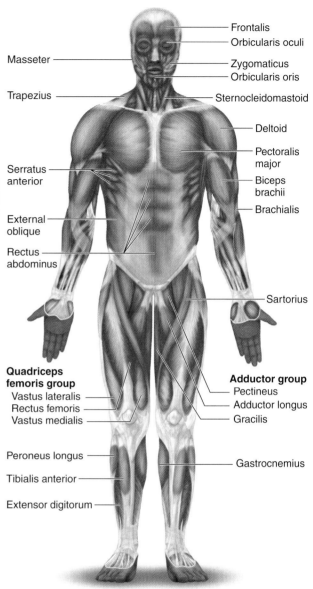

Frontalis
Orbicularis oculi
Masseter
Zygomaticus
Orbicularis oris
Trapezius
Sternocleidomastoid
Deltoid
Pectoralis major
Serratus anterior
Biceps brachii
Brachialis
External oblique
Rectus abdominus
Sartorius

Quadriceps femoris group
Vastus lateralis
Rectus femoris
Vastus medialis

Adductor group
Pectineus
Adductor longus
Gracilis

Peroneus longus
Tibialis anterior
Extensor digitorum

Gastrocnemius

Figure 4-9 Major muscles of the body.

skull protects the brain, the vertebrae protect the spinal cord, and pelvic bones protect the bladder and other organs.

There are several different types of muscles:

☑ Skeletal muscles attach to bones to create body movements and also produce heat **(Figure 4-9).**

☑ Voluntary muscles are those under a person's control to move.

☑ Smooth muscles such as in the heart, esophagus, and blood vessels are involuntary.

☑ The diaphragm is a thin muscle below the lungs that does the primary work of breathing.

☑ All muscle activity is controlled by the nervous system.

In addition:

☑ **Tendons** are fibrous tissues that connect muscles to bones.

☑ **Ligaments** are tough bands of tissue that join bones together at joints.

Emergency Care Related to the Musculoskeletal System

Need to Recognize

Musculoskeletal injuries include fractures, dislocations, sprains, and strains:

◆ Although *fractures* can be serious injuries, particularly when nearby organs or blood

vessels are damaged by broken bone ends, most fractures are not life-threatening.

◆ In a *dislocation*, one or more bones move out of their normal position in a joint, preventing the joint from functioning as usual.

◆ A *sprain* is damage to ligaments and other structures in a joint.

◆ A *strain* is a tearing of muscle or tendon tissue usually caused by overexerting the muscle.

Musculoskeletal injuries are often associated with other injuries.

◆ Vertebral fractures are likely to injure the spinal cord and cause nervous system damage.

- Fractures of the femur often cause much soft-tissue damage and bleeding.
- A fracture of the pelvis may damage the bladder or other organs in the pelvic cavity.
- A skull fracture may cause brain damage.

Do You Understand?

1. Describe how the body looks in the anatomical position.

_____

2. The main function of the respiratory system is to allow oxygen to enter the blood from air breathed in and to remove _____.

3. What condition occurs when vital organs are not receiving enough oxygen due to blood loss?

_____

4. When can fractures be life-threatening?

_____

Nervous System

✓ Need to Know

The **nervous system** has three general sets of functions:

- ☑ Sensory nerves throughout the body gather information and send this information to the brain.
- ☑ The brain integrates and analyzes information, both consciously and automatically, for immediate and future uses.
- ☑ Motor nerves carry signals from the brain to control movement and other actions.

The nervous system controls the actions of most other body systems. For example, when nervous system receptors find a low level of oxygen in the blood, the brain directs the muscles of breathing to speed up the respiratory rate and the heart to beat faster to ensure the body gets enough oxygen.

The brain controls the nervous system (**Figure 4-10**). The brain connects directly with the spinal cord, the pathway to and from nerves throughout the body. The brain and spinal cord form the **central nervous system**. The spinal cord is encased inside vertebrae, the bones of the spine, from which nerves extend throughout the body in the peripheral nervous system.

Emergency Care Related to the Nervous System

◼ Need to Recognize

Injury or illness affecting the nervous system may have general or specific effects on the body.

- Head and spinal injuries can have serious or life-threatening effects.
- If the respiratory center in the brain is damaged, the person may stop breathing.
- Damage to the spine may cause paralysis of a part of the body.
- Head injuries may also cause bleeding or swelling of the brain, with widespread effects.

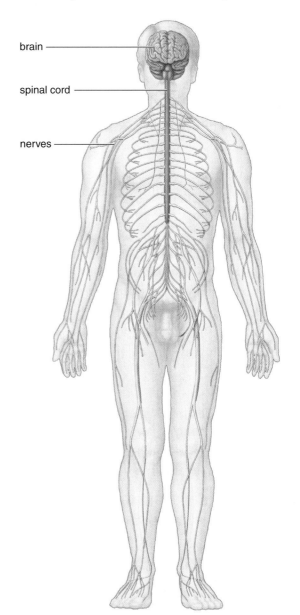

brain

spinal cord

nerves

Figure 4-10 The nervous system.

The Human Body 49

Brain functions can be more generally affected by injury or illness. **Altered mental status** describes changes in a person's responsiveness, such as becoming dizzy, disoriented, lethargic, or comatose. Altered mental status may result from:

- Head injuries.
- Any injury causing reduced oxygenation.
- Sudden illness, such as stroke, seizure, or diabetic emergencies.
- Poisoning or drug overdose.

Injuries elsewhere in the body and some illnesses also affect the nervous system. Because pain results from damage to nerve fibers in many areas of the body, pain is always assessed as a symptom that may reveal something about an injury or illness.

- A crushing pain in the chest may be caused by a heart attack.
- Abdominal pain that begins in the area of the umbilicus and then settles into the lower abdomen on the right side may be a sign of appendicitis, which can become a medical emergency.

Although pain is not always present with serious conditions, pain should always be taken seriously.

The Skin

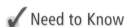 Need to Know

The primary function of the skin is to protect the body from the external environment (temperature extremes, pathogens, and other substances). Other functions include:

- ☑ The skin helps regulate body temperature. When the body becomes hot, blood vessels in the skin dilate (widen) to bring heat to the surface to dissipate; sweating also helps cool the skin. When the body becomes cold, blood vessels constrict to conserve heat.
- ☑ The skin helps prevent water loss from the body (dehydration).
- ☑ Nerve sensors in the skin react to touch, pressure, pain, and temperature.

Emergency Care Related to the Skin

■ Need to Recognize

Skin is frequently damaged by traumatic injuries.

- Cuts and scrapes are common causes of bleeding. The blood vessels in the skin are

relatively small, and bleeding from the skin seldom involves as much blood loss as from deeper blood vessels.

- Any openings in the skin, however, may allow pathogens into the body, including blood-borne pathogens that can cause very serious illnesses. Whenever exposed to a victim's body fluids, First Responders must take BSI precautions.
- Exposure to temperature extremes can damage the skin, such as occurs with frostbite or burns. With temperature extremes, regulatory mechanisms may not be able to keep the body at its normal temperature. The skin of a victim of hypothermia (whole body cooling) often looks pale and cool. In heatstroke, a life-threatening condition in which the body becomes overheated, sweating stops and the skin is flushed and very hot to the touch.
- Serious burns destroy tissue, let pathogens into the body, and may allow a loss of body heat and body fluid.

The skin often reveals important information about the condition of the body. For example:

- When blood oxygen levels are low, the skin may look bluish, especially at the lips, under the nails, and around mucous membranes. This is called cyanosis. The skin of a victim in shock is often cool, clammy or sweating, and pale or bluish, or ashen in a dark-skinned person.
- Sweating and pale skin are also signs of a possible heart attack.
- Many sudden illnesses cause sweating and skin color changes (flushed or pale).

Other Body Systems

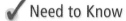 Need to Know

Gastrointestinal System

The primary function of the **gastrointestinal system** is to digest food and extract energy and nutrients to meet the body's needs. Food and fluids pass through the esophagus to the stomach and then the small and large intestines, where nutrients are absorbed into the bloodstream to be transported to body cells. Accessory organs of digestion include the pancreas and liver, which produce substances that aid in digestion, and the gallbladder, which stores bile made by the liver. The pancreas is also an endocrine system organ (discussed in a later section).

The abdominal cavity is not protected by bones, so gastrointestinal organs may be easily injured by traumatic forces.

☑ In a closed abdominal injury, the skin is not broken. Pain or tenderness along with a swollen or rigid abdomen may suggest the internal injury.

☑ In an open abdominal wound, internal organs may be exposed to the outside, raising the risk of infection.

The gastrointestinal system may also be involved in a number of sudden illnesses and conditions:

☑ An ingested poison is absorbed in the same manner as nutrients from food and enters the bloodstream to affect the body.

☑ Various illnesses may cause vomiting or diarrhea. If either continues, the victim may develop dehydration, a serious condition in which the body loses needed water. Infants especially can lose significant body fluid from diarrhea, which quickly becomes a medical emergency.

☑ Vomiting blood is likely a sign of a serious internal injury.

Urinary System

The **urinary system** functions to remove metabolic wastes from the body in urine and to help the body maintain fluid and electrolyte balances. The blood transports wastes to the kidneys, which filter them out and produce urine. Urine is stored temporarily in the bladder.

☑ Traumatic injury may damage the bladder or kidneys, possibly resulting in blood in the urine.

☑ Blood in the urine is always a sign of a problem requiring medical attention.

☑ Changes in urination may also indicate the presence of a health problem.

☑ A long period without urination in an infant may be a sign of dehydration, a medical emergency.

Reproductive System

Different **reproductive system** organs in males and females produce the sperm and eggs necessary for reproduction. Other female functions relate to gestation (pregnancy), childbirth, and lactation (milk production).

☑ Abdominal injuries may damage the genitals or reproductive organs. Such wounds may require special care. Care should include concern for the victim's privacy and be performed with sensitivity.

☑ In rare situations, a pregnant woman may develop complications. Childbirth may occur unexpectedly away from a healthcare facility, in which case a First Responder may need to assist.

Endocrine System

The **endocrine system** includes a series of glands in various body areas that produce hormones. Hormones affect the functioning of organs throughout the body. The pancreas, an important endocrine organ, produces the hormone insulin, which is needed for the control of blood sugar levels.

☑ All hormones affect a person's health, and the over- or under-production of each can cause disease.

☑ Most hormonal problems develop slowly and seldom cause a need for emergency care.

☑ **Diabetes** is an endocrine disorder affecting over 16 million Americans. It may cause very high or very low blood sugar levels that can quickly progress to a medical emergency. One form of diabetes results when the pancreas does not produce enough insulin; another form occurs when the body does not effectively use the insulin produced.

Lymphatic System and Immune System

The **lymphatic system** consists of lymph nodes and lymphatic vessels throughout the body and other organs. The primary function of the lymphatic system is to help defend against disease as part of the **immune system.**

The concept of **immunity** is important in emergency care.

☑ Once you have had certain infectious diseases, such as chickenpox, you are immune to that disease, which means you cannot contract it again.

☑ Immunity for some diseases can be acquired also by receiving a **vaccine.**

☑ A vaccine is available for hepatitis B. Healthcare workers and professional rescuers often receive this vaccine due to the risk of acquiring this bloodborne infection when frequently caring for victims of injury.

☑ Tetanus vaccine, given in a booster at least every 10 years, is also recommended to prevent a tetanus infection when the skin is broken.

Do You Understand?

1. Changes in a patient's responsiveness, including dizziness and disorientation, are called

_____ .

2. True or false: Skin condition may reveal a problem with oxygenation.

3. Prolonged vomiting or diarrhea may result in
   a. dehydration.
   b. fever.
   c. infectious disease.
   d. increased blood pressure.

Conclusion

Because body systems are interrelated, illness and injury can have many different effects. You will learn more about specific injuries and medical emergencies in later chapters. You will also learn more about how to interpret different conditions that produce patterns of signs and symptoms because of effects on different body systems.

Key Terms

abdomen (p. 42)

abdominal cavity (p. 42)

abdominal quadrants (p. 42)

acute myocardial infarction (p. 46)

airway (p. 44)

airway obstruction (p. 44)

altered mental status (p. 49)

alveoli (p. 44)

anatomical position (p. 42)

anterior (p. 42)

arteries (p. 45)

atria (p. 45)

blood pressure (p. 45)

body system (p. 43)

bronchi (p. 44)

capillaries (p. 46)

cardiac arrest (p. 46)

central nervous system (p. 48)

choking (p. 44)

circulatory system (p. 45)

contraction (p. 45)

diabetes (p. 50)

diaphragm (p. 42)

distal (p. 42)

dysrhythmia (p. 46)

endocrine system (p. 50)

epiglottis (p. 44)

esophagus (p. 44)

extremities (p. 41)

fibrillation (p. 46)

gastrointestinal system (p. 49)

immune system (p. 50)

immunity (p. 50)

inferior (p. 43)

lateral (p. 42)

ligaments (p. 47)

lymphatic system (p. 50)

medial (p. 42)

midline (p. 42)

musculoskeletal system (p. 46)

myocardium (p. 45)

nervous system (p. 48)

organ (p. 43)

pelvic cavity (p. 42)

pelvis (p. 42)

Review Questions

1. Inside the thoracic cavity are located the
   a. gallbladder and intestines.
   b. heart and lungs.
   c. spinal cord and brainstem.
   d. stomach and liver.

2. In reference to the anatomical position, "superior" refers to
   a. toward the head.
   b. toward the front of the body.
   c. lying faceup.
   d. away from the midline of the body.

3. What structure prevents solids and liquids from entering the trachea?
   a. Esophagus
   b. Pharynx
   c. Alveoli
   d. Epiglottis

4. The diaphragm is made of
   a. bone tissue.
   b. muscle tissue.
   c. lung tissue.
   d. ligaments and tendons.

5. An acute myocardial infarction is commonly known as
   a. a stroke.
   b. a heart attack.
   c. an asthma attack.
   d. shock.

6. Respiratory rate is primarily controlled by which body system?
   a. Respiratory
   b. Circulatory
   c. Nervous
   d. Musculoskeletal

7. When skin is destroyed by a serious burn, what may result?
   a. Dehydration
   b. Heart attack
   c. Heat stroke
   d. Stroke

8. Diabetes is a disorder in which body system?
   a. Musculoskeletal
   b. Gastrointestinal
   c. Lymphatic
   d. Endocrine

9. A vaccine is available to prevent infection by
   a. hepatitis B.
   b. hepatitis C.
   c. HIV.
   d. TB.

10. Which of these body systems can produce heat in the body?
    a. Immune
    b. Respiratory
    c. Musculoskeletal
    d. Endocrine

Lifting and Moving Patients

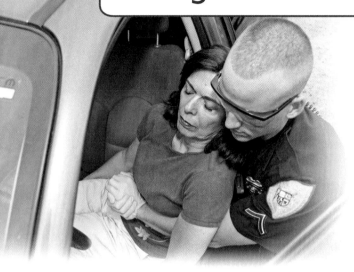

Chapter Preview

- Body Mechanics and Lifting Techniques
- Patient Positioning
- Emergency Moves
- Nonemergency Moves
- EMS Equipment for Moving Patients

You Respond To . . .

a scene at an industrial plant where an explosion has occurred. When you are sure the scene is safe, you enter with your partner and find three patients unresponsive on the floor, one of whom is lying on top of another. You know you need to assess all three quickly before beginning care, but you cannot access the one without moving the patient on top of him.

Introduction

In most circumstances, patients should not be moved but should be treated where they are found. Movement can cause additional injury or aggravate an injury or illness. Wait for responding EMS personnel, who are trained to move and transport a patient safely. In some emergency situations, however, you must move a patient in immediate danger before completing your assessment and treatment. In addition, you may need to assist other EMS personnel in moving patients. This chapter describes how to move or position a patient safely to prevent further injury and how to avoid injury yourself when doing so.

Body Mechanics and Lifting Techniques

▶ Need to Do

Back injury is an occupational hazard for First Responders and EMS personnel. To minimize the possibility of back injury, it is important to use good body mechanics and follow proper lifting techniques. **Body mechanics** are the principles of using your body most safely to prevent strains and other injuries caused by lifting or other stresses **(Figure 5-1)**.

▸ **Know your physical ability and limitations.** Do not try to lift or move a patient whose weight exceeds your ability to move the patient safely. In an awkward situation that would require twisting or unnatural movements, wait for additional personnel to help. If you have any doubt whether you can safely lift the patient, call for more personnel.

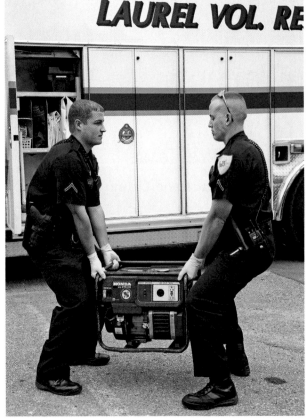

Figure 5-1 Good body mechanics when lifting include keeping the back straight and lifting with the legs.

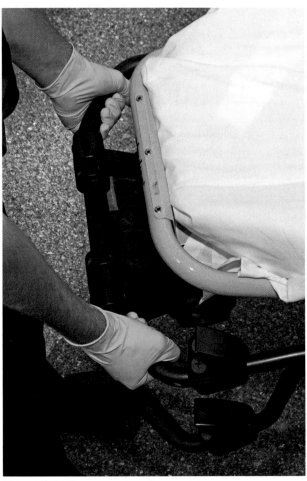

Figure 5-2 The power grip.

- **Plan the lift.** If the patient is heavy or in an awkward location, wait for additional rescuers. Time spent planning a lift helps minimize the risk of back injury.

- **Ensure that you have a good grip.** Before beginning the lift, get a good grip on the patient or equipment. Latex medical exam gloves can become slippery, especially after wearing them for some time. Be careful when lifting while wearing latex gloves. Lift using the "power grip" with palms up **(Figure 5-2).**

- **Test the load.** Before you completely undertake the lift, test the load. If it appears that you or other rescuers will be overburdened, stop and rethink the lift.

- **Position your feet properly before starting the lift.** Stand on a firm surface with feet shoulder-width apart. Take special care if the surface is slippery or not level.

- **Lift with your legs.** Always lift with your legs and not with your back. Your leg muscles are stronger and more stable than your back. Tightening your abdominal muscles pro-

vides additional support during the lift. Bend your knees and keep your back straight, then straighten your legs as you lift.

- **Keep the patient's weight as close to your body as possible.** This minimizes the strain on your arms and back. Try to lift straight up.

- **Avoid twisting your back during the lift.** Twisting your back decreases the stability of the spine and increases the risk of injury. If you must turn, pivot with your feet. Plan any turning or pivoting before starting the move. When lifting with one hand only, do not lean to the side.

- **Communicate clearly and frequently with your partner and other EMS providers.** This helps ensure everyone lifts at the same time to prevent a strain on one rescuer.

Practice lifting and moving techniques to move patients safely in an emergency. Your instructor will show you equipment used in your local EMS system for moving patients so that you can practice with it.

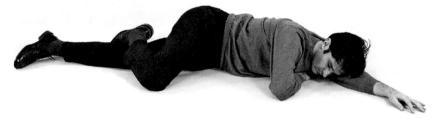

Figure 5-3 The recovery position.

Patient Positioning

▶ Need to Do

Generally, a patient should be repositioned only when necessary for treatment. Follow these positioning guidelines:

1. Reposition a breathing unresponsive patient who is not a trauma patient in the **recovery position,** preferably on the left side **(Figure 5-3).** The recovery position helps keep the airway open and allows fluids to drain from the mouth.

2. Do not move or reposition a trauma patient unless it is clearly necessary to treat a life-threatening condition. Wait until additional EMS personnel can evaluate and stabilize the patient. If it is necessary to reposition a patient on the back to give care such as CPR, support the patient's head and neck during the move with the multiple-rescuer **log roll** technique.

3. If a responsive patient is experiencing pain or difficulty breathing, allow the patient to assume a position of comfort, often in a sitting or semi-reclined position.

4. Allow a responsive patient who is nauseated or vomiting to remain in a position of comfort, but stay nearby in a position from which you can appropriately manage the airway.

Recovery Position

✓ Need to Know

An unresponsive patient who is breathing and who is not suspected to have a spinal injury should be put in the recovery position. This position is used for several reasons:

- ☑ It helps keep the airway open.
- ☑ It allows fluids to drain from the mouth.
- ☑ It prevents the patient from inhaling stomach contents if the patient vomits.

▶ Need to Do

If possible, unless it could worsen the patient's injury, put the patient on his or her left side. Because of anatomical differences, the left side reduces the chances of the patient vomiting. The modified HAINES (High Arm IN Endangered Spine) position is recommended because it reduces movement of the neck in case of potential spinal injury **(see Skill 5-1).** Once the patient is in the recovery position, continue to monitor the ABCs.

For an unresponsive breathing infant:

- ◗ Hold the infant face-down over your arm with his or her head slightly lower than the body **(Figure 5-4).**

- ◗ Support the head and neck with your hand and keep the nose and mouth clear.

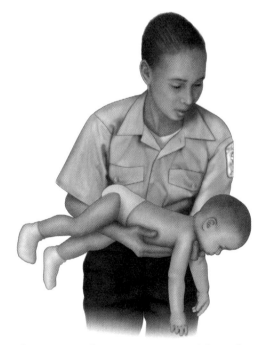

Figure 5-4 The recovery position for infants.

Skill 5-1   **Modified HAINES Recovery Position**

1 Extend the patient's arm that is farther from you above the patient's head.

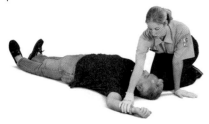

2 Position the patient's other arm across the chest.

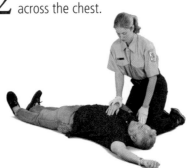

3 Bend the patient's nearer leg at the knee.

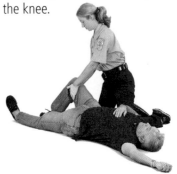

4 Put your forearm that is nearer the patient's head under the patient's nearer shoulder with your hand under the hollow of the neck.

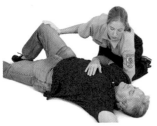

5 Carefully roll the patient away from you by pushing on the patient's flexed knee and lifting with your forearm while your hand stabilizes the head and neck. The patient's head is now supported on the raised arm.

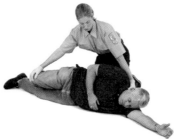

6 While continuing to support the head and neck, position the patient's hand palm down with fingers under the armpit of the raised arm. The patient's forearm should be flat on the surface at 90 degrees to the body.

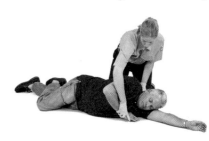

7 With the patient now in position, check the airway and open the mouth to allow drainage.

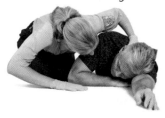

Log Roll

✓ Need to Know

The log roll is used to move a patient from a prone position to a supine position to assess and treat the patient when necessary.

☑ The log roll can be used to move a patient into a supine position on the ground for treatment or to move the patient onto a **backboard.**
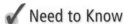

☑ Three to five rescuers are required to safely roll the patient without twisting the spine (**Skill 5-2**).

☑ For a trauma patient who may have a spinal injury, one rescuer must stabilize the head in line with the body throughout the move.

🖐 Do You Understand?

1. What is the best way to lift a heavy weight?
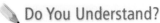

Skill 5-2   Log Roll

1 The rescuer at the patient's head holds the head in line with the body as two or three additional rescuers take position with hands at the patient's lower and upper leg, hip and torso, and shoulder.

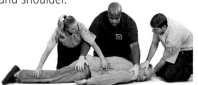

2 At the direction of the responder at the head, the rescuers in unison roll the patient toward them, with the head held in line and the spine straight.

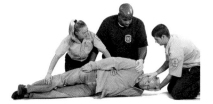

3 The rescuers complete the log roll, positioning the patient on the back with head and neck still in line with the body.

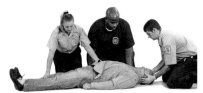

2. When lifting or carrying a patient, keep the patient _____ your body.

3. True or false: Allow a responsive patient to choose the most comfortable position.

4. List three benefits of the recovery position for an unresponsive breathing patient without a spinal injury.

_____

_____

_____

Emergency Moves

■■ Need to Recognize

An **emergency move** is an immediate move of the patient before assessment or treatment. The patient is moved *only* for two circumstances:

1. The patient faces an immediate danger if not moved, such as:
   - Fire is present or likely to occur
   - Explosives are present or there is a danger of explosion (e.g., a natural gas leak)
   - The patient cannot be protected from other hazards at the scene
   - You are unable to gain access to other patients who need lifesaving care
   - You cannot make the scene safe (e.g., a structure about to collapse)

2. You cannot give lifesaving care because of the patient's location or position (e.g., a cardiac arrest patient is slumped in a chair or lying on a bed)

The greatest danger in moving a patient quickly is the possibility of aggravating a spinal injury. Take care with all emergency moves to keep the head and neck in line with the spine as much as possible during the move. It is impossible to protect the spine while removing a patient from a vehicle quickly.

- In some EMS systems, First Responders may be trained in the rapid **extrication** (removal) of patients from a vehicle using a cervical collar and inline stabilization of the head and neck.
- Follow your local protocol.
- In most situations, wait for EMTs trained in special techniques for extrication from a vehicle.

One-Rescuer Emergency Drags

▶ Need to Do

With all emergency moves:

- Make every effort to pull or drag the patient in the direction of the long axis of the body to provide as much protection for the spine as possible.
- Do not drag the patient sideways, and avoid twisting the neck or trunk.
- Never pull the patient's head away from the neck and shoulders.
- The risk of spinal injury can be minimized by using a blanket, rug, board, or similar device when available.

The choice of which drag to use depends on the materials at hand, the patient's condition, and the situation. The firefighter's drag is used to stay low to the floor in a smoke-filled room. **Skill 5-3** shows several common one-rescuer emergency drags.

Skill 5-3   One-Rescuer Emergency Drags

Clothing Drag: Pull on the patient's clothing in the neck and shoulder area, supporting the head with your forearms.

Blanket Drag: Put the patient on a blanket and drag the blanket, supporting the patient's head with the blanket gathered in your hands.

Shoulder Drag: Put your hands under the patient's armpits and drag backward, supporting the head between your forearms and elbows.

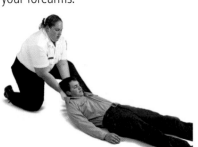
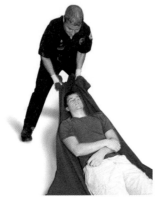
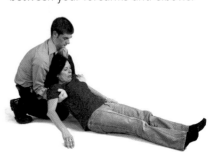

Firefighter's Drag: Tie the patient's wrists together, straddle the patient with your head under the wrists, and crawl forward on your hands and knees.

Upper Extremity Drag: Put your hands under the patient's armpits, grasp the patient's forearms, and drag the patient, supporting the head between your arms.

Upper Extremity Drag for Rapid Extrication: Support the head as best you can leaning back against your chest and chin. Note: Use only in an emergency when alone.

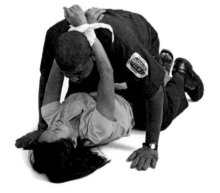
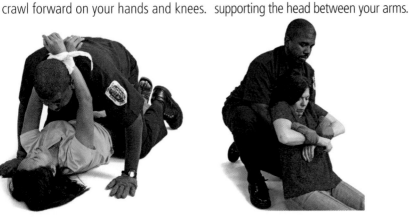
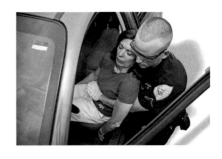

Emergency Carries

✓ Need to Know

Emergency carries, like emergency drags, are used when a patient must be moved immediately. One or more rescuers may carry the patient using different methods depending on the patient's size and condition and the situation:

- ☑ The walking assist is used for patients able to bear some weight and move with help.

- ☑ The cradle carry is used for lighter patients.
- ☑ Multiple-rescuer techniques are safer and less stressful for both the patient and rescuers and should be used whenever two or more responders are present.

▶ Need to Do

With all emergency carries:

- ◆ Remember to use good body mechanics and lifting techniques.

◆ Do not try to lift or carry an injured person before checking for injuries, unless you are sure that there is no injury to the neck or spine. Use an emergency drag instead.

Skills 5-4 and 5-5 show common emergency carries.

 Do You Understand?

1. What are the two reasons for moving a patient before assessment or treatment?

_____   _____

Skill 5-4 **One-Rescuer Emergency Carries**

Packstrap Carry: Pull the patient's arms over your shoulders and cross them over your chest as you bend forward and pull the patient onto your back.

Cradle Carry: Lift the patient with one arm under the patient's knees and the other under the patient's back.

Piggyback Carry: Support the patient's weight with your arms under the patient's thighs. If able, have the patient clasp hands and lean forward; if not able, grasp the patient's hands with yours to keep patient from falling back.

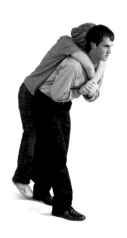 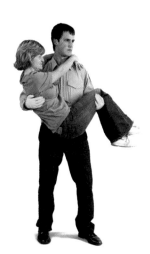 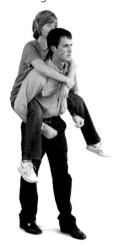

One-Rescuer Assist: Place one arm around the patient's waist a nd, with your other arm, hold the patient's hand after passing the patient's arm around your neck.

Firefighter's Carry: Support the patient's weight on your shoulders while holding the patient's thigh and arm.

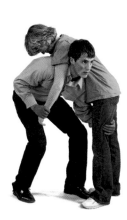 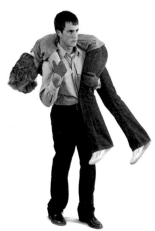 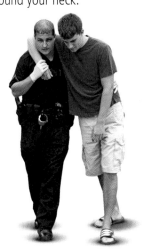

Skill 5-5 Two-Rescuer Emergency Carries

Two-Rescuer Cradle Carry: Both rescuers clasp arms behind the patient's back and under the legs.

Two-Rescuer Extremity Carry: To carry a patient down steps, the forward rescuer grasps patient's legs under the knees while the rear rescuer reaches under patient's armpits from behind to grasp the patient's forearms.

Two-Rescuer Assist: Both rescuers position the patient's arms over their shoulders. Each rescuer grasps the patient's wrist, with the other arm around the patient's waist.

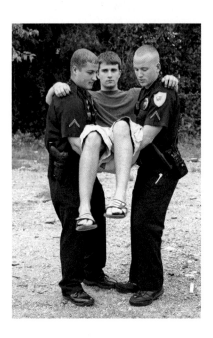

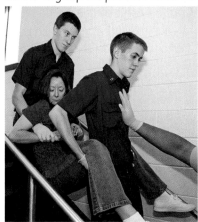

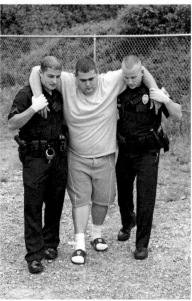

2. How can you support a patient's head when using the shoulder drag?

   _____

3. Which emergency carry is best for carrying a patient down stairs?
   a. Piggyback
   b. Firefighter's
   c. Two-rescuer extremity
   d. Two-rescuer cradle

Nonemergency Moves

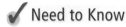 Need to Know

Nonemergency moves are used to move the patient when there is no threat to the patient's life. These moves are conducted by multiple rescuers.

They are not used if the patient has a suspected spinal injury, internal bleeding, or uncontrolled external bleeding.

Ideally, all patients should be stabilized before being moved. In addition, steps should be taken to minimize any chance of aggravating the patient's illness or injury. Although these moves are usually performed by responding EMS personnel, you must be familiar with the common techniques for moving patients. Before using a nonemergency move, you must:

☑ Complete the primary and secondary assessment

☑ Correct any life-threatening problems

☑ Immobilize all suspected fractures and dislocations

☑ Ensure there are *no* signs or symptoms of neck or spinal injury

Direct Ground Lift

▶▶ Need to Do

The direct ground lift is a nonemergency move for patients without suspected neck or spinal injuries. It is typically used to lift and carry a supine patient from the ground to a **stretcher.** The patient's arms should be crossed on the abdomen or chest. At sig-

nals from the rescuer at the head, the rescuers work in unison to lift and carry the patient **(Skill 5-6).**

Extremity Lift

▶▶ Need to Do

The extremity lift is a two-rescuer technique commonly used for patients without a suspected neck

---

Skill 5-6   **Direct Ground Lift**

1 The rescuers kneel on one side of the patient. Preferably all rescuers kneel on the same knee. The patient's arms are placed on his or her chest or abdomen if possible.

2 The rescuer at the head places one arm under the patient's neck and shoulder and cradles the patient's head. This same rescuer places the other arm under the patient's lower back. The second rescuer places one arm under the patient's waist and one arm under the thighs just below the buttocks. The third rescuer places one arm under the patient's knees and the other under the lower legs. Note: If there are only two rescuers, the second rescuer places one arm under the patient's knees and one arm above the patient's buttocks.

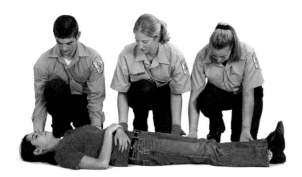

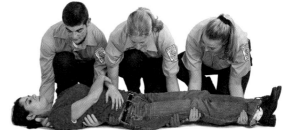

3 On signal, the rescuers lift the patient to their knees and roll the patient in toward their chests.

4 On signal, the rescuers stand and move the patient to the stretcher. The patient is lowered by reversing the steps.

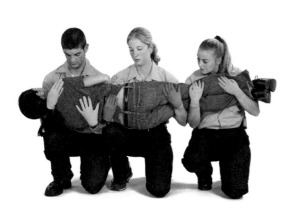

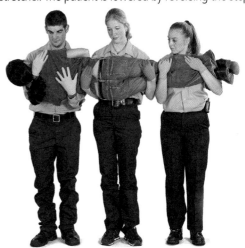

Skill 5-7   Extremity Lift

1 The first rescuer kneels at the patient's head and the second rescuer kneels by the patient's feet. The rescuer at the head places one arm under each of the patient's shoulders while the rescuer at the feet positions the patient's arms.

2 The rescuer at the head then slips his or her hands under the patient's armpits and grasps the patient's wrists and crosses them on the patient's chest. The rescuer at the feet turns around and reaches his or her hands back and under the patient's knees.

3 Both rescuers move to a crouching position and assess their grip on the patient.

4 On a signal from the rescuer at the head, the rescuers stand up simultaneously and move forward with the patient.

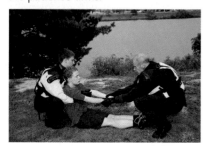 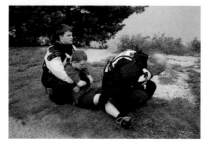 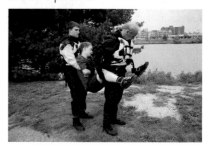

or spinal injury or injuries of the arms or legs **(Skill 5-7).** This lift may be used with a responsive or an unresponsive patient. It may be used, for example, to carry a patient a short distance or to move the patient from a chair to the ground or a stretcher. The extremity lift may also be used as an emergency move to carry a patient through a tight space such as a narrow hallway.

BOX 5-1

EXTREMITY LIFT—ALTERNATIVE POSITION

Skill 5-7 describes a common way the extremity lift is used to lift and move a patient. This method is generally preferred if the rescuers must move some distance or up or down an inclined surface. An alternate position for the second rescuer is shown in the figure here, with the rescuer at the patient's feet facing the patient and other rescuer. This method can be used to move a patient to the side or a short distance but can be dangerous if the rescuer must walk backwards over any surface that is not level and unobstructed.

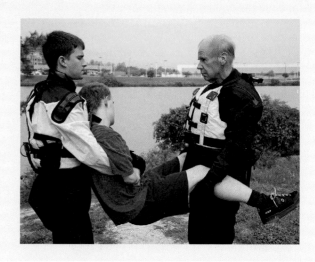

Transfer from Bed to Stretcher

▶▶ Need to Do

You may be called upon to assist EMS personnel in transferring the patient from a bed to a stretcher using either the direct carry or the draw sheet technique **(Skills 5-8 and 5-9).** These techniques are not used with a patient with a suspected spinal injury.

EMS Equipment for Moving Patients

✓ Need to Know

First Responders often assist EMTs and other EMS personnel with packaging and moving patients, using a wide range of commercial devices. Different equipment is used in different areas, and you

---

Skill 5-8   Direct Carry

1 Position the stretcher at a right angle to the bed, ideally, with the head end of the stretcher at the foot of the bed. Unbuckle the straps and remove other items from the stretcher. Both rescuers stand between the bed and the stretcher, facing the patient.

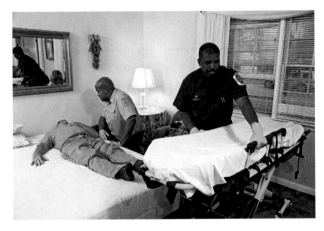

2 The rescuer at the head slides one arm under the patient's neck and cups the patient's farther shoulder. The second rescuer slides one arm under the patient's hips and lifts slightly. The rescuer at the head slides his or her other arm under the patient's back, and the second rescuer places his or her other arm underneath the patient's knees. Together, both rescuers slide the patient to the edge of the bed.

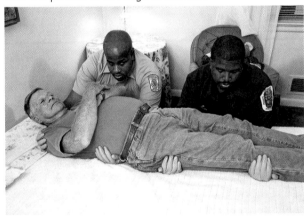

3 On a signal of the rescuer at the head, the rescuers lift and curl the patient toward their chests.

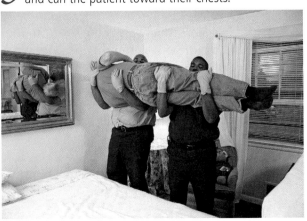

4 The rescuers step back, rotate toward the stretcher, and place the patient gently on the stretcher.

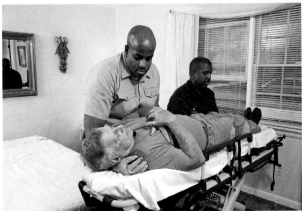

Skill 5-9   **Draw Sheet Transfer**

1 Loosen the bottom sheet of the bed and roll its edge on the side where you will place the stretcher.

2 Position the stretcher alongside the bed. Prepare the stretcher: Adjust the height, lower the rails, and unbuckle the straps. Both responders reach across the stretcher and grasp the rolled sheet edge firmly at the level of the patient's head, chest, hips, and knees.

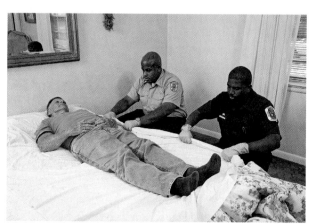

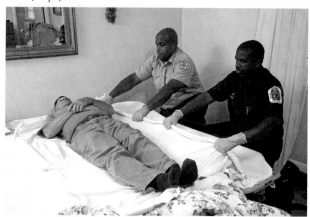

3 Slide the patient gently onto the stretcher.

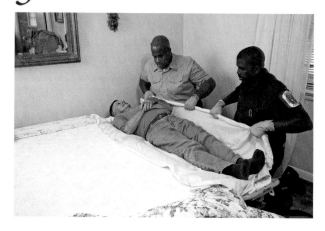

should learn the devices that you are likely to encounter in your area. **Table 5-1** describes common standard devices used for packaging and moving or transporting patients.

Do You Understand?

1. List three or four things you should do before moving the patient using a nonemergency move.

_____   _____

_____   _____

2. Which rescuer usually gives the signal to lift or move a patient in a multiple-rescuer nonemergency move?

_____

3. A short backboard is typically used for a

    a. short patient.

    b. patient without a spinal injury.

    c. patient inside a vehicle.

    d. patient receiving CPR.

BOX 5-2

DRAW SHEET TRANSFER— ALTERNATIVE METHOD

Skill 5-9 describes a common way the draw sheet transfer is used to move a patient from a bed to a stretcher, using the sheet already under the patient as a draw sheet. In an alternate method, the rescuers first roll the patient onto one side, and one rescuer holds the patient in that position while the second positions a sheet with rolled edge beneath the patient, as shown here. Then the patient is rolled back into the original position and the rescuers together pull on the sheet to slide the patient onto the stretcher.

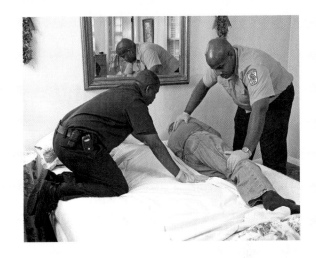

Conclusion

Always remember the most important principle for moving a patient: Move the patient only if necessary to escape danger or to position the patient for lifesaving care. In both emergency and nonemergency moves, use good body mechanics to prevent injury to both you and the patient.

Table 5-1

Typical Equipment for Packaging and Moving Patients

Long Backboard: Up to 7 feet long, long backboards are used for patients found lying down with suspected spinal injuries. The patient is immobilized on the board with straps.

Short Backboard: Typically less than 4 feet long, a short backboard is used to stabilize a sitting patient's back before the patient is moved. A short backboard is typically used in the extrication of a patient with suspected spinal injury from a vehicle. The patient is later moved onto a long backboard or other immobilization device.

Vest Extrication Device: An alternative to a short backboard for extricating patients from a vehicle or other sitting position in a confined space, the vest extrication device wraps around the patient to help stabilize the head and spine.

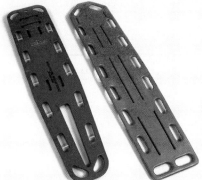

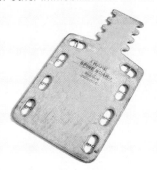

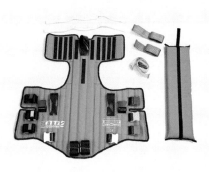

Table 5-1 Continued

Standard Stretcher: The standard stretcher, also called a **cot** or gurney, has wheels and rails and is used to move and transport patients. Most models have folding legs that collapse as the stretcher is pushed into the ambulance.

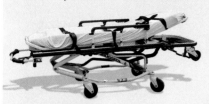

Portable Stretcher: Portable stretchers may be used in situations where a standard stretcher cannot be maneuvered or in multiple-casualty incidents.

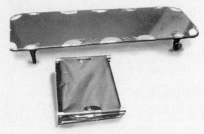

Orthopedic Stretcher: Also called a **scoop stretcher**, the orthopedic stretcher splits in two or four sections, which are slid under the patient from the sides to "scoop" the patient into the stretcher. It is then reassembled and locked into a rigid structure. The patient can easily be transferred to a standard stretcher.

Basket Stretcher: Also called a wire basket or Stokes basket, the basket stretcher is used to transport a patient over rough terrain or in other special rescue situations.

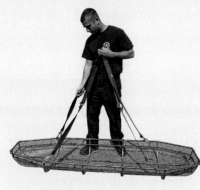

Stair Chair: A stair chair is used in situations where it is impractical to use a stretcher, such as down long flights of stairs or through narrow, twisting passageways. Stair chairs are designed to be carried easily down stairs and wheeled over flat surfaces.

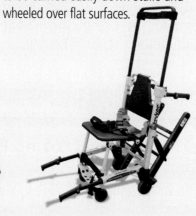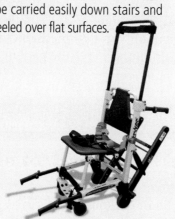

Key Terms

backboard (p. 56)

body mechanics (p. 53)

cot (p. 66)

emergency move (p. 57)

extrication (p. 57)

log roll (p. 55)

nonemergency move (p. 60)

orthopedic stretcher (p. 66)

recovery position (p. 55)

scoop stretcher (p. 66)

stair chair (p. 66)

stretcher (p. 61)

vest extrication device (p. 65)

Review Questions

1. In most circumstances, patients should be treated
   a. where they are found.
   b. on their backs.
   c. on a stretcher.
   d. in the recovery position.

2. What maneuver should you *avoid* when lifting a patient?
   a. Bending your knees
   b. Spreading your feet apart
   c. Twisting your back
   d. Tightening abdominal muscles

3. If possible, position an unresponsive breathing patient without a spinal injury on his or her
   a. back.
   b. stomach.
   c. right side.
   d. left side.

4. In the HAINES recovery position, the patient's head is supported on
   a. the patient's upraised arm.
   b. the rescuer's hand.
   c. the ground.
   d. a rolled blanket.

5. How many rescuers are needed to safely log roll a patient with a suspected spinal injury?
   a. 1
   b. 1 or 2
   c. 3 to 5
   d. At least 6

6. What is the greatest risk when moving a patient quickly using an emergency move?
   a. Injuring your own back
   b. Aggravating a spinal injury
   c. Provoking cardiac arrest
   d. Causing abdominal organ injury

7. A walking assist is used to move
   a. a responsive patient with altered mental status.
   b. a responsive patient who can bear some weight.
   c. an unresponsive patient with a spinal injury.
   d. an unresponsive patient without a spinal injury.

8. A direct ground lift is used as
   a. a nonemergency move for a patient without a spinal injury.
   b. a nonemergency move for a patient with a spinal injury.
   c. an emergency move for a patient who is vomiting.
   d. an emergency move for a patient who needs CPR.

9. To transfer a patient from a bed to a stretcher, use
   a. a two-rescuer cradle carry or direct carry.
   b. a draw sheet transfer or an extremity lift.
   c. a direct ground lift or piggyback carry.
   d. a direct carry or draw sheet transfer.

10. An orthopedic stretcher is used primarily for
    a. moving patients found lying down.
    b. moving patients with preexisting back problems.
    c. transferring patients from the EMS stretcher to a hospital bed.
    d. air-lifting patients from rough terrain.

Unit 2

Patient Assessment

Chapter 6: Patient Assessment

Patient Assessment

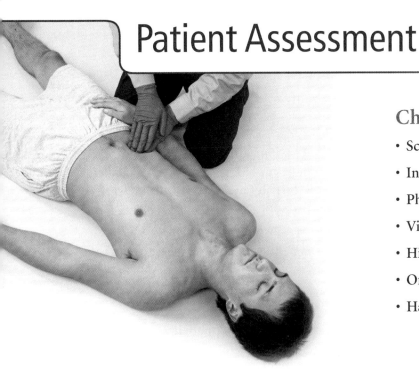

Chapter Preview

- Scene Size-Up
- Initial Assessment
- Physical Examination
- Vital Signs
- History
- Ongoing Assessment
- Hand-Off Report

You Respond To . . .

a nearby park where a teenage boy has just been pulled out of the water. It has been only two minutes since you got the call. While approaching, you have the general impression that he is not breathing, and you know time is a crucial factor. You've already planned your next actions even before you reach him and confirm unresponsiveness.

Introduction

Patient assessment involves some of the most important skills that First Responders practice. As the first one on the scene, you quickly act to ensure the scene is safe, assess the patient, and care for immediate threats to life. The care you pro-

vide before EMTs and other personnel arrive is always based on your patient assessment.

Scene Size-Up

■ Need to Recognize

As soon as you receive a call from dispatch, think about the scene you are headed for and factors that may affect safety for you, bystanders, and the patient. The dispatcher's information may alert you to hazards or special precautions that will be needed. As you arrive, begin the **scene size-up** before you exit your vehicle and while approaching the patient. Look for:

- Appropriate BSI precautions to take
- Any hazards at the scene
- Clues to help you better understand the nature of the emergency

BSI Precautions

▶ Need to Do

In preparation for providing patient care, put on medical exam gloves as you approach the patient. Observe the scene and patient to determine whether to use other personal protective equipment:

☑ Protective eyewear

☑ Gown and mask

☑ Turn-out gear for protection against hazards

Remember also to follow standard precautions to protect yourself against possible disease transmission (Chapter 2).

Scene Safety

■ Need to Recognize

Before you enter the scene, and again while approaching the patient, continue to observe for any hazards present in the scene **(Figure 6-1)**. Look for:

Vehicle crashes

▸ Traffic hazards

▸ Downed wires

▸ Risk of fire or explosion

▸ Unstable vehicles

▸ Hazardous materials

Potential violence

▸ Crime scenes

▸ Potentially violent patient or bystanders

▸ Guard dogs, wild animals

Environmental dangers

▸ Unstable surfaces

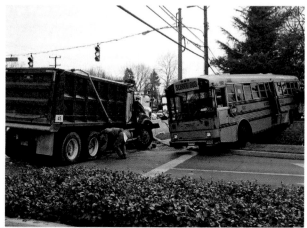

Figure 6-1 Size up the scene for potential hazards before approaching.

▸ Water, ice

▸ Weather extremes

Hazards within structures

▸ Low-oxygen areas

▸ Toxic substances, fumes

▸ Risk of collapse

▸ Risk of fire or explosion

▶ Need to Do

Chapter 18, EMS Operations, describes in more detail the dangers of hazardous materials incidents and multiple-casualty incidents. In all emergencies, follow the same general principles:

▸ Enter the scene only if it is safe.

▸ If the scene is unsafe, make it safe if you can or stay away.

▸ Protect bystanders and other rescuers from hazards at the scene.

▸ If it is safe to reach the patient, protect the patient from environmental threats such as temperature extremes, rain, and so on.

Mechanism of Injury

■ Need to Recognize

Often, but not always, you will know from the dispatch call whether the emergency involves a **trauma patient** (someone who is injured) or a **medical patient** (someone with signs and symptoms of illness). With a trauma patient, the scene size-up includes evaluating the scene for clues about the **mechanism of injury**—how the patient was injured. The mechanism of injury will help you understand the forces involved and the likelihood of serious injury or the presence of internal injuries **(Figure 6-2)**. Consider:

▸ What specifically caused the injury?

▸ Was there an impact with a blunt or sharp object?

▸ What body area received the impact? What organs may be injured?

▸ How much force may have been involved?

▸ Might the force have been transferred from one body area to another?

For example:

▸ A vehicle collision may cause head and spinal injuries. If an unrestrained driver struck the steering wheel, chest and internal organ injuries may be present.

- ◆ A fall from a height may cause extremity fractures. A fall from a great height may also include chest, spinal, and other injuries.
- ◆ A blunt impact to the abdomen may cause a closed injury and internal bleeding.
- ◆ A diving incident may cause a spinal injury.
- ◆ A gunshot may cause extensive internal damage not apparent from the appearance of the outside wound.
- ◆ A fall forward onto a hand may transfer force up the arm and cause a shoulder dislocation.

▶ Need to Do

Remember that you are quickly considering the mechanism of injury during the scene size-up as you approach the patient. Do not delay the patient assessment to examine the scene in detail, but think about the mechanism of injury as you come up to the patient. Later, after the initial assessment, you can consider the mechanism of injury more fully while gathering the history and performing a physical exam.

Nature of Illness

■ Need to Recognize

With a medical patient, consider the nature of the illness, rather than a mechanism of injury, during the scene size-up.

- ◆ Until you are certain the patient has no immediate threat to life, do not stop to talk to family members or bystanders. However, listen to what they tell you as you approach the patient and begin your assessment.
- ◆ Observe the patient's position and demeanor as you approach for clues about the nature of the illness or the patient's signs and symptoms.
- ◆ Use all your senses to observe anything unusual in the scene, such as medicine containers or unusual odors. Note the temperature of the environment.

If the patient may be unresponsive, move immediately to the initial assessment and ask questions afterwards. If the patient appears responsive, unless you observe an immediate threat, you can now ask the patient, family members, or bystanders why EMS was called.

Number of Patients

▶ Need to Do

During the scene size-up, also determine how many patients are involved. Observe for clues as you approach—such as the possibility that someone may have been thrown from a vehicle during a crash—and ask those present if everyone is accounted for.

- ◆ Be certain you know how many patients are involved before you begin patient care.
- ◆ Call for additional help immediately for multiple patients.
- ◆ Once you begin patient care, it will be more difficult to stop and call.

If more patients are present than responders, triage the patients first rather than performing a detailed assessment of any one patient (Chapter 19).

Additional Resources

■ Need to Recognize

Finally, the scene size-up should also include consideration of whether additional resources may be needed at the emergency scene. Depending on the original call to EMS, such resources may already be on the way or you may need to call dispatch immediately. Always describe the injuries of patient(s) to the dispatcher in detail, so an Advanced Life Support (ALS) ambulance can be sent to the scene if needed.

Consider:

- ◆ The number of patients and the types and seriousness of injuries
- ◆ The possible need for air transport (Chapter 18)
- ◆ The potential for fire or explosion
- ◆ The potential presence of hazardous materials (Chapter 18)
- ◆ Any need for extrication
- ◆ Any need for law enforcement or traffic control
- ◆ Damage to power lines or other utilities

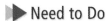 Do You Understand?

1. Name at least three things you look for in the scene size-up.

   _____

   _____

   _____

2. True or false: Take all the time you need to analyze the mechanism of injury before approaching the patient.

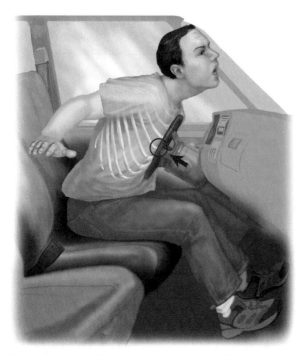

Direct forces often injure that impacted area of the body; the larger the force, the more likely is a serious injury such as a fracture or damage to internal organs.

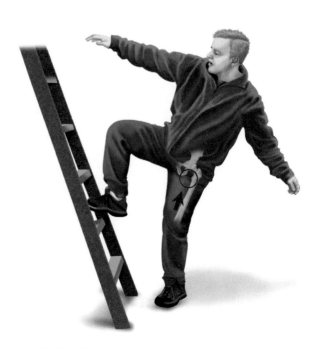

An **indirect force** may also be transferred up or down an extremity, as when falling on one leg. Similarly falling on an outstretched arm may cause dislocation of shoulder bones.

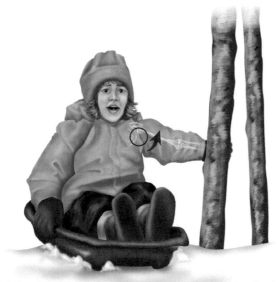

Twisting forces occur when the body moves in one direction but a force keeps some part of an extremity from moving with the rest of the body. Twisting forces may cause fractures or dislocations of bones at joints.

Figure 6-2 Common mechanisms of injury.

Initial Assessment

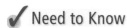 **Need to Know**

The **initial assessment** is the first patient assessment, performed as soon as you reach the patient, to identify any immediate threats to life.

☑ The initial assessment is a rapid means to determine the patient's general condition and set initial priorities for care.

☑ The initial assessment begins with your initial impression of the patient and proceeds in an orderly manner through a check of the patient's **responsiveness,** airway, breathing, and circulation status.

Need to Do

In completing a patient assessment:

- Perform the initial assessment of all patients after the scene size-up.
- If the scene is safe, perform the assessment before moving the patient.

General Impression

Need to Recognize

As you approach the patient, you should already be forming a **general impression** of the patient's condition based on what you observe. Consider these factors:

- Is the patient ill or injured?
- What is the patient's **chief complaint**? (Ask the patient what is wrong. If the patient is unresponsive or cannot say, the chief complaint is the reason EMS was called.)
- Does the patient's appearance give clues about his or her condition (skin color, behavior, etc.)?
- Are there signs of a serious problem: a gaping wound, blood pooling under the body, neck or extremities twisted, and so on?
- Note the patient's sex and approximate age, which may be relevant to assessment or treatment choices.

Your impression may influence your later actions, but the following steps of the initial assessment should always be performed in the same order regardless of your initial impression.

Responsiveness

Need to Recognize

As you approach, you may notice immediately whether the patient is responsive:

- *Responsive* means a person is conscious and awake. A patient who is speaking, coughing, crying, or purposefully moving is responsive.
- Even if the patient cannot talk because of an injury, he or she may be able to move and thereby signal responsiveness.

- A patient who cannot talk or move may be paralyzed but may still be able to respond through purposeful eye movements or other signs.

Need to Do

Begin this assessment by speaking to the patient: State your name and say that you are a First Responder and are here to help.

- If the patient is not speaking, making other sounds, or moving, tap the person gently on the shoulder and ask, "Are you okay?" **(Figure 6-3)**.
- Be careful not to move the patient in any way when assessing responsiveness. Do not shake the patient's shoulder or touch the head or neck. The patient may have a spinal injury that any movement could worsen.
- Always suspect a spinal injury in a trauma patient and take steps to stabilize the patient's head and neck (Chapter 15).

Unresponsiveness may be a sign of an urgent life-threatening problem (such as not breathing) or it may result from a less urgent problem. You cannot yet know, so continue your assessment by checking the airway, breathing, and circulation (ABCs) (described later). Regardless of its cause and whether other life-threatening problems are present, unresponsiveness is considered a life-threatening emergency. For example, if the patient is lying on his or her back, the tongue may move back in the throat and block the airway, preventing breathing.

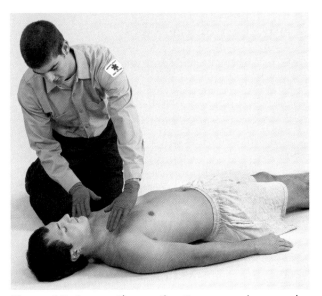

Figure 6-3 Assess the patient's responsiveness by tapping the shoulder and asking "Are you okay?"

The degree of a patient's responsiveness is frequently assessed using the **AVPU scale (Box 6-1)**. This scale is useful for noting changes in a patient's responsiveness during the time you are providing care and for communicating this information to other arriving EMS personnel.

- Make a mental note of the patient's level of responsiveness or write it down along with the time.
- A change in a patient's level of responsiveness, especially deterioration toward unresponsiveness, generally indicates a serious condition.

Responsiveness in Pediatric Patients

▇ Need to Recognize

Infants and young children, even when alert, may respond differently from older children and adults:

- Look for age-appropriate responses, such as following your movements with their eyes, crying, responding to parents or family members, or making purposeful movements.
- Assess an apparently unresponsive infant by flicking the bottom of the feet and noting the infant's response.

BOX 6-1

THE AVPU SCALE

A = **Alert.** The patient is oriented to time and place.

V = Responds to **Verbal** stimuli. The patient is not clearly oriented to time and place but responds when spoken to.

P = Responds to **Painful** stimuli. The patient does not respond when spoken to but moves or responds to pain. Firmly rub the patient's sternum, if no chest injury, or gently pinch the skin between the neck and shoulder to try to elicit a response.

U = **Unresponsive** to all stimuli. The patient's eyes are closed and there is no movement or other response to painful stimuli.

Checking the ABCs

✓ Need to Know

After checking responsiveness, the initial assessment continues with checking the **ABCs**:

A = Airway
B = Breathing
C = Circulation

This check identifies immediate life threats that must be corrected before patient assessment continues.

Airway

▶ Need to Do

The **airway** is the route air moves from the mouth and nose through the throat (pharynx) and down to the lungs. The airway may be blocked by something stuck in the throat, by swollen airway tissues in a patient with a severe allergic reaction or neck injury, or by an unresponsive patient's own tongue **(Figure 6-4)**. Because the airway must be patent (open) for the patient to breathe, you must confirm that it is **patent** or take action to open it or clear an obstruction.

- If a responsive patient is talking, crying, or coughing, the airway is open.
- A patient with a very weak, wheezing cough may have a partially blocked airway and not be breathing normally, which also is an emergency. Chapter 7 describes techniques to clear an airway obstruction.
- In an unresponsive patient, you may need to open the airway. If the patient is lying supine (face up), you must prevent the tongue from obstructing the airway by positioning the patient's head to open the airway.

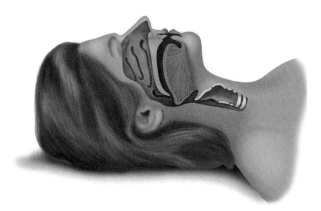

Figure 6-4 The tongue may block the airway in an unresponsive victim.

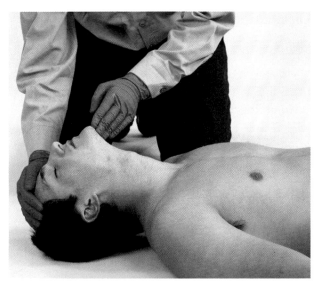

Figure 6-5 Head tilt–chin lift.

- Open the airway with the head tilt–chin lift if the patient does not have a potential spinal injury, or with the jaw thrust if a spinal injury may be present.

The **head tilt–chin lift** is performed by tilting the head back and lifting the chin with the fingers as shown in **Figure 6-5**. This position moves the tongue away from the opening into the throat to allow air to pass through the airway.

- Use your fingers, not your thumb, to lift the chin.
- Do not press deeply into the soft tissues of the chin.
- Ensure the mouth stays open.

With the **jaw thrust,** do not tilt the head back to open the airway. Instead, only lift the jaw upward, using both hands **(Figure 6-6)**.

- The jaw thrust is more difficult and fatiguing but is effective.
- If the lips close, open the lower lip with your gloved thumb.

When in doubt, use the jaw thrust. If you cannot successfully open the airway with the jaw thrust, then switch to the head tilt-chin lift method, because opening the airway is more important than the risk of spinal damage caused by the small movement of the neck when the head is tilted back.

If there is evidence of trauma to the head or the patient has vomited, inspect the mouth for blood, loose teeth, vomit, or anything else that may obstruct the airway. Use a gloved finger or suction if needed to clear the airway (Chapter 7).

If you find an unresponsive person in a position other than lying supine, do not immediately roll the patient onto his or her back to open the airway:

- Do not move a patient unnecessarily. Doing so may cause additional injury, especially if the patient may have a spinal injury.
- Try to determine whether the patient's airway is open by looking, listening, and feeling for breathing through the nose or mouth without moving the patient **(Figure 6-7)**.
- A patient who is clearly breathing has an open airway. You should not move this patient unless it is necessary for providing other care.
- If you are unable to determine whether an unresponsive patient is breathing, you will need to move the patient into the supine (face-up) position to open the airway and check for breathing.
- Support the head and neck when moving a trauma patient, as described in Chapter 15. Then open the airway.

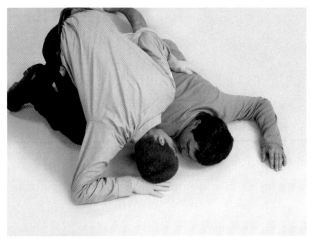

Figure 6-7 Check a patient's breathing in the position found.

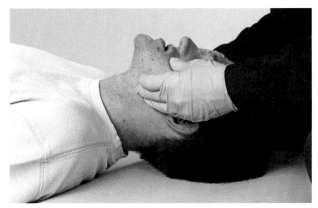

Figure 6-6 The jaw thrust.

Breathing

▄▄ Need to Recognize

The next step is to check the patient's breathing. In a responsive adult, check for adequate breathing. Inadequate breathing is characterized by diminished mental status and any of the following:

- Difficult or labored breathing
- Wheezing or gurgling sounds with breathing
- Pale skin (ashen skin in a dark-skinned patient) or a blue (cyanotic) color of the lips and nail beds
- A respiratory rate slower than 8 or greater than 30 breaths a minute

▶ Need to Do

In an unresponsive adult with the airway open, check for breathing **(Figure 6-8)**:

1. Lean over with your ear close to the person's mouth and nose and look at the patient's chest to see if it rises and falls with breathing.
2. *Listen* for any sounds of breathing.
3. *Feel* for breath on your cheek.

- If you do not detect any signs of breathing within 10 seconds, assume the person is not breathing.
- Lack of breathing may be caused by an obstructed airway (choking) or other causes.
- If the patient is not breathing, you must immediately give ventilations as described in the next chapter.

It is difficult to assess a breathing child's adequacy of respiration, so check for the presence or absence of breathing the same as in an unresponsive adult.

Circulation

▄▄ Need to Recognize

Next, check for circulation, which means checking that the heart is beating and blood is moving through the body (circulating):

- If the patient's heart has stopped or the patient is bleeding profusely, vital organs are not receiving enough oxygen to sustain life.
- If the patient is responsive or breathing, his or her heart is beating.

▶ Need to Do

To check circulation, feel for a **pulse:**

- In a responsive adult or child, check the **radial pulse,** located in the wrist just proximal to the base of the thumb. Note whether the pulse is irregular or very slow or very fast. Take note also of the patient's skin color and condition. Pale or ashen skin that is cool and clammy may indicate a circulation problem and a condition such as shock (Chapter 12).
- To check the pulse in an unresponsive adult, use the **carotid pulse** in the neck. Holding the patient's forehead with one hand to keep the airway open, put the index and middle fingers of your other hand on the side of the patient's neck nearer you. Find the Adam's apple and then slide your fingertips toward you and down the patient's neck to the groove at the side of the neck **(Figure 6-9)**. Pressing gently, feel for a pulse for at least 5 but not more than 10 seconds.

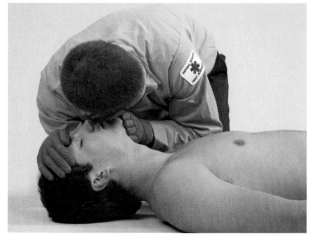

Figure 6-8 Look, listen, and feel for breathing.

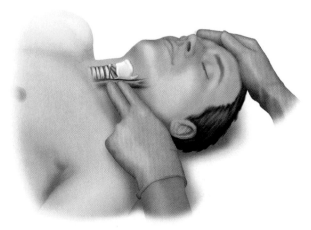

Figure 6-9 Check the carotid pulse in an unresponsive adult.

- In an unresponsive child, check either the carotid or **femoral pulse.** The femoral pulse is located in the center of the groin crease.

- To check the pulse in an infant, use the **brachial pulse** in the inside of the upper arm instead of the carotid pulse. With one hand on the infant's forehead to maintain head position for an open airway, put your fingers of your other hand about midway between the shoulder and elbow on the inside of the arm and press gently, feeling for no more than 10 seconds (**Figure 6-10**).

In the initial assessment, do not take the time to count the pulse, but note whether the pulse is irregular or very slow or very fast. These may be signs that the patient is not stable.

- Lack of a definite pulse along with the absence of adequate breathing signifies the heart has stopped or is not beating effectively enough to circulate blood.

- If the patient lacks a pulse and is not breathing adequately, start cardiopulmonary resuscitation (CPR) as described in Chapter 9.

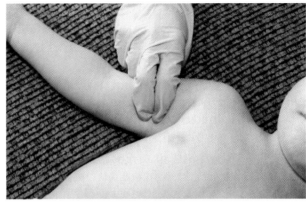

Figure 6-10 Check the brachial pulse in an unresponsive infant.

Check for Serious Bleeding

■■ Need to Recognize

The second part of the circulation check is to look for serious bleeding, which is life threatening.

- Bleeding from an injured artery is usually most serious. The blood is bright red and spurts or pulses from the wound.

Skill 6-1 **Initial Assessment of an Unresponsive Patient**

1 Check responsiveness.

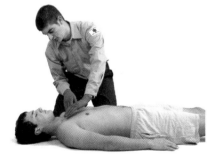

2 Open the airway.

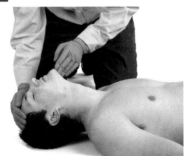

3 Look, listen, and feel for breathing.

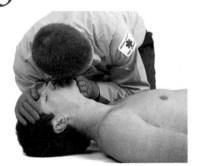

4 Check for a pulse.

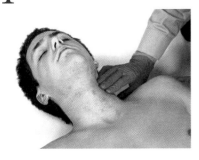

5 Look for severe bleeding.

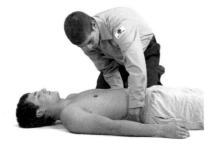

◆ Bleeding from a vein is generally slower, and the blood is dark red and flows more steadily. Venous bleeding also can become life-threatening over time.

◆ Do not remove the patient's clothing to check the whole body for bleeding. Instead, look for blood-saturated clothing and blood pooling beneath the patient's body (**Figure 6-11**).

◆ During the initial assessment, do not yet address minor bleeding or wounds because the patient may have more serious injuries that require your immediate attention.

◆ If you find serious bleeding, control it immediately with direct pressure on the wound as described in Chapter 12. **Skill 6-1** summarizes the steps of the initial assessment.

Patient Priority

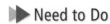 Need to Do

The results of the initial assessment determine whether the patient may have a critical condition and the steps you will need to take:

◆ Unresponsiveness or any problem with the airway, breathing, or circulation indicates the patient is a high priority. Stabilize the patient or arrange for immediate transport.

◆ Continue to reassess the patient and treat life-threatening conditions while waiting for additional EMS personnel to arrive.

◆ Call the responding EMT unit with an update of the patient's condition.

Report to EMS

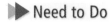 Need to Do

Following the initial assessment, call the responding EMS unit and provide an update report on the

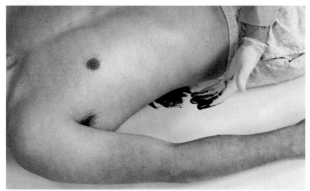

Figure 6-11 Assess for serious bleeding.

patient and the results of your assessment. Provide this information:

◆ Number of patients

◆ Age and gender of patients

◆ The patient's chief complaint

◆ The patient's level of responsiveness

◆ The patient's airway, breathing, and circulation status

Ask the responding unit their estimated time of arrival, and continue to care for the patient accordingly.

Do You Understand?

1. How do you begin to assess responsiveness in a patient who is not moving or speaking?

_____

2. How do you open the airway of an unresponsive trauma patient?

_____

3. Look, _____, and feel for breathing.

4. In a responsive adult, check the _____ pulse; in an unresponsive adult, check the _____ pulse.

5. True or false: Control any bleeding found in the initial assessment.

Physical Examination

✓ Need to Know

Following the initial assessment, unless you are caring for a life-threatening condition, perform a **physical examination** and question the patient, family members, or bystanders to gather additional information about the patient's condition. The purpose of the physical exam is to find and assess the signs and symptoms of illness or injury. Do not interrupt care for a serious problem to carry out the exam. Information gained from the exam and history may help you care for the patient and be of value to arriving EMS personnel.

As a general rule, complete the physical exam of an unresponsive patient or a patient with a significant mechanism of injury; this is called a **rapid trauma assessment.** With a responsive medical patient or a trauma patient with only a minor injury, the exam should focus on that area and need not be complete; this is called a **focused physical exam.** In addition to the general physical exam

BOX 6-2

DCAP-BTLS

While the acronym DOTS is used by many First Responders to guide the physical examination, a more detailed memory aid is used by some other emergency care professionals and responders:

D = Deformities
C = Contusions
A = Abrasions
P = Punctures
B = Burns
T = Tenderness
L = Lacerations
S = Swelling

As with DOTS, each area of the body is examined for the presence of these injuries and signs of injury.

and history described here, later chapters on specific injuries and illness describe other assessments to make and questions to ask the patient or family.

▶ Need to Do

In performing a physical exam, do the following:

- Allow a responsive patient to remain in the position he or she finds most comfortable while performing the physical exam. The patient does not need to be moved to the supine position as shown in the illustrations.

- Ask a responsive patient for consent to do a physical examination. Describe what you are about to do before touching the patient.

- Do not start the exam with a painful area. For example, if one knee hurts, start the exam on the other leg. Do not touch or manipulate any body area the patient tells you is very painful.

- Watch for a patient's facial expression or stiffening of a body part, which may reveal pain or tenderness the patient does not tell you about.

- In a responsive patient, begin with the area of the chief complaint and examine other body areas only as appropriate; perform a focused examination.

- With an unresponsive patient, examine the patient from head to toe in a systematic

manner, looking for any signs or symptoms of injury or illness.

- A **sign** is an objective observation or measurement such as warm skin or a deformed extremity.

- A **symptom** is a subjective observation reported by the patient, such as pain or nausea.

A systematic head-to-toe approach helps prevent overlooking important parts of the examination:

- Begin at the head because injuries here are more likely to be serious than injuries in the extremities or lower in the body.

- With responsive children, you may choose to begin at the feet and work up the body. Children are often alarmed when a stranger immediately begins an examination of their head. Beginning lower and working up can help you gain the child's confidence.

As a general rule, look and **palpate** (feel) for the following signs and symptoms of injury or illness throughout the body, comparing one side of the body to the other when appropriate. The acronym **DOTS** is a reminder of what to look for in a trauma patient:

D = Deformities
O = Open injuries
T = Tenderness (pain)
S = Swelling

The following examination sequence is described for a trauma patient with a significant mechanism of injury (**Skill 6-2**).

Head

- Gently feel the scalp and note any deformities, depressions, or lacerations.

- As you feel the scalp, periodically look at your gloved hands. Any blood on the gloves may hint at the presence of an open injury on the back of the head.

- Examine the face and note any swelling, discoloration, bleeding, deformity, or open wounds. Check the eyes for any obvious injuries, swelling, inflammation, or bleeding.

- Inspect the pupils for size, equality, and reaction to light, using a penlight.

- Examine the ears and note any laceration or bleeding of the outer ear. Look for any blood or clear or blood-tinged watery fluid coming from the ear canal. Watery fluid from either the ears or nose may indicate a skull fracture.

Skill 6-2 Detailed Physical Examination

1 Palpate and inspect the scalp and face.

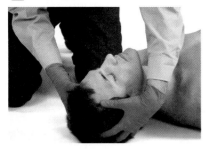

2 Check for eye injuries and assess the pupils.

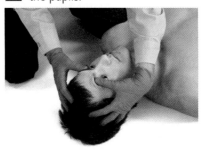

3 Check the ears for bleeding or leaking fluid.

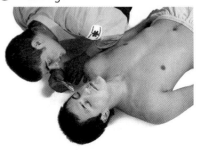

4 Check the mouth for injury, bleeding, and potential airway obstructions.

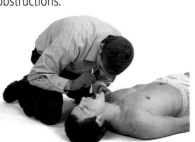

5 Remove upper body clothing and palpate and inspect the neck in front and back.

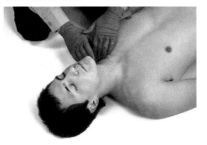

6 Palpate and inspect the chest, and observe chest movement with breathing.

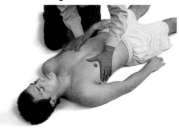

7 Palpate and inspect the four quadrants of the abdomen.

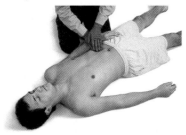

8 Reach under the patient to palpate the back and check for bleeding.

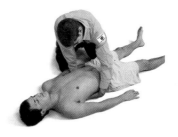

9 Remove lower body clothing and palpate the pevis.

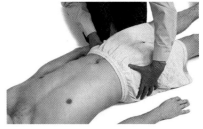

10 Palpate and inspect each upper and lower leg.

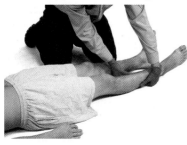

11 Check the pulse in each foot.

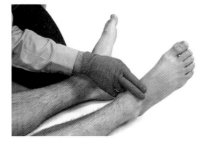

12 Check each foot for movement and sensation.

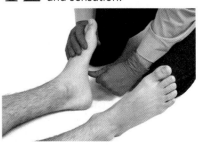

13 Palpate and inspect upper extremities from the clavicle to the shoulder and down the arm.

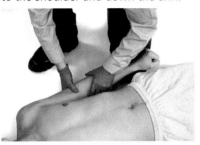

14 Check the radial pulse in each arm.

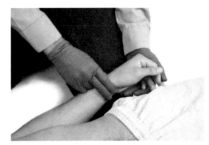

15 Check each hand for movement and sensation.

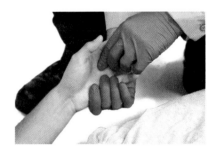

- Examine the nose and note any deformity, swelling, bleeding, or discoloration.
- Examine the mouth and note any missing teeth or open injuries. The presence of blood or other substances in the mouth can potentially threaten the patient's breathing.

Neck and Cervical Spine

- Assume that any patient with a head injury may also have a neck injury. With a head or neck injury, immobilize the cervical spine.
- Gently feel the back of the neck without moving it, looking for deformity, wounds, swelling, or tenderness. If any of these signs is present, immobilize the neck immediately.
- Examine the front of the neck and note any wounds, swelling, or discoloration. Look for a breathing hole, called a **stoma,** which may result from past neck surgery. Usually a stoma is detected in the initial assessment. If present, protect the stoma at all times from clothing, blood, or vomitus.

Chest

- Visually inspect the chest looking for any wounds, including sucking chest wounds, contusions (bruising), or deformities.
- Feel the chest with gentle pressure along the sides of the chest wall. Note the presence of any fractures or pain.
- Observe the expansion of the chest with breathing, normally equal on both sides.

Unequal chest expansion may be caused by a problem with the lungs or with the chest wall. If it appears that a segment of the chest moves with breathing in a direction opposite that of the remainder of the chest (flail chest), document this and report it to arriving EMTs.

- With a female patient, provide adequate privacy or a blanket to cover the breasts.

Abdomen

- Inspect the abdomen, looking for any swelling, bloating, rigidity, or the presence of wounds.
- If the patient complains of abdominal pain, ask where the pain is located. Then gently feel each of the four abdominal quadrants, leaving the quadrant with the pain last. If abdominal tenderness is noted, document its location.
- Do not repeatedly examine the abdomen.
- Assess any obvious bleeding or injury to the genitalia after ensuring privacy for the patient. In the male patient, note any bleeding or injury on the penis, scrotum, or groin. In a female patient, note the severity of the bleeding and provide a pad for placement over the genitalia. Otherwise, examination of the genitalia is usually deferred until the patient is in the emergency department.

Back

- Unless a head or spinal injury is suspected, roll the patient onto the side to examine the back. If a head or neck injury is suspected, do not move the patient but slide your gloved hand under the back and feel with your hand. Be careful to avoid broken glass and other sharp objects. Note any blood on your gloves after examining the back.

◆ Sweep the entire lower back, looking at the fingertips of your gloved hands for any bleeding.

◆ Treat any tenderness, swelling, or deformity of the lower part of the spine as a sign of a spinal injury and do not move the patient.

Pelvis

◆ Place your hands on the upper anterior aspect of the pelvis and gently press downward toward the patient's back. Note any tenderness or instability. Do not rock the pelvis.

◆ Then gently compress the pelvis toward the midline, again noting any tenderness or instability.

Extremities

◆ Inspect both legs for any obvious bleeding or deformity.

◆ Unless there is an obvious fracture or deformity, ask the patient to lift or move the legs.

◆ Palpate each leg, starting at the thigh and progressing downward.

◆ Palpate the knee and the kneecap (patella).

◆ Examine the lower leg and foot and note any swelling, deformity, or bleeding.

◆ Check the pulses in both feet. This pulse, the dorsalis pedis pulse, is located on the top of the foot.

◆ If a fracture is not suspected, check the feet for motor function by asking a responsive patient to wiggle the toes.

◆ Gently brush the patient's foot lightly to test for normal sensation.

◆ Examine the upper extremities in the same manner as the legs.

◆ Inspect the arms, looking for deformity, bleeding, or swelling.

◆ Unless there is an obvious fracture or deformity, ask the patient to lift or move the arms.

◆ Palpate both upper extremities, beginning with the collarbone (clavicle). Feel the bone, starting at the sternum and moving outward. Then feel the shoulder, noting any tenderness or swelling.

◆ Examine the arm and elbow, moving toward the fingers.

◆ Feel the radial pulse at the wrist.

◆ If fracture or dislocation is not suspected, ask the patient to squeeze your hands and compare the strength of both of the patient's hands.

◆ Lightly brush the fingers, asking the patient where you are touching. Document any deficiency.

Do You Understand?

1. True or false: A rapid trauma assessment involves only the airway, breathing, and circulation.

2. DOTS stands for:

   Deformities

   O_____

   Tenderness

   S_____

3. What is a clear fluid leaking from the ears a sign of?

   _____

4. In addition to DOTS, assess the extremities for a pulse, _____, and _____.

Vital Signs

✓ Need to Know

Some First Responders are trained to check the patient's **vital signs** as part of the physical examination. Vital signs assessed by First Responders include:

☑ Breathing rate, rhythm, depth, and ease

☑ Pulse rate, rhythm, and strength

☑ Skin color, temperature, and condition

☑ Pupil size, equality, and reaction to light

☑ Blood pressure

Vital signs reveal additional information about the patient's condition.

☑ Changes in a patient's vital signs, from the first set you take (called **baseline** vital signs), are important and should be documented.

☑ Changes may show the patient deteriorating or improving with treatment.

Table 6-1 lists the normal ranges for vital signs in different age groups. Remember that individuals vary significantly in terms of what is normal for them. Vital signs are also affected by stress, activity, and many other variables.

Table 6-1

Normal Vital Signs

Patient	Normal Respiratory Rate at Rest	Normal Pulse Rate at Rest	Normal Blood Pressure (systolic/diastolic)
Infant	20–30	80–150	84–106/56-70
Child	18–30	70–130	98–124/50-80
Adult	12–20	60–100	118–140/60-90

Breathing

 ### Need to Do

To assess the patient's respiration:

1. Do not tell a responsive patient that you are assessing breathing because the rate may change. Count respirations while holding the patient's wrist draped across the chest as if taking a pulse **(Figure 6-12)**. Observe or feel for the chest rising and falling (one cycle equals one breath).

2. Count the number of breaths in 30 seconds and multiply by two.

3. Note whether the patient is making an effort to breathe (normal breathing is effortless), is short of breath, or is using abdominal muscles in breathing. Also note whether breathing is noisy.

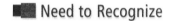 ### Need to Recognize

As a First Responder, you need to recognize the characteristics of respiratory distress:

- Gasping or wheezing
- Very fast or slow respiratory rate
- Very shallow or very deep breathing
- Shortness of breath, difficulty speaking

Pulse

 ### Need to Do

To assess the patient's pulse:

1. Have a responsive patient sit or lie down.

2. Take a radial pulse in an adult or child. If you cannot find a radial pulse in an adult, take a carotid pulse, or a brachial pulse in a child. Always take a brachial pulse in an infant.

3. Count the beats for 30 seconds and multiply by two.

4. Note the strength of the pulse (strong or weak).

5. Note the rhythm of the pulse (regular or irregular).

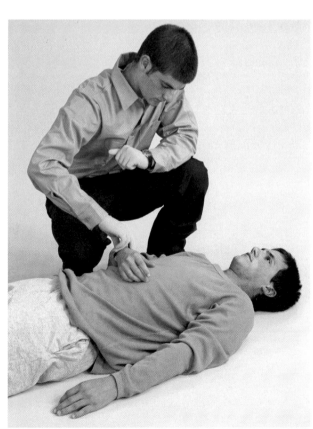

Figure 6-12 Assess a responsive patient's respiratory rate as if taking the pulse.

◼️ Need to Recognize

As a First Responder, you need to recognize the characteristics of a possible circulation problem:

♦ Very fast or very slow pulse

♦ Very weak or strong, bounding pulse

♦ Very weak and fast pulse (called a thready pulse)—may indicate shock

♦ Irregular rhythm—may indicate a cardiac problem

♦ Unequal pulses at different sites

Skin

▶️ Need to Do

To assess the patient's skin temperature and condition:

1. Assess skin temperature using the back of your hand on the patient's skin.

2. Assess skin color.

3. Assess skin moisture.

4. In a young child, assess capillary refill. Press on the patient's fingernail or skin with your finger and time how long it takes for color to return when the pressure is released.

◼️ Need to Recognize

As a First Responder, you will need to recognize the skin characteristics that may indicate a possible problem:

♦ Skin temperature:
  ◦ Cool skin—may indicate shock or hypothermia
  ◦ Very warm skin—may indicate heat stroke or fever

♦ Unusual coloration:
  ◦ Pale skin may indicate shock or hypothermia.
  ◦ A blue hue (**cyanosis**) of the nail beds or mouth may result from cardiac problems, respiratory problems, or hypothermia.
  ◦ A mottled appearance to the skin may occur with shock or cardiac failure.
  ◦ A reddish skin color may result from heat exposure, carbon monoxide poisoning, or a burn.
  ◦ Yellow skin may indicate a liver problem.

♦ Skin condition:
  ◦ Moist skin (except normal sweating in a warm environment)—may indicate shock or other emergencies

  ◦ Abnormally dry skin—may indicate dehydration or heat stroke

  ◦ Capillary refill time longer than 2 seconds—may indicate shock or diminished blood flow

Pupils

▶️ Need to Do

To assess the patient's pupils (**Figure 6-13**):

1. Assess the size of the patient's pupils. In bright light, they will be smaller than normal. In a dark area, they will be larger.

2. Assess the pupils for equality. Note any difference.

3. Assess reactivity to light by shining a penlight briefly in the eye; the pupil should constrict. In a very bright environment, cover the eyes instead and observe for dilation (expansion) followed by constriction (contraction) when uncovered.

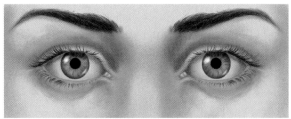

Normal pupils

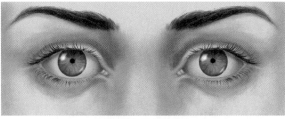

Constricted pupils

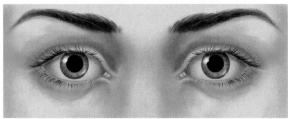

Dilated pupils

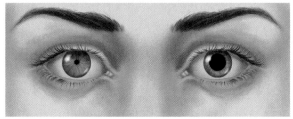

Unequal pupils

Figure 6-13 Assess pupils for size and equality.

■■ Need to Recognize

As a First Responder, you will need to recognize the pupil characteristics that may indicate a problem:

- Dilated or constricted pupils—may indicate drug use, poisoning, or a nervous system condition
- Unequal pupils—may indicate a brain injury, stroke, or other conditions
- Nonreactive pupils—may result from medication or a brain injury

Blood Pressure

✓ Need to Know

Some First Responders are trained to take the patient's blood pressure. **Blood pressure** is the force of the blood pressing against the arterial wall as a result of the heart's pumping action, somewhat like water pressure in a hose. When the heart contracts, the pressure is higher (**systolic pressure**), and the pressure falls lower when the heart relaxes between beats (**diastolic pressure**). Blood pressure measures both types of pressure. It is always recorded as systolic pressure over diastolic pressure, such as 130/90.

Measuring Blood Pressure by Auscultation

▶ Need to Do

Blood pressure is usually measured by **auscultation**, which involves using a stethoscope to listen for the sound of the pulse **(Skill 6-3)**:

1. Choose the correct size cuff to encircle the patient's upper arm **(Figure 6-14)**. Position the cuff with the lower edge an inch or more above the elbow crease, with the bladder centered over the brachial artery. Do not wrap it too tightly.

Skill 6-3 **Measuring Blood Pressure by Auscultation**

1 Position the cuff on the patient's arm.

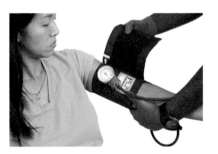

2 Position stethoscope diaphragm and inflate the cuff 30 mmHg beyond where the sound disappears.

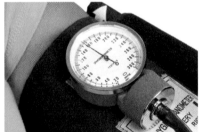

3 Watching the gauge, slowly deflate the cuff at 2 to 3 mmHg per second.

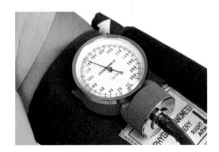

4 Note the pressure when the pulse tapping sound returns (systolic pressure).

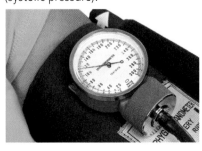

5 As the cuff deflates, note the reading when the tapping disappears (diastolic pressure).

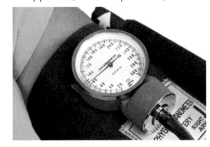

6 Deflate the cuff and record the pressure (systolic/diastolic).

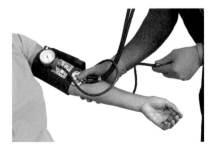

When you do not know the patient's normal blood pressure before the injury or medical emergency, it is difficult to interpret this vital sign because of the wide variation among individuals. Repeated measurements, however, provide important information about a possible trend in the patient's condition. The drop of blood pressure in shock usually develops as a late sign.

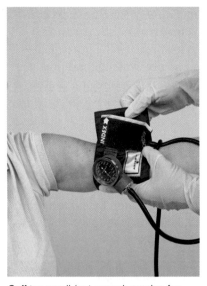 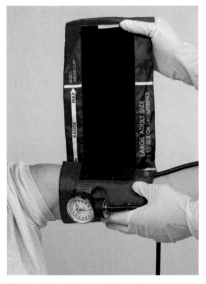 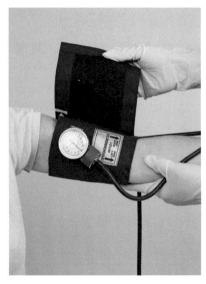

Cuff too small (not enough overlap for closure without being too tight).   Cuff too large (too much overlap, covers too much of patient's upper arm).   Correct cuff size (just right).

Figure 6-14 Choose the correct size blood pressure cuff.

2. Place the stethoscope over the brachial artery below the cuff. Pump the bulb until the pulse sound disappears and inflate the cuff 30 mmHg beyond this point. Alternatively, feel the radial pulse and inflate the cuff 30 mmHg beyond the point where you stop feeling the pulse.

3. Hold the stethoscope diaphragm over the brachial artery. While watching the gauge, open the valve to slowly deflate the cuff at a rate of 2 to 3 mmHg per second.

4. Note the pressure on the gauge when you first hear the pulse tapping sound return. This is the systolic pressure.

5. Continue to let the cuff deflate and note the reading when the tapping sound disappears. This is the diastolic pressure.

6. Deflate the cuff completely, remove it, and record the pressure (systolic/diastolic).

Measuring Blood Pressure by Palpation

If you do not have a stethoscope or the scene is too noisy to hear the pulse tapping sounds, you can measure systolic blood pressure by palpation rather than auscultation.

▶ Need to Do

Measuring blood pressure by palpation:

1. While palpating the radial pulse, inflate the cuff 30 mmHg beyond the point where you stop feeling the pulse.

2. While watching the gauge, open the valve to slowly deflate the cuff.

3. Note the pressure when you feel the radial pulse return. This is the systolic pressure. (You cannot measure diastolic pressure by palpation.)

4. Record the pressure as systolic pressure and include the word palpated (e.g., "130 palpated" or "130/Palp").

✎ Do You Understand?

1. List three or four signs of respiratory difficulty.

   _____   _____

   _____   _____

2. Shock may be indicated by skin characteristics that include _____ and _____ skin.

3. What are the three assessments of the pupils?

   _____   _____

   _____

History

✓ Need to Know

Patient assessment includes learning the patient's **history.** This information is gained from the patient and others about his or her condition and potentially related other factors.

☑ Although the history should focus on the specific or chief complaint, it should be complete when possible to ensure valuable information is not overlooked.

☑ With responsive medical patients, you may take the history before performing the physical exam.

☑ With trauma patients and any unresponsive patient, perform the physical exam first.

▶ Need to Do

♦ Talk to a responsive patient.

♦ With an unresponsive patient, talk to family members or bystanders about what they know or saw.

♦ Look for a medical alert insignia or other medical identification. In the home, also look for medication bottles and a Vial of Life, a medical information form often kept on or in the refrigerator.

♦ With a trauma patient, try to assess the forces involved. For example, a patient who fell from a height or was struck in the head by a heavy object is at greater risk of having a spinal injury and must not be moved during assessment or care.

♦ When taking the history of a responsive patient with a sudden illness, ask fully about the patient's situation to learn possible causes. For example, in a case of poisoning, the patient may not immediately associate present symptoms with something ingested an hour or more ago. Similarly, a patient could be experiencing the effects of carbon monoxide breathed inside a building, even though you encountered the patient outside.

Use the SAMPLE format to ensure you cover the patient's full history:

S = Signs and symptoms. What can you observe about the patient (signs)? Ask the patient how he or she feels (symptoms) and to describe any pain felt. Ask why the patient called EMS.

A = Allergies. Ask the patient if he or she has any allergies to foods, medicines, insect stings, anything in the environment, or other substances. Look for a medical alert ID.

M = Medications. Ask the patient if he or she is currently taking or recently has taken any prescribed medications or over-the-counter products, including vitamins, supplements, and herbal remedies.

P = Pertinent past medical history. Ask the patient if he or she has experienced anything like this before or is seeing a healthcare provider for any illnesses. Ask if the patient has ever been in the hospital. Again, a medical alert ID may indicate the patient has a condition such as diabetes or epilepsy.

L = Last food or drink. Ask the patient what he or she last ate or drank. Ask when and how much.

E = Events. Ask the patient what happened and try to identify the events that led to the current situation. When did the patient first begin to experience the problem?

♦ If the patient is unresponsive, ask family members or bystanders whether they know the answers to these questions.

♦ Check the scene for clues of what may have happened. The patient may have just taken a medication, for example, or you may see something like a syringe that could indicate possible drug abuse. A nearby container of a poisonous household product could indicate a possible poisoning.

♦ Consider the environment: A very cold or hot environment may produce a temperature-related emergency or contribute to sudden illness.

♦ Consider the patient's age. A younger person who slips on ice and falls may have only a bruise, whereas an elderly person who falls is more likely to have a broken bone.

The information from the **SAMPLE history** may help you give the right initial emergency care. When additional EMS personnel arrive, give them the information you gathered. It will help them to provide the appropriate medical care.

✎ Do You Understand?

1. How can you gather a history if the patient is unresponsive?

_____

2. True or false: The M in the SAMPLE history refers to prescription medications only.

3. What kinds of allergies should you ask about in the history?

_____

Ongoing Assessment

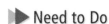 Need to Do

While awaiting additional EMS resources and giving any emergency care, continue to assess the patient. Calm and reassure the patient while reassessing the ABCs and repeating the physical examination as needed.

Repeat the initial assessment:

- Every 15 minutes for a stable patient
- Every 5 minutes for an unstable patient

Remember to:

- Reassess mental status.
- Maintain an open airway.
- Monitor breathing for rate and quality.
- Reassess pulse for rate and quality.
- Monitor skin color, temperature, and condition.
- Repeat the physical exam as needed.

The **ongoing assessment** also allows you to check that your interventions are effective or perform additional treatments as needed.

Hand-Off Report

Need to Do

When EMS personnel arrive, give them a hand-off report with detailed information about the patient's:

- Age and gender
- Chief complaint

- Responsiveness
- Airway and breathing status
- Circulation status

Also include:

- Your physical exam findings
- Results of your SAMPLE history
- Interventions you have provided and the patient's response to them

You may also complete a written report containing the same information.

Conclusion

The patient assessment is just the beginning of your care for an emergency patient. If you find a threat to life, care for it immediately as described in the following chapters on the airway and circulation. If there are no immediate threats to life, continue with a fuller physical examination and history and care for conditions you find, as described in later chapters.

Key Terms

ABCs (p. 74)

airway (p. 74)

auscultation (p. 85)

AVPU scale (p. 74)

baseline (p. 82)

blood pressure (p. 85)

brachial pulse (p. 77)

carotid pulse (p. 76)

chief complaint (p. 73)

cyanosis (p. 84)

diastolic pressure (p. 85)

DOTS (p. 79)

femoral pulse (p. 77)

focused physical exam (p. 78)

general impression (p. 73)

hand-off report (p. 88)

head tilt–chin lift (p. 75)

Review Questions

1. Check the emergency scene to ensure all patients have been noted
   a. during the initial scene size-up.
   b. after you check the most critical patient's ABCs.
   c. after the initial assessment.
   d. before checking for scene hazards.

2. Suspect a potential spinal injury in
   a. all unresponsive patients.
   b. patients with significant blood loss.
   c. all trauma patients.
   d. all patients.

3. Using the AVPU scale, a patient who does not respond to your voice but who moves when pinched is classified as
   a. A.   c. P.
   b. V.   d. U.

4. Inadequate breathing in an adult may be characterized by a respiratory rate slower than _____ or greater than _____ breaths a minute.
   a. 8, 20   c. 8, 30
   b. 12, 20   d. 12, 30

5. Check for breathing for no longer than _____ seconds.
   a. 5   c. 15
   b. 10   d. 20

6. Which pulse is checked in an unresponsive infant?
   a. Carotid
   b. Femoral
   c. Radial
   d. Brachial

7. How is the back checked in the physical exam of an unresponsive trauma patient?
   a. Slide your gloved hand under the patient's back.
   b. Support the head and roll the patient face down.
   c. Look for blood running out from under the body on either side.
   d. The back is not checked in an unresponsive trauma patient.

8. The pulse is assessed for rate,
   a. rhythm, and strength.
   b. pressure, and equality.
   c. rhythm, and equality.
   d. rhythm, and depth.

9. Capillary refill is abnormal in a child if color returns only after more than _____ second(s).
   a. 1   c. 3
   b. 2   d. 4

10. Reassess the ABCs in an unstable patient every
    a. minute.
    b. 2 minutes.
    c. 5 minutes.
    d. 15 minutes.

Unit 3
Airway

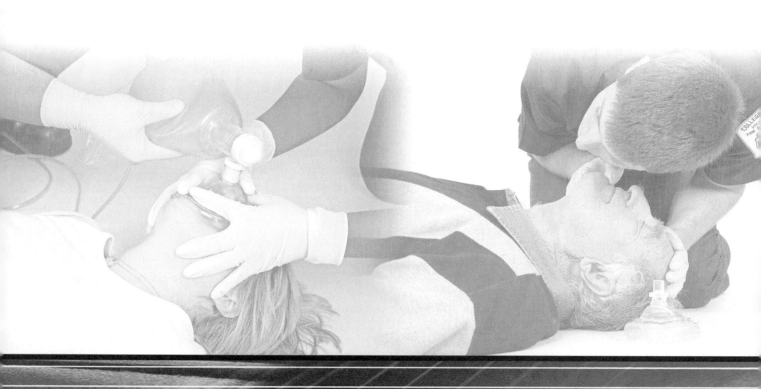

Chapter 7

The Airway and Breathing Emergencies

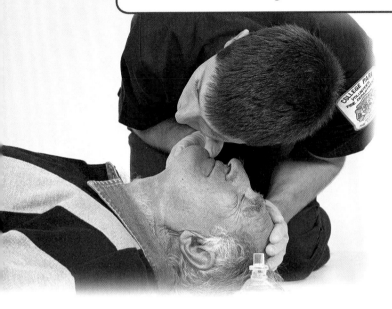

Chapter Preview

- Anatomy and Physiology Review
- The Airway
- Breathing
- Foreign Body Airway Obstructions (FBAO)

You Respond To ...

the scene where an elderly woman is lying on the floor. Your assessment reveals she is unresponsive, and when you open her airway, you cannot detect breathing. A family member present says it has been about 4 minutes since she collapsed, and you know you need to act quickly.

Introduction

Emergencies involving the airway or breathing are common and are among the most critical patient situations you will encounter. If you discover in the initial assessment that the patient's airway is not open or that the patient is not breathing, it is crucial to act immediately because cells in vital organs begin to die within minutes without oxygen. Any illness or injury that impairs the airway or breathing is a respiratory emergency.

Anatomy and Physiology Review

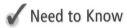 Need to Know

The primary organs of the respiratory system are the structures of the airway and the lungs (**Figure 7-1**):

☑ The **airway** is the path air takes from the nose and mouth to the lungs.

☑ Air entering the nose or mouth passes through the **pharynx.**

☑ The **nasopharynx** is the upper section of the airway from the nasal cavity.

☑ The **oropharynx** is the lower section (throat) from the oral cavity (**Figure 7-2**).

☑ Air passes through the pharynx to the **trachea** (windpipe), the top section of which is the larynx (voicebox).

☑ Below the neck the trachea branches into the left and right **bronchi** (singular: bronchus), the passageways into the lungs.

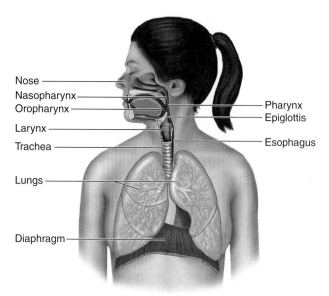

Figure 7-1 Structures of the respiratory system.

☑ The bronchi branch into smaller tubular passages in the lungs and eventually end in the **alveoli,** the tiny air sacs where oxygen and carbon dioxide pass into and out of capillaries.

Because the pharynx also leads to the **esophagus,** the tube that carries food to the stomach, another structure, called the epiglottis, is very important for breathing.

☑ The **epiglottis** is a leaf-shaped tissue flap that prevents solids and liquids from entering the trachea and blocking the airway or reaching the **lungs.**

☑ The epiglottis directs food and drink to pass from the throat to the esophagus and stomach.

Breathing depends on muscular movements under the control of the nervous system.

1. When the **diaphragm** (the large muscle below the lungs) contracts and moves down, the thoracic cavity and lungs expand, decreasing the pressure within the lungs **(Figure 7-3)**.

2. Air flows into the lungs because the pressure is lower.

3. When the diaphragm relaxes and moves up, the size of the thoracic cavity is reduced and air flows back out of the lungs.

The main function of the respiratory system is to bring oxygen into the body when the person inhales and to remove carbon dioxide, a waste product, when the person exhales.

☑ In the lungs, oxygen enters the blood from the inhaled air, and carbon dioxide leaves the blood into the air breathed out

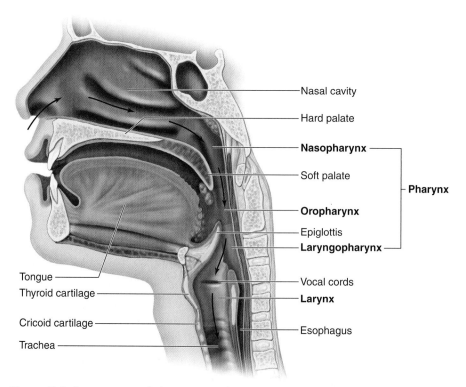

Figure 7-2 Structures of the upper airway.

Inhalation   **Exhalation**

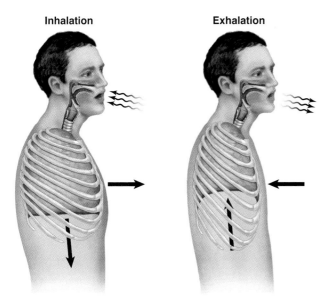

Figure 7-3 The mechanics of breathing.

(exhaled). This process in the lungs is called **external respiration.**

☑ **Internal respiration** is the process of oxygen and carbon dioxide moving into and out of the blood within internal body tissues.

The Airway Anatomy of Infants and Children

✓ Need to Know

Important differences to remember in infants and children airway management include the following:

☑ Airway structures are smaller and more easily obstructed by foreign bodies.

☑ The tongue takes up proportionally more space in the mouth than in adults. It also more easily obstructs the airway in an unresponsive patient.

☑ Because the trachea is more flexible in infants and children, care must be taken not to hyperextend the neck by pushing the head back too far when opening the airway in an unresponsive patient.

The primary cause of cardiac arrest in infants and children is an uncorrected respiratory problem.

🖎 Do You Understand?

1. The _____ prevents food from entering the trachea.

2. The large muscle that does most of the work of breathing is the _____ .

3. The airway of an infant or young child is more easily obstructed by either the _____ or a _____ .

The Airway

▰ Need to Recognize

The airway is the first thing you check in the initial assessment of a patient. You may need to open the airway, maintain its patency, or clear it when it is compromised, as described in the following sections. A later section describes care for a foreign body obstruction of the airway.

Opening the Airway

▶ Need to Do

Opening the airway of an unresponsive patient in the initial assessment is described in Chapter 6. Remember that the tongue is the most common cause of airway obstruction in an unresponsive patient because when the muscle relaxes, gravity may pull the tongue back in the pharynx, which blocks the airway.

▸ If a spinal injury is not suspected, use the head tilt–chin lift to lift the tongue from the back of the throat and open the airway.

▸ In a trauma patient, use the jaw lift instead to open the airway.

Assessing the Airway

▰ Need to Recognize

Any factor that impedes the flow of air in and out of the lungs can affect respiration and become life threatening.

▸ An **airway obstruction** is a physical blockage of the airway that prevents the flow of air.

▸ A person who is eating may have a piece of food lodged in the pharynx, a condition called **foreign body airway obstruction (FBAO),** or **choking.**

▸ An injury to the head or neck may cause the soft tissues of the upper airway to swell and obstruct the airway.

All of these are life-threatening situations.

Another potential problem with the airway is a failure of the epiglottis to prevent substances from entering the trachea. The swallowing reflex normally prevents this, but in an unconscious person, this reflex may not function, which allows liquids or solids to enter the trachea and lungs. If an unresponsive patient lying on his or her back vomits, the vomit may flow back down the throat and into the trachea and lungs, blocking or limiting respiration and possibly causing a severe lung infection.

> ◗ After opening the airway, assess that it is **patent** (open) and clear of any fluids or solids that may compromise the airway.
>
> ◗ Assess the airway in all unresponsive patients and responsive patients with injuries or altered mental status who may not be able to protect their own airway.
>
> 1. Open the patient's mouth with a gloved hand.
> 2. Listen for sounds indicating a liquid in the airway, such as gurgling or **stridor** (a high-pitched sound on inhaling caused by an obstruction).
> 3. Look inside the airway for any fluids, solids, or objects such as broken teeth or dental appliances that may compromise the airway.
> 4. Clear the airway using a finger sweep or suction.

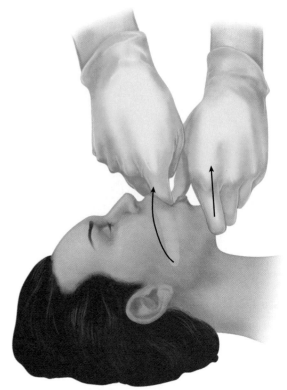

Figure 7-4 Use the finger sweep to remove a solid object from the airway.

Clearing a Compromised Airway

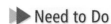 Need to Do

A compromised airway in an unresponsive patient can be cleared by either a finger sweep or the use of suction. Suction requires equipment and is described in the following chapter along with other devices used for the airway and ventilation. Perform the finger sweep quickly.

1. Perform a finger sweep only if you see fluids or solids in the mouth or airway. Never perform a blind finger sweep.
2. Unless the patient is injured, roll the patient onto one side (preferably the left side).
3. With a dressing or cloth over your index and middle fingers, wipe liquids or semi-liquids from the mouth.
4. To remove solid objects, hook your index finger and sweep the object to the side and out of the mouth. Be careful not to force the object deeper into the airway (**Figure 7-4**).

Maintaining an Open Airway

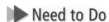 Need to Do

> ◗ As long as the patient is positioned supine, the airway must be kept open by maintaining

either the head tilt–chin lift or the jaw thrust. One First Responder may do this while others perform other care.

> ◗ An airway adjunct may also be used to help maintain an open airway; these devices are described in the next chapter.
>
> ◗ If you are alone with a patient who is breathing effectively, and you must attend to other care, you can move the patient into the **recovery position** to keep the airway open.

Recovery Position

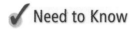 Need to Know

The recovery position is used for an unresponsive patient who is breathing and who is not suspected to have a spinal injury. It offers several benefits:

> ☑ It helps keep the airway open so that you do not need to maintain the head tilt–chin lift or jaw–thrust maneuver.
>
> ☑ Unrecognized airway obstructions are less likely to occur.
>
> ☑ It allows fluids to drain from the mouth so that the patient does not choke on blood, vomit, or other fluids.

☑ It prevents the patient from inhaling stomach contents if the patient vomits.

▶ Need to Do

Unless this position could worsen a patient's injury, put the patient on his or her left side; this side reduces the chances of the patient vomiting.

The modified HAINES (High Arm IN Endangered Spine) position is now recommended because it reduces movement of the neck in case of potential spinal injury (Skill 7-1).

Use the HAINES position for adults and children. For an unresponsive breathing infant, hold the infant facedown over your arm with his or

Skill 7-1 | Modified HAINES Recovery Position

1 Extend the patient's arm that is farther from you, above the patient's head.

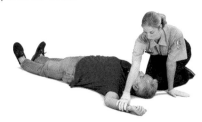

2 Position the patient's other arm across the chest.

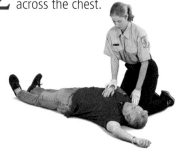

3 Bend the patient's nearer leg at the knee.

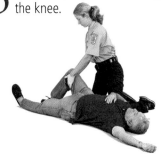

4 Put your forearm that is nearer the patient's head under the patient's nearer shoulder with your hand under the hollow of the neck.

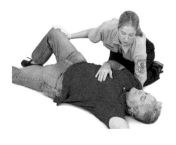

5 Carefully roll the patient away from you by pushing on the patient's flexed knee and lifting with your forearm while your hand stabilizes the head and neck. The patient's head is now supported on the raised arm.

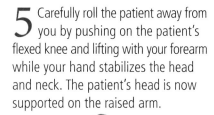

6 While continuing to support the head and neck, position the patient's hand palm down with fingers under the armpit of the raised arm, with the patient's forearm flat on the surface at 90 degrees to the body.

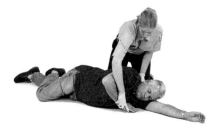

7 With the patient now in position, check the airway and open the mouth to allow drainage.

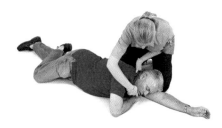

8 Once the patient is in the recovery position, continue to monitor the patient's breathing while waiting for advanced help to arrive.

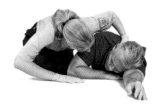

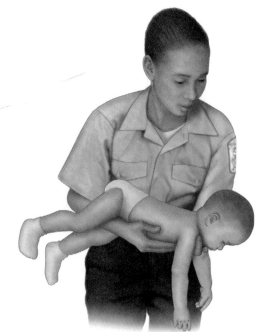

Figure 7-5 Infant recovery position.

her head slightly lower than the body **(Figure 7-5)**. Support the head and neck with your hand and keep the nose and mouth clear.

✎ Do You Understand?

1. Use the jaw thrust to open the airway in any _____ patient.

2. True or false: Sweep the mouth with your finger in any patient whose airway may be obstructed.

3. List at least three benefits of using the recovery position for an unresponsive patient who is breathing.

_____

_____

_____

Breathing

Assessing Breathing

▰ Need to Recognize

Remember the ABCs: Immediately after opening an unresponsive patient's airway, check for breathing. Ask a responsive patient, "Are you choking?" The ability to cough strongly, talk, or make vocal sounds indicates that the patient is breathing.

With an unresponsive patient, place your ear close to the patient's mouth and nose and assess for breathing for no more than 10 seconds:

- Look for the rise and fall of the chest.
- Listen for air escaping during exhalation.
- Feel for air coming from the mouth and nose.

Even if an airway obstruction is present, you may briefly observe movement of the chest as an unresponsive patient makes an effort to breathe, but this does not last long and you will not hear or feel air movement. As well, some reflex gasping (**agonal respirations**) may be present just after cardiac arrest; this should not be confused with breathing.

As you determine the presence of breathing, also assess the effort or work of breathing:

- Breathing should be effortless.
- Breathing should be relatively quiet.
- Observe the chest for adequate rise and fall.
- Look for the movement of **accessory muscles** to breathe (movement of the abdomen and neck area).

Breathing emergencies include respiratory distress (difficulty breathing) and respiratory arrest or inadequate breathing.

Respiratory Distress

▰ Need to Recognize

A patient in respiratory distress is breathing but may be

- gasping for air
- panting
- breathing faster or slower than normal
- making wheezing or other sounds with breathing
- using accessory muscles in the effort to breathe

Typically, the patient cannot speak a full sentence without pausing to breathe. The patient's skin may look pale and be cool and moist; the lips and nail beds may be bluish (**cyanosis**). Lowered oxygen levels in the blood may make the patient feel dizzy or disoriented. The patient may feel extreme distress. The patient may be sitting and leaning forward, hands on knees, in what is called the **tripod position (Figure 7-6)**.

- Because respiratory distress in an infant or child may rapidly progress to arrest, it is crucial to act quickly when an infant or child has trouble breathing.

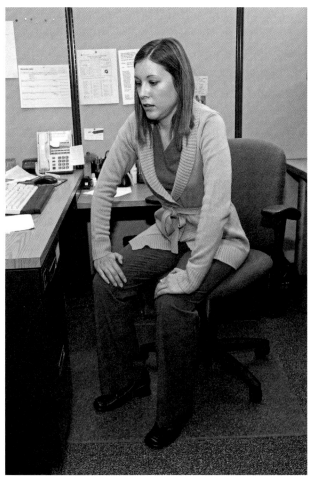

Figure 7-6 The tripod position typically assumed by responsive patients in respiratory distress.

◗ In addition to the signs and symptoms seen in adults, an infant or child may have flaring nostrils and more obvious movements of chest muscles with the effort to breathe.

▶ Need to Do

Respiratory distress is a medical emergency. Unless the patient's condition progresses to inadequate breathing or respiratory arrest, ventilation is not needed, although the patient will benefit from supplemental oxygen. The care of respiratory distress is described in Chapter 11.

Inadequate Breathing and Respiratory Arrest

▰ Need to Recognize

Respiratory arrest or inadequate breathing is a life-threatening emergency:

◗ **Respiratory arrest** is the condition of not breathing at all.

◗ **Inadequate breathing** is a condition in which the patient is not getting enough oxygen because of breathing too slowly or too weakly.

◗ In both situations the patient needs **ventilation.**

If an adult patient is breathing at a rate less than 10 breaths per minute, take this as a sign of inadequate breathing—the patient is not receiving sufficient oxygen. The patient will likely have altered mental status and may have a cyanotic appearance. In an adult who is not breathing adequately, do not wait for respiratory arrest before beginning to provide rescue breathing, or ventilations.

When you check the ABCs in a child or infant, look only for the presence or absence of breathing, because a child may be breathing slowly but still adequately.

Ventilation

✔ Need to Know

A patient who is not breathing or whose breathing is inadequate needs ventilation. Ventilation, also called rescue breathing, is the process of moving air or oxygen into the patient's lungs either from the First Responder or through a device such as a bag mask.

☑ If the patient's heart is still beating, ventilation provides oxygen for the blood circulating to vital tissues, keeping the patient alive until breathing starts again spontaneously or advanced care is given.

☑ If the patient has no pulse, ventilation is combined with chest compressions in CPR to help circulate the oxygenated blood to vital organs (see Chapter 9).

Without special equipment, provide ventilation with your own exhaled air. Air contains about 21% oxygen, and the breath we exhale is about 16% oxygen—still enough oxygen to increase the oxygen level in the patient's blood to maintain life. This chapter describes ventilation given by mouth; Chapter 8 describes ventilation using special equipment and oxygen.

Masks and Barrier Devices

Barrier devices are always recommended when giving ventilation by mouth. Two common types are pocket masks and face shields **(Figure 7-7):**

☑ Both devices offer personal protection from the patient's fluids, as well as from the patient's exhaled air when equipped with a one-way valve.

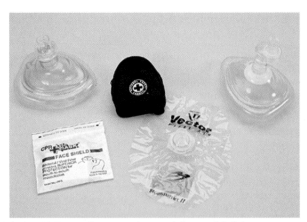

Figure 7-7 Pocket masks and face shields.

☑ With either device, keep the patient's head positioned to maintain an open airway as you deliver breaths through the device.

Face Masks

The **resuscitation mask,** also called a pocket face mask or a face mask, seals over the patient's mouth and nose and has a port through which you blow air to give ventilations.

☑ A one-way valve allows your air in through the mouthpiece, but the patient's exhaled air exits the mask through a different opening.

☑ When using a face mask, it is essential to seal the mask well to the patient's face while maintaining an open airway.

☑ Use the bridge of the nose as a guide for correct placement. Mask position is critical because a poorly positioned mask may leak.

How you hold the mask depends on

☑ your position by the patient

☑ whether the head tilt–chin lift or jaw–thrust technique is used to open the airway

☑ whether you have one hand or two hands free to seal the mask

The following hand positions assume you have both hands free to seal the mask.

▶ Need to Do

From a position at the patient's side (when giving CPR) using the head tilt-chin lift:

1. With the thumb and index finger of your hand closer to the top of the patient's head,

seal the top and sides of the mask to the patient's head as shown in **Figure 7-8a.**

2. Put the thumb of your second hand on the lower edge of the mask.

3. Put the remaining fingers of your second hand under the jaw to lift the chin.

4. Press the mask down firmly to make a seal as you perform a head tilt–chin lift to open the airway.

From a position at the top of the patient's head (with two rescuers or when not giving CPR) using the head tilt–chin lift:

1. Put your thumbs on both sides of the mask as shown in **Figure 7-8b.**

2. Put the remaining fingers of both hands under the angles of the patient's jaw on both sides.

3. As you tilt the head back, press the mask down firmly to make a seal as you lift the chin with your fingers.

From a position at the top of the patient's head using the jaw thrust:

1. Without tilting the patient's head back, position your thumbs on the mask the same as for the head tilt–chin lift from the top of the patient's head, with fingers under the angles of the jaw.

2. Lift the jaw to open the airway as you press down with your thumbs to seal the mask, without tilting the head back **(Figure 7-8c).**

Face Shield

▶ Need to Do

Like a mask, a **face shield** is positioned over the patient's mouth as a protective barrier. The patient's nose, however, must be pinched closed when giving a ventilation to prevent the air from coming out the nose instead of entering the lungs **(Figure 7-9).** A face mask is generally preferred to a face shield because air may leak around the shield.

If No Barrier Device Is Available

▶ Need to Do

If no barrier device is available, give ventilations directly from your mouth to the patient's mouth; nose; or stoma, if present. The risk of disease transmission is still very low.

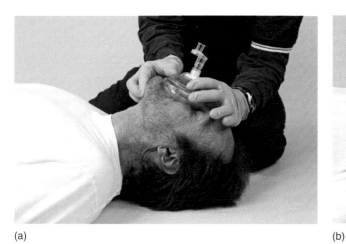

(a)

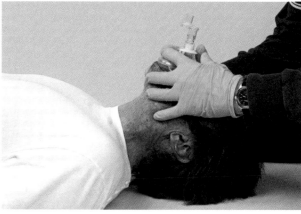

(b)

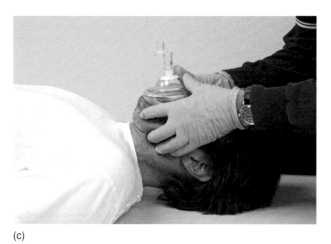

(c)

Figure 7-8   (a) Face mask hand position with rescuer at patient's side. (b) Face mask hand position with rescuer at patient's head. (c) Face mask hand position when using the jaw-thrust technique. Do not tilt the head back.

Mouth to Mouth

- Gently pinch the patient's nose shut and seal your mouth over the patient's mouth.
- Blow into the patient's mouth for about 1 second, watching the chest rise to confirm the air going in.
- Remove your mouth to let the air escape.

Mouth to Nose

- If the patient's mouth cannot be opened or is injured or if you cannot get a good seal with

your mouth over the patient's mouth, give ventilations through the nose.

- Hold the patient's mouth closed, seal your mouth over the nose to blow in, and then allow the mouth to open to let the air escape.

Mouth to Stoma

Because of past illness or injury, some people breathe through a hole in their lower neck called a **stoma.**

- During your check of the ABCs, check this hole when assessing breathing.
- To give ventilations, cup your hand over the patient's nose and mouth to prevent your air

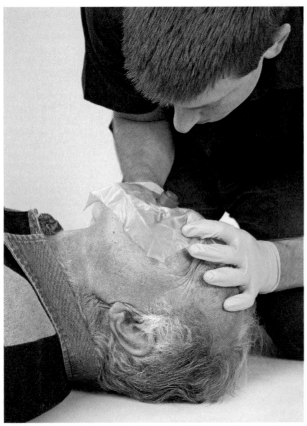

Figure 7-9 Position the face shield over the patient's mouth and pinch the nose.

from leaving by the nose and mouth instead of going to the lungs.

- Then seal your mouth or barrier device over the stoma, and give breaths as usual.

Mouth to Nose and Mouth

Because of their smaller size, infants and very small children are generally given ventilations through both their mouth and nose.

- Seal your mouth over both the nose and mouth and give gentle breaths as usual.
- Watch to see the chest rise with each breath.

Techniques of Ventilation

▶ Need to Do

With the patient supine, open the airway with the head tilt–chin lift or the jaw thrust. Use a face mask or other barrier device but do not delay ventilation to get one.

- Use the basic technique to blow air into the patient while watching the chest rise to make sure your air is going into the lungs.
- Do not try to rush the air in or blow too forcefully.

- Do not take a big breath to exhale more air into the patient; take a normal breath.
- Give each breath over about 1 second.
- If the breath does not go in, you feel resistance, or you do not see the patient's chest rise, then try again to open the airway.
- If your breath still does not go in, then the patient has an airway obstruction and needs care for choking (see later section).
- If your initial breath goes in, give a second breath over 1 second.

Always give 2 breaths immediately after discovering the patient is not breathing or is breathing inadequately.

- If your breaths go in, check for a pulse (the C in the ABCs).
- If the patient has a pulse but is not breathing, continue ventilations at a rate of 1 breath every 5-6 seconds in an adult or every 3-5 seconds for a child. **Skill 7-2** describes the sequence of steps for giving breaths.
- Use the same steps with a face shield, mouth-to-mouth ventilation, or other techniques with the nose or a stoma.

Ventilating Infants

▶ Need to Do

Ventilating infants is similar to the technique for adults and children, with these differences:

- Gently tilt the head back to open the airway and check breathing—do not overextend the neck.
- If the correct size barrier device is not available, cover both the mouth and nose with your mouth to give breaths. (Use the mouth or nose only if you cannot cover both.)
- Give 1 breath every 3-5 seconds.

Cricoid Pressure

✓ Need to Know

Cricoid pressure, also called the Sellick maneuver, is a technique used by some First Responders that prevents the air given during ventilation from passing through the esophagus to the stomach.

- ☑ Air in the stomach can cause vomiting, which interrupts ventilation and may cause **aspiration,** the movement of vomit or other fluids or solids into the lungs, which can cause a serious infection and other problems.

Skill 7-2 **Mouth-to-Mask Ventilation**

1 Open the airway. Look, listen, and feel for adequate breathing for no more than 10 seconds.

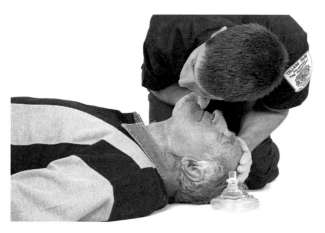

2 If not breathing adequately, position the mask or barrier device and give 2 breaths over 1 second each, watching the chest rise and letting it fall.

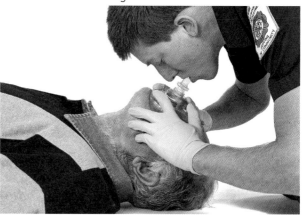

3 If the first breath does not go in, try again to open the airway and give another breath. If it still does not go in, the patient may be choking. Proceed to care for a foreign body airway obstruction.

4 If your first 2 breaths go in, check the patient for no more than 10 seconds for a pulse. If there is a pulse but no adequate breathing, continue ventilations. For an adult, give each breath over 1 second at a rate of 10 to 12 breaths per minute (1 breath every 5-6 seconds). For an infant or child, give each breath over 1 second at a rate of 12 to 20 breaths per minute (1 breath every 3-5 seconds). For all patients, recheck for a pulse about every 2 minutes. If there is no pulse, start CPR beginning with chest compressions.

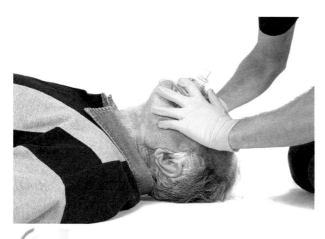

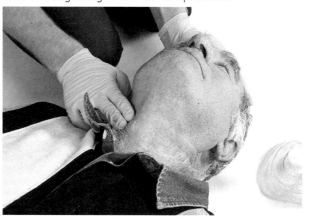

(ALERT)

- • Do not blow harder than is needed to make the chest rise.
- • After each breath, remember to let the air escape and the chest fall.
- • Blowing in too forcefully or for too long is ineffective and may put air in the stomach, which may cause vomiting.
- • Do not blow in too frequently.

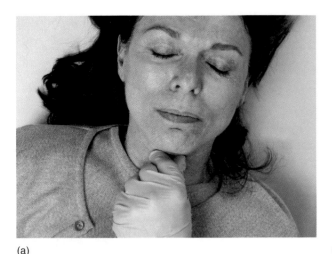
(a)

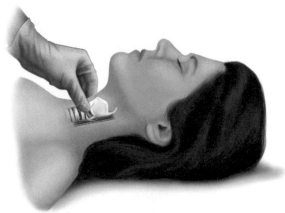
(b)

Figure 7-10   (a) The hand position for cricoid pressure. (b) Cricoid pressure compresses the esophagus against the spine.

☑ Cricoid pressure put on the trachea squeezes the esophagus closed, preventing air from traveling to the stomach **(Figure 7-10)**.

▶ **Need to Do**

Cricoid pressure is performed only on unresponsive patients, only by a rescuer trained in this technique, and only by an additional rescuer who uses the technique while other rescuer(s) perform ventilation and/or CPR chest compressions. You can apply cricoid pressure to an adult, a child, or an infant, using less pressure for smaller patients. Follow these steps:

1. With your index finger, locate the patient's Adam's apple (thyroid cartilage).

2. Slowly slide your finger down the patient's neck. Feel the indentation just past the bottom of the thyroid cartilage and, just below this, the higher cricoid cartilage. In an obese patient, it may be easier to begin at the sternum and move upward to find the cricoid ring as the first solid structure in the neck. Take care not to mistake the thyroid cartilage for the cricoid cartilage.

3. With index finger and thumb, apply moderate pressure down on the cricoid cartilage. Maintain this pressure continuously while ventilation is being given.

Special Circumstances for Ventilation

✓ **Need to Know**

In some circumstances, you may have to adjust how you give ventilations or respond to a chang-

ing situation. These circumstances include the patient's vomiting, a patient with dentures, and a patient with facial injuries.

Vomiting

Usually, if the head is positioned correctly to open the airway and ventilations are not given too forcefully or too fast, the air will move through the trachea into the lungs rather than down the esophagus to the stomach. In some cases, air may move into the stomach:

☑ If the airway is not sufficiently open

☑ If breaths are given too quickly

☑ If you continue to blow in air even after the lungs have expanded and the chest has risen

In these cases, air may be forced into the stomach, making vomiting more likely. Vomiting presents two problems. If an unresponsive patient vomits, you have to roll the patient onto the side to drain the mouth and clear the airway before continuing ventilation. Vomiting also increases the risk of aspiration. Although a patient may vomit even with correct ventilation technique, take steps to help prevent vomiting:

1. Open the airway before giving a breath.

2. Blow steadily over 1 second.

3. Watch the chest rise as you give each breath.

4. Stop each breath when the chest rises rather than continuing to blow.

5. Let the chest fall between breaths.

Dentures

☑ A patient's dentures are usually left in place during ventilation.

☑ If they are loose and make it difficult to give breaths or may fall back in the mouth and block the airway, remove dentures before ventilating the patient.

Facial Injuries

If the patient's mouth cannot be opened or is injured, or if you cannot get a good seal with your mask or mouth over the patient's mouth, give ventilations through the nose.

1. Hold the patient's mouth closed.
2. Seal your mouth over the nose to blow in.
3. Allow the mouth to open to let the air escape.

A patient with injuries may have blood in the mouth, which needs to be cleared before giving ventilations.

Do You Understand?

1. An adult patient breathing fewer than _____ breaths per minute is breathing inadequately.

2. Which type of barrier device is preferred for giving a patient ventilations?

_____

3. How much time should each ventilation take?

_____

4. An adult patient who has a pulse but is not breathing should receive 1 ventilation every _____ seconds.

5. List at least three incorrect actions that may lead to a patient's vomiting during ventilation.

_____

_____

_____

Foreign Body Airway Obstructions (FBAO)

✓ Need to Know

A foreign body airway obstruction (FBAO) occurs when some object blocks the airway.

☑ A severe airway obstruction means the patient is getting no air at all and consequently no oxygen into the blood.

☑ This patient will soon become unresponsive, and the heart will soon stop.

☑ Care is urgently needed to clear the airway and then to provide ventilation or CPR as needed.

With a mild obstruction, the patient is still getting some air into the lungs. The patient may be able to cough out the obstructing object.

Assessing An Airway Obstruction

Need to Recognize

♦ Most cases of choking in adults occur while eating.

♦ Most cases of choking in infants and children occur while eating or playing. Hot dogs are a common food causing choking in children.

♦ Often someone is present and recognizes the choking event while the patient is still responsive.

With a *mild obstruction,* a responsive patient is usually coughing forcefully in an attempt to expel the object:

♦ The patient is getting some air and may be making wheezing or high-pitched sounds with breaths, along with coughing.

♦ Do not interrupt the person's coughing or attempts to expel the object.

With a *severe obstruction,* the patient is getting very little or no air:

♦ The person may look frantic and be clutching at his or her throat.

♦ The person cannot speak.

♦ You may notice a pale or bluish coloring around the patient's mouth and nail beds.

♦ A patient who is coughing very weakly and silently, or not coughing at all, is unlikely to expel the obstructing object.

♦ Ask the patient if he or she is choking.

♦ If the patient cannot answer but indicates that he or she is choking, begin care for an airway obstruction in a responsive patient (**Figure 7-11**). This is an urgent situation that requires immediate care.

In an unresponsive patient, an airway obstruction is assessed when the ABCs are checked as usual:

1. If the patient's head is positioned to open the airway but the patient is not breathing, give 2 ventilations.

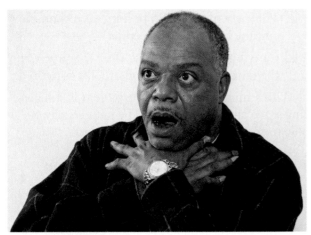

Figure 7-11 The universal sign of a responsive, choking patient.

2. If your first breath does not go into the patient and make the chest rise, try again to open the airway and give a second breath.

3. If it still does not go in, assume that the patient has an obstructed airway.

▶▶ Need to Do

Care for an FBAO depends on whether the patient is responsive or unresponsive and whether, in a responsive patient, the obstruction is mild or severe:

⬧ For a *responsive, choking patient who is coughing,* encourage the coughing to clear the object. Stay with the patient and call for additional EMS resources if the object is not immediately expelled.

⬧ For a *responsive, choking patient who cannot speak or cough forcefully,* give abdominal thrusts as described in **Skill 7-3**.

⬧ For an *unresponsive patient with an FBAO,* if your ventilations do not go in, ensure additional EMS personnel have been summoned and begin CPR.

Management of Severe Airway Obstructions in Responsive Patients

▶▶ Need to Do

With a responsive patient, after quickly saying who you are, asking for consent, and telling the patient what you intend to do, give abdominal thrusts:

1. Stand behind the patient and reach around his or her abdomen. Having one leg forward between the patient's legs helps you brace in case the patient becomes unresponsive and falls. Keep your head slightly to the side

in case the patient's head snaps back if the patient becomes unresponsive.

2. Make a fist with one hand and place the thumb side of the fist against the patient's abdomen just above the navel. Grasp the fist with your other hand.

3. Thrust inward and upward into the patient's abdomen with quick jerks. The pressure of each jerk serves to force air from the lungs up the trachea to expel the object. Pause only briefly after each abdominal thrust to see if the patient is able to breathe or cough. If not, continue with additional thrusts. If abdominal thrusts are not effective, consider using chest thrusts.

If you are giving abdominal thrusts to a child or someone much shorter than you, kneel behind the patient. If the patient is much taller than you, ask the patient to kneel or sit because it is important that your thrusts are upward as well as inward, which is impossible if you have to reach up to the patient's abdomen.

⬧ Abdominal thrusts may sometimes cause internal injury, so a patient treated with abdominal thrusts is recommended to be examined by a healthcare provider.

⬧ When a severe obstruction is not cleared, the patient will become unresponsive within minutes. Quickly and carefully lower the patient to lie on his or her back on the floor and provide care for an FBAO in an unresponsive patient.

Management of Airway Obstructions in Unresponsive Patients

▶▶ Need to Do

If a responsive, choking patient becomes unresponsive, or if you find an unresponsive patient with an FBAO:

1. Make sure additional EMS personnel have been called.

2. Provide CPR.

3. Begin by opening the airway.

4. When you open the patient's mouth to give a ventilation, look first for an object in the mouth.

5. If you see an object in the patient's mouth, remove it with a finger sweep.

6. Then give 2 breaths and check for a pulse.

If your breaths do not go in, the chest compressions given in CPR may expel the foreign object (Chapter 9). While giving CPR, each time you open the patient's mouth to give breaths, check first to see if an object is visible, and remove it if so.

Skill 7-3 **Severe Foreign Body Airway Obstruction in a Responsive Adult or Child**

1 Stand behind an adult patient with one leg forward between the patient's legs. Keep your head slightly to one side. With a small child, kneel behind the child. Reach around the abdomen.

2 Make a fist with one hand and place the thumb side of the fist against the patient's abdomen just above the navel. Grasp your fist with your other hand.

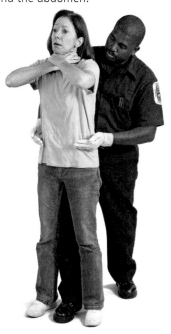

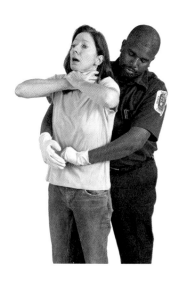

3 Thrust inward and upward into the patient's abdomen with quick jerks. Continue abdominal thrusts until the patient can expel the object or becomes unresponsive. If abdominal thrusts do not succeed in clearing the object from the airway, you may try chest thrusts.

4 For a responsive pregnant patient or any patient you cannot get your arms around, give chest thrusts in the middle of the breastbone from behind the patient. Take care not to squeeze the ribs with your arms.

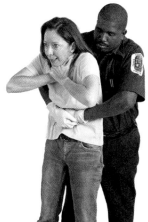

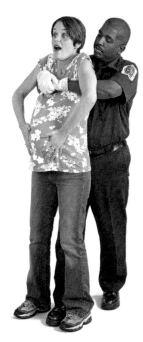

Foreign Body Airway Obstructions in Infants and Children

✓ Need to Know

The great majority of childhood deaths from FBAOs occur in children below the age of 5, most of these in infants. Foreign bodies include:

- ☑ Toys and other small objects
- ☑ Pieces of popped balloons
- ☑ Food such as hot dogs, round candies, nuts, and grapes

▪ Need to Recognize

Suspect an FBAO in an infant or child with a sudden onset of respiratory distress associated with coughing, gagging, stridor, or wheezing. If a responsive choking infant can cry or cough, watch carefully to see if the object comes out.

If the infant is responsive but cannot cry or cough:

- ◆ Ensure that additional EMS personnel have been summoned.
- ◆ Give the infant alternating back slaps and chest thrusts to attempt to expel the object.

▶ Need to Do

1. Support the infant held in one hand against your thigh as you kneel or sit, keeping the infant's head lower than the body.
2. To prevent spinal injury, support the infant's head and neck during these maneuvers.
3. The steps for back slaps and chest thrusts are described in the **Skill 7-4**.

If a responsive infant to whom you are giving choking care becomes unresponsive:

1. Give CPR, starting with chest compressions.
2. Check for an object in the mouth before you give a breath, and remove any object you see. Never perform a finger sweep of the mouth if you do not see an object, because this could force an object deeper into the throat.

When you encounter an unresponsive infant:

1. Open the airway first and check for breathing as usual.
2. If the infant is not breathing when you have opened the airway, give 2 breaths.
3. If your first breath does not go in and the infant's chest does not rise, try again after repositioning the head to open the airway.
4. If the second breath does not go in, assume that the infant has an airway obstruction and provide CPR, checking the mouth for an object each time you open it to give a ventilation.

✎ Do You Understand?

1. Describe the signs of a severe FBAO in a responsive patient (list as many as possible).

   _____

   _____

   _____

2. How many abdominal thrusts do you give a responsive adult with a severe FBAO?

   _____

3. What care is given to an unresponsive infant with a severe FBAO?

   _____

4. True or false: Give a pregnant woman with a severe FBAO chest thrusts instead of abdominal thrusts.

Conclusion

Assisting patients with airway or breathing emergencies is a common and critical First Responder function. Time is crucial when breathing stops or becomes inadequate—this is why checking the airway and breathing are the first steps in the ABCs. This chapter discusses airway and breathing assessment and the care you can provide without any special equipment. This care includes clearing and maintaining an open airway, recognizing and treating respiratory arrest and distress, and clearing an FBAO.

Skill 7-4 Severe Foreign Body Airway Obstruction in Responsive Infant

1 Support the infant's head in one hand, with the torso on your forearm and your thigh. Give up to 5 back slaps between the shoulder blades.

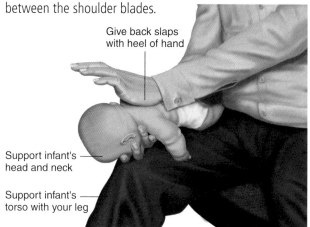

Give back slaps with heel of hand

Support infant's head and neck

Support infant's torso with your leg

2 Check for the expelled object. If not present, continue with next step.

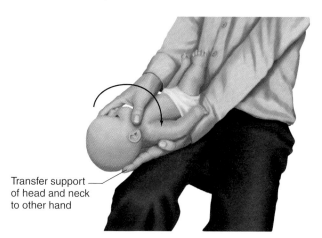

Transfer support of head and neck to other hand

3 With other hand on back of infant's head, roll the infant face up.

4 Give up to 5 chest thrusts with two fingers on sternum. Check the infant's mouth for the expelled object.

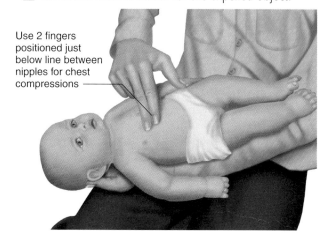

Use 2 fingers positioned just below line between nipples for chest compressions

5 Repeat steps 1-4, alternating back slaps and chest thrusts and checking the mouth. If you are alone and EMS personnel have not already been summoned, call after 1 minute. Continue until the object is expelled or the infant becomes unresponsive. If the infant becomes unresponsive, give CPR. After each cycle of compressions, look inside the mouth before giving breaths and remove any object you see.

Key Terms

accessory muscles (p. 96)

agonal respirations (p. 96)

airway (p. 91)

airway obstruction (p. 93)

alveoli (p. 92)

aspiration (p. 100)

barrier device (p. 97)

bronchi (p. 91)

choking (p. 93)

cricoid pressure (p. 100)

cyanosis (p. 96)

diaphragm (p. 92)

epiglottis (p. 92)

esophagus (p. 92)

external respiration (p. 93)

face shield (p. 98)

foreign body airway obstruction (FBAO) (p. 93)

inadequate breathing (p. 97)

internal respiration (p. 93)

lungs (p. 92)

nasopharynx (p. 91)

oropharynx (p. 91)

patent (p. 94)

pharynx (p. 91)

recovery position (p. 94)

respiratory arrest (p. 97)

resuscitation mask (p. 98)

stoma (p. 99)

stridor (p. 94)

trachea (p. 91)

tripod position (p. 96)

ventilation (p. 97)

Review Questions

1. The most common cause of airway obstruction in an unresponsive patient is
   a. the tongue.
   b. food.
   c. a toy.
   d. vomit.

2. An airway obstruction may cause stridor, which is
   a. the total absence of breathing.
   b. a gurgling sound.
   c. a high-pitched sound on inhaling.
   d. the aspiration of blood.

3. In the recovery position, the patient's head is supported on
   a. your knee.
   b. the back of your hand.
   c. the patient's arm.
   d. the floor.

4. Assess a responsive patient's breathing by asking
   a. "Can your breathe?"
   b. "Are you choking?"
   c. "What is your name?"
   d. "Does it hurt when you breathe in?"

5. Cyanosis, which may occur with inadequate breathing or respiratory distress, is
   a. movement of the accessory muscles of breathing.
   b. gasps that occur with cardiac arrest.
   c. fast, irregular breathing.
   d. a bluish color seen in the lips and nail beds.

6. Breathing at a rate less than _____ breaths per minute is one of the signs of inadequate breathing in an adult.

    a. 6

    b. 8

    c. 10

    d. 12

7. The one-way valve in a face mask prevents

    a. your air from going anywhere but into the patient's lungs.

    b. the patient from vomiting.

    c. the patient's air from exiting through the mouthpiece.

    d. oxygen from escaping from the mask.

8. The best way to give mouth-to-mask ventilations is to

    a. watch the chest rise to make sure your air is going into the lungs.

    b. take a big breath to exhale more air into the patient.

    c. give each breath over about 2 seconds.

    d. blow forcefully until you feel resistance.

9. For an infant who has a pulse but is not breathing, give ventilations at a rate of _____ breaths per minute.

    a. 5 to 6

    b. 5 to 10

    c. 12 to 16

    d. 12 to 20

10. The treatment for an FBAO in an unresponsive infant is

    a. back slaps and chest thrusts.

    b. CPR.

    c. continued ventilations.

    d. abdominal thrusts.

Ventilation Devices and Oxygen

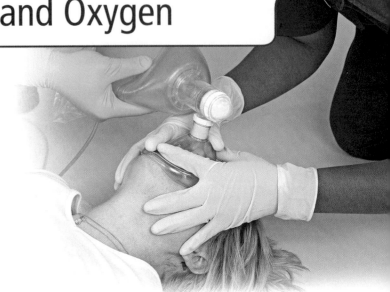

Chapter Preview

- Suctioning
- Airway Adjuncts
- Bag Mask Ventilation
- Bag Mask Ventilation with Children and Infants
- Supplemental Oxygen

You Respond To ...

a home where a man is lying injured on the ground after falling from the roof. You and your partner have a full kit, including ventilation equipment and oxygen. Your assessment reveals he is not breathing after you open the airway, and when you give the first ventilation through your resuscitation mask, you feel resistance and hear the gurgling of blood or other material in his airway.

Introduction

In most emergencies, First Responders can provide care for the airway and breathing without specialized equipment or supplies beyond basic personal protective equipment such as medical exam gloves and a resuscitation mask. Several adjunctive devices, however, can enhance the effectiveness of resuscitation. These devices include suction devices to help keep the patient's airway clear, oral and nasal airways to help ensure air reaches the patient's

lungs, bag mask units for more effective ventilation, and supplemental oxygen. The resuscitation adjuncts you may use depend on your training and job. These devices may not always be available, so it is essential to be able to perform ventilation without special equipment, as described in Chapter 7. Care should never be delayed while waiting for adjunctive equipment.

Suctioning

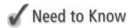 Need to Know

Suction is used to clear blood, vomit, and other substances from a patient's airway. Although different types of suction devices are available, their use is similar.

- ☑ Manual devices develop suction with a hand-pumping action.
- ☑ Some suction devices are powered by a battery or pressurized oxygen.
- ☑ Soft rubber **bulb syringes** are used for suctioning infants.

Suction devices for adults and children have a clear plastic tip that is inserted into the mouth or nostrils to suck out fluids and small solids.

☑ Different suction tips are available, varying from small, soft plastic tips, more effective with fluids, to larger, more rigid tips (a "tonsil tip"), more effective for removing vomit and particulate matter in an unresponsive patient.

☑ Some devices have a suction control port at the base of the tip that you cover with your finger to produce suction.

☑ Be familiar with the specific equipment you may use in an emergency.

Suction is useful if a patient's airway is fully or partially obstructed by body fluids, vomitus, or other matter and cannot be cleared with draining the mouth and using a finger sweep. Most suction units are inadequate for removing solid objects like teeth, foreign bodies, and food.

▶ Need to Do

♦ If the patient vomits during ventilation, or if secretions or blood accumulate and impede ventilation, stop and quickly suction the mouth and/or nose and then continue the resuscitation.

♦ You usually know the airway needs suctioning when you hear gurgling sounds during breathing or ventilation.

The patient's head is turned to the side to help drain vomit or fluids before suctioning. If the patient may have a spinal injury, the patient must be turned on the side with the head and body inline as a unit, with the help of other responders. (See **Skills 8-1** and **8-2**.)

Safety Precautions When Suctioning

▶ Need to Do

♦ Because many suction devices generate strong suction pressures, be careful with the suction tip.

♦ Prolonged contact with mucous membranes in the mouth and nose can cause bruising, swelling, or bleeding.

♦ Never insert the suction tip farther than you can see or deeper than the base of the tongue.

♦ Because prolonged suctioning can decrease the amount of air reaching the patient's lungs, do not suction more than:
   ◦ 15 seconds at a time for adults
   ◦ 10 seconds at a time for children
   ◦ 5 seconds at a time for infants

♦ Watch for a decreased heart rate in infants, and if the pulse is slow, stop suctioning and provide ventilation.

♦ Vigorous suctioning may stimulate the patient's gag reflex, causing vomiting.

♦ Be especially careful not to suction too deep in an infant.

♦ Always suction an infant's mouth before the nostrils, because suctioning the nose may stimulate the infant to breathe in and thereby inhale fluid or secretions from the mouth.

♦ Follow standard precautions against disease transmission through body fluids. After the emergency, dispose of any contents in the reservoir of the suction device and clean the device according to the manufacturer's recommendations.

✎ Do You Understand?

1. True or false: Never insert the suction tip deeper than the base of the tongue.

2. In an adult, never suction longer than _____ seconds at a time, or _____ seconds in a child.

3. When using a bulb syringe to suction an infant's mouth, do you squeeze the bulb before, after, or during insertion into the mouth?

Airway Adjuncts

✔ Need to Know

Oral and nasal **airways** are devices that help keep a patient's airway open during resuscitation or until the patient receives advanced medical attention, although they are not definitive airway control devices.

☑ An airway adjunct device helps prevent the problem of the tongue obstructing the airway.

☑ An airway helps keep the airway open more easily than the head position alone during ventilation or when caring for a breathing patient.

☑ Supplemental oxygen can be given through a resuscitation mask or bag mask with an airway in place.

Skill 8-1 Suctioning—Adult or Child

1 Confirm the suction device is working and produces suction.

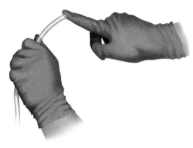

2 Turn the patient's head to one side and open the mouth (with a spinal injury, support the head and turn it with the body as one unit).

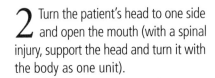

3 Sweep out solids and larger amounts of fluid with your finger.

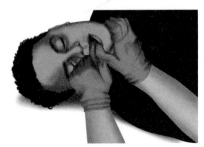

4 Determine the maximum depth of insertion by measuring the catheter tip from the earlobe to the corner of the mouth.

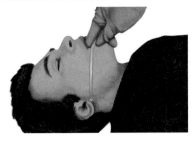

5 Turn on the suction or pump handle to create suction.

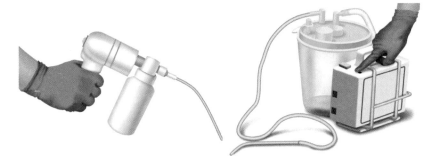

6 Insert the catheter tip carefully into the patient's mouth. Put your finger over the proximal opening to begin suctioning, and move the tip about as you withdraw it.

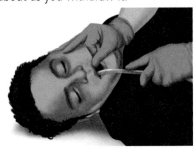

7 Reposition the patient's head with the airway open, and begin or resume ventilation if needed.

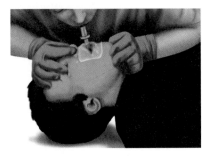

Skill 8-2 Suctioning—Infant

1 Hold the infant in position for suctioning, with the infant's head lower than the body and turned to one side.

2 Squeeze the suction bulb first and then gently insert the tip into the infant's mouth.

3 Gradually release the bulb to create suction as you withdraw the tip from the mouth.

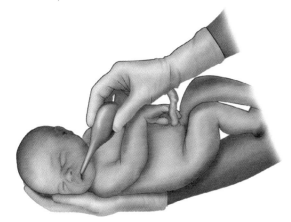 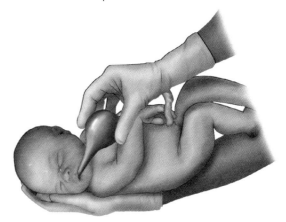

4 Move the bulb aside and squeeze it with the tip down to empty it.

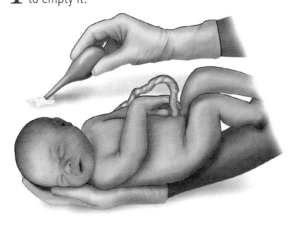

5 Repeat steps 2-4 until the airway seems clear, up to 3 times.

6 Repeat the suctioning process for each nostril.

7 Begin or resume ventilation if needed.

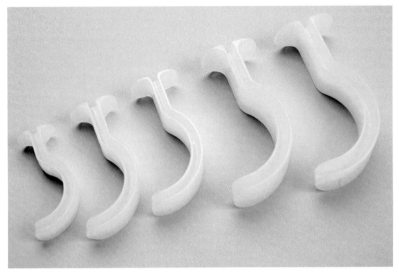

Figure 8-1 Oral airways.

Oral Airways

Oral airways, also called **oropharyngeal airways (OPAs),** are used only in unresponsive patients who do not have a gag reflex.

- ☑ If inserted into a responsive patient or one who still has a gag reflex, an oral airway can cause vomiting.

- ☑ The patient's airway must be opened before the airway device is inserted; the device does not open the airway itself but will help to keep it open.

- ☑ An oral airway can be used in an unresponsive patient who is breathing or who is receiving ventilations.

Proper sizing and placement of the oral airway is essential:

- ☑ An improperly placed airway device can compress the tongue into the back of the throat and further block the airway.

- ☑ Oral airways are curved so that they fit the natural contour of the mouth. They are available in various sizes to assure a proper fit **(Figure 8-1)**.

- ☑ An oral airway that is too big can cause vomiting and may prevent a face mask from sealing well.

- ☑ An airway adjunct that is too small can slide into the back of the pharynx and obstruct the airway **(Figure 8-2)**.

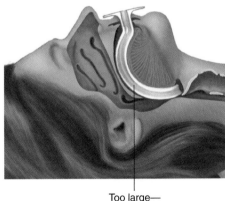
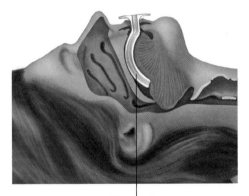

Too large—
device blocks airway

Too small—
device causes tongue to obstruct airway

Figure 8-2 An oral airway that is too large or too small will obstruct the airway.

▶▶ Need to Do

Remember to open the patient's airway before inserting the oral airway, as described in **Skill 8-3**. Periodically reassess the oral airway to confirm that it remains in the proper position. A patient can be suctioned with an oral airway in place.

The following steps are an alternate technique for inserting an oral airway in infants and children:

1. Select the proper size: Measure from the corner of the patient's lips to the bottom of the earlobe or angle of jaw.
2. Open the patient's mouth.

Skill 8-3 Oral Airway Insertion

1 Choose the correct oral airway size. Measure from the corner of the patient's lips to the tip of the earlobe or angle of the jaw.

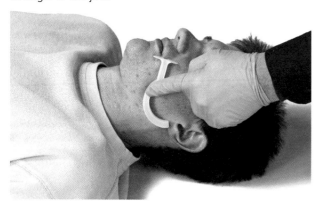

2 Open the patient's airway with head tilt–chin lift or jaw thrust, and open the mouth.

3 Insert the airway device with the tip pointing toward the roof of the mouth.

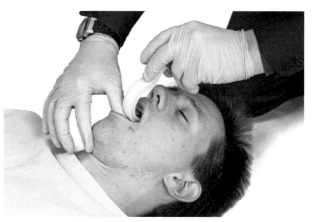

4 When the tip reaches the back of the mouth and you feel resistance, rotate the airway 180 degrees.

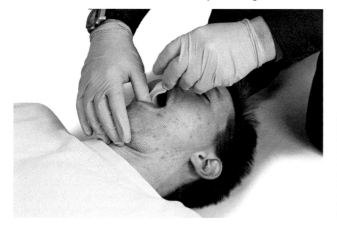

5 Continue to insert the airway device to the final position (with the flange resting on the patient's lips).

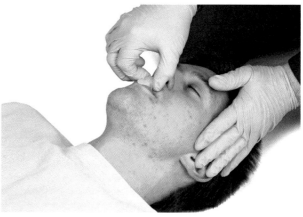

3. Use a tongue blade to press tongue down and out of the way.

4. Insert the airway in the upright (anatomic) position.

Nasal Airways

✓ Need to Know

A **nasal airway,** also called a **nasopharyngeal airway (NPA),** like an oral airway, helps maintain an open airway **(Figure 8-3).**

- ☑ A nasal airway can be used in a responsive patient or an unresponsive patient with a gag reflex.

- ☑ Nasal airways are also effective for unresponsive patients with mouth or jaw injuries or tightly clenched teeth that prevent the use of an oral airway.

- ☑ Nasal airways are less likely to cause gagging and vomiting than oral airways.

- ☑ A disadvantage is that nasal airways are too narrow to suction effectively.

- ☑ Although the tube is lubricated, insertion still causes some patients pain and may cause significant bleeding in some patients.

▶ Need to Do

Insert a nasal airway as described in **Skill 8-4,** and continue to keep the patient's airway open with the head tilt–chin lift or jaw thrust. If needed, suction through a nasal airway using a small flexible suction catheter.

✎ Do You Understand?

1. True or false: Because an oral airway will open the patient's airway, you do not need to position the patient's head to open the airway before inserting the oral airway.

2. In an adult, an oral airway is inserted with the tip pointing toward _____.

3. List two disadvantages of using a nasal airway.

_____   _____

Bag Mask Ventilation

✓ Need to Know

A **bag mask** protects a First Responder like a face mask but is more effective for providing ventilations to a nonbreathing patient.

- ☑ The patient receives air from the atmosphere (21% oxygen) rather than air the responder exhales (16% oxygen).

- ☑ The more oxygen delivered to the lungs, the more oxygen that will reach the patient's vital organs to maintain life.

Several different types of bag mask units are available, but all have at least three components **(Figure 8-4):**

- ☑ The self-inflating bag holds the air or oxygen delivered to the patient when the bag is squeezed.

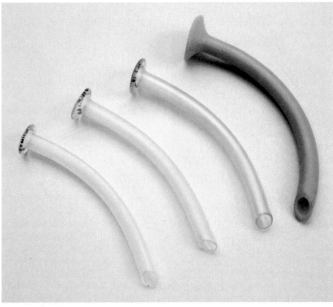

Figure 8-3 Nasal airways.

☑ The one-way valve allows air or oxygen to flow from the bag to the patient but prevents the patient's exhaled air from returning to the bag.

☑ The mask is similar to a resuscitation mask and is connected to the bag and valve; the proper size mask must be used for a proper fit.

☑ An oxygen reservoir bag may also be attached to the other end of the bag when supplemental oxygen is used.

▶▶ **Need to Do**

To use the bag mask on a nonbreathing patient:

◗ Position yourself above the patient's head, open the airway, and position the mask on the patient's face.

◗ If you are alone, hold the mask with one hand and squeeze the bag with the other **(Figure 8-5)**. To hold the mask in place with one hand, use

---

Skill 8-4 **Nasal Airway Insertion**

1 Choose the correct nasal airway size, measuring from the tip of the nose to the tip of the patient's ear. The diameter of the airway should not be so large that it causes tissue around the nostril to turn white from the pressure.

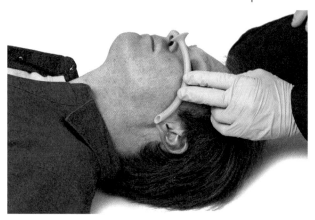

2 Coat the nasal airway with water-soluble lubricant.

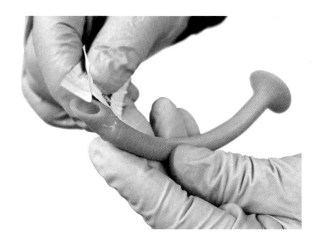

4 Insert the nasal airway straight back, sliding it along the floor of the nostril. If the airway cannot be inserted into one nostril, try the other nostril; do not force this airway.

3 Insert the nasal airway in the right nostril with the bevel toward the base of the nostril or the septum.

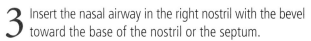

5 Insert the nasal airway until the flange rests against the nose.

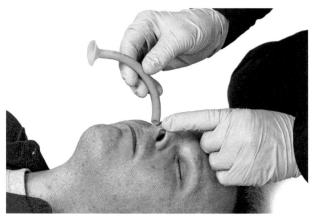

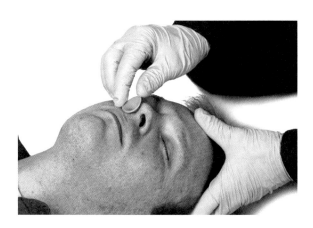

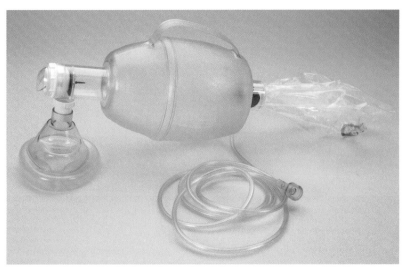

Figure 8-4 A typical bag mask (BVM) unit.

the C-clamp technique, with your thumb and index finger on the edges of the mask while your other fingers lift the jaw into the mask.

▶ When a second responder is available to help, one responder holds the mask in place using both hands.

▶ Two-rescuer use of the bag mask is recommended whenever possible because of the difficulty one person may have sealing the mask on the patient's face with one hand while squeezing the bag with the other.

▶ With the mask sealed in place, ventilations are delivered by squeezing the bag. Squeeze a 1-liter adult bag about 1/2-2/3 of its volume. Squeeze a 2-liter adult bag about 1/3 its volume.

▶ Squeeze the bag over 1 second, watching the patient's chest rise.

▶ Give a ventilation every 5-6 seconds in an adult (or every 3-5 seconds in an infant or child), the same as with ventilating by mouth or resuscitation mask.

Monitor the effectiveness of ventilations:

▶ Be careful to give ventilations at the usual rate and not to overventilate the patient.

▶ Watch for the rise and fall of the patient's chest, and feel for resistance as you squeeze the bag. Increased resistance may mean that there is blood or vomit in the airway or that the airway is no longer open.

▶ A problem may occur with sealing the mask to the patient's face, especially when a single First Responder must do this with

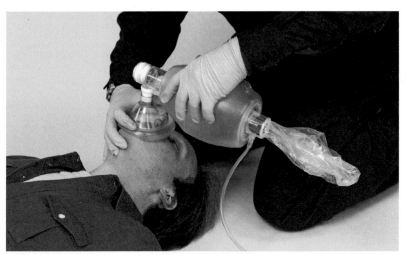

Figure 8-5 A single responder can use the bag mask to provide ventilation, although use by two rescuers is recommended.

one hand. If air is escaping around the mask, try repositioning the mask and your fingers.

♦ If you cannot obtain an adequate seal and the patient's chest does not rise with ventilations, or there are any other problems with using the bag mask, then use an alternate technique, such as a resuscitation mask.

See **Skill 8-5**.

Skill 8-5 **Bag Mask for Ventilation—2 Rescuers**

1 Rescuer 1 assembles the bag mask with the correct size mask and puts the mask over the patient's mouth and nose.

2 Rescuer 2 positions his or her hands: Thumbs and index fingers circling each side of the mask, other three fingers behind the lower jawbone. Pull the jaw up into the mask rather than pushing the mask down on the jaw.

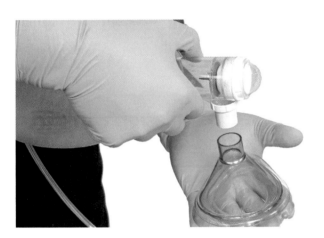

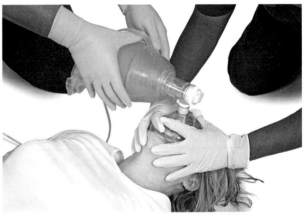

3 Rescuer 2 opens the airway and seals the mask to the patient's face.

4 Rescuer 1 squeezes the bag to provide ventilations:
• 1 ventilation over 1 second in an adult, every 5-6 seconds (10-12 per minute).
• 1 ventilation over 1 second in a child or an infant, every 3-5 seconds (12-20 per minute).

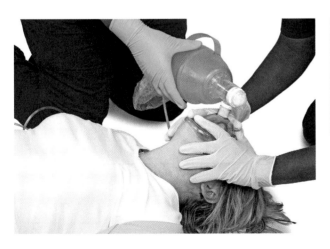

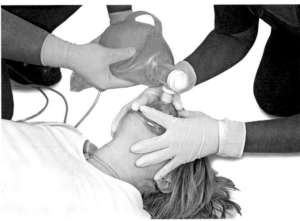

(continued)

Skill 8-5 continued

5 Recheck the patient's pulse about every 2 minutes. If there is no pulse, call for an AED and start CPR.

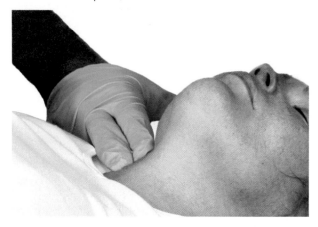

Bag Mask Ventilation with Oxygen

✓ Need to Know

If available, supplemental oxygen should be used with the bag mask:

- ☑ An **oxygen reservoir** bag is attached to the valve on the bag, and the oxygen tubing is attached to the bag.

- ☑ The device is used the same way to give ventilations, only now it is oxygen rather than air being delivered to the patient. The reservoir holds oxygen being delivered to the device so that the bag always fills with oxygen to be delivered in the next ventilation.

- ☑ When two First Responders are present, the second sets up the oxygen equipment and prepares to connect it to the bag mask while the first begins ventilations with the bag mask alone.

Bag Mask Ventilation with Children and Infants

✓ Need to Know

The bag mask can be used with a nonbreathing infant in the same manner as with an adult or child. Be sure to choose the correct size mask and a smaller bag than the 1600 mL bag for adults:

- ☑ About 500 mL for newborns
- ☑ 750 mL for infants and small children
- ☑ 1200 mL for large children and adolescents

▶ Need to Do

With an infant or child, squeeze the bag only enough to make the chest rise, avoiding forceful squeezing or overinflation that may lead to vomiting.

Do You Understand?

1. True or false: Using a bag mask not connected to supplemental oxygen provides the patient with the same percentage of oxygen as using a pocket mask.

2. Squeeze the bag of a bag mask until
   a. the chest rises.
   b. the bag is empty.
   c. you can squeeze it no farther.
   d. the patient coughs.

3. How often are ventilations given to an adult when using a bag mask?

---

4. If you arrive alone at a scene where a patient needs ventilation, should you take the time to assemble the bag mask and oxygen equipment?

Supplemental Oxygen

✓ Need to Know

Supplemental oxygen, when available, should always be used for ventilation. In many other emergency situations including heart attack, stroke, and seizures, an injured or ill patient will benefit from receiving oxygen. Depending on the oxygen delivery device used, the patient can receive oxygen at concentrations up to 100%, compared to 21% oxygen in the air. The equipment involved in giving supplemental oxygen includes:

☑ A pressurized cylinder, which typically stores the oxygen source. When full, cylinders have a pressure of 2,000 pounds per square inch (psi). They come in various sizes and are usually painted green, although some stainless steel cylinders are not.

☑ The **pressure regulator** reduces the pressure of oxygen leaving the tank to a safe level and has a gauge that shows the pressure remaining within the cylinder. If the gauge reads 2,000 psi, the tank is full; if it reads 1,000 psi, it is half full, and so on. The pressure regulator is designed so that it works only with oxygen tanks.

☑ The **flow meter,** used to adjust the rate of oxygen delivery, is usually built into the pressure regulator. The flow of oxygen reaching the patient is set by turning the calibrated flow valve.

☑ Oxygen tubing connects the cylinder to the delivery device. Connecting tubes are typically 4 to 5 feet long and have an adapter at each end.

☑ An **oxygen delivery device,** such as a face mask or nasal cannula, provides the flowing oxygen to the patient.

Safety Around Oxygen

Need to Do

Although oxygen does not burn, it vigorously supports combustion and creates a hazardous situation if used near an ignition source. Follow these guidelines:

▶ Never allow smoking or an open flame near the oxygen source.

▶ Never use grease, oil, or adhesive tape on the cylinder, pressure regulator, or delivery device, because these are combustible.

▶ Never expose an oxygen cylinder to a temperature over 120°F (48.9°C).

▶ Never drop a cylinder or let it fall against another object. Oxygen cylinders should never be left standing. Instead, place the cylinder on its side so that it cannot fall over. If the valve is dislodged, the cylinder can become a dangerous projectile powered by the compressed gas.

▶ Never try to use a non-oxygen regulator on an oxygen cylinder.

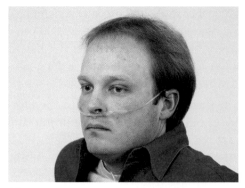

(a)

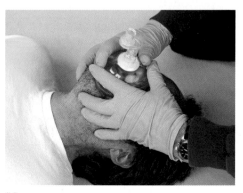

(b)

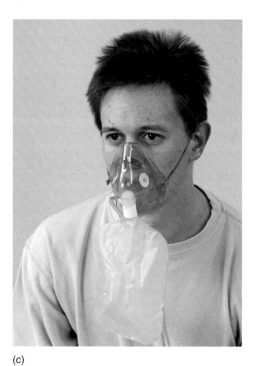

(c)

Figure 8-6 Oxygen delivery devices: (a) nasal cannula, (b) resuscitation mask, and (c) nonrebreathing mask.

Oxygen Delivery Devices

✔ Need to Know

Different oxygen delivery devices have different advantages and disadvantages. The following devices are most frequently used in emergency situations **(Figure 8-6)**:

☑ **Nasal cannulas,** sometimes called nasal prongs, are used with breathing patients who do not require a high concentration of oxygen. The device has two small prongs that fit shallowly into the nostrils. The nasal cannula is easy to use and comfortable for the patient. The oxygen concentration delivered depends on the flow rate (1 to 6 hr. /min) and the patient's breathing rate and ranges from about 24% to 50%.

☑ Some resuscitation masks have a special port for oxygen, which can be used for breathing patients who need oxygen. The mask can be secured to the patient's head by an elastic band. A typical plastic face mask provides an oxygen concentration of 30% to 60% with a flow rate of 10 liters per minute.

☑ **Nonrebreathing masks** have a mask and a reservoir bag and are used with breathing patients. The oxygen fills the reservoir, which empties partially as the patient inhales. The patient's exhaled air escapes through a valve. With a minimum oxygen flow rate of 8 liters per minute, the oxygen concentration ranges from 80% to 95%. The flow rate is adjusted to prevent the reservoir from completely collapsing when the patient inhales. A firm mask fit is needed to prevent atmospheric air from entering the mask.

☑ Bag mask units can deliver oxygen through a tube connecting to the bag or an oxygen reservoir. Oxygen concentrations delivered to a nonbreathing patient by a bag mask with a reservoir can approach 100%. A breathing patient can also use a bag mask with a reservoir to receive oxygen; unless the patient is having difficulty breathing, the bag is not squeezed.

Administration of Oxygen

▶▶ Need to Do

Skill 8-6 describes the steps for setting up the oxygen equipment and administering oxygen to the patient. Remember to follow safety principles when working with oxygen.

- ◆ If you are alone with a patient, do not stop providing ventilations to set up oxygen equipment.

- ◆ Give ventilations and care for other life-threatening problems first.

- ◆ Wait until the patient is relatively stable and breathing independently or until another responder can help with the oxygen equipment.

- ◆ Once the patient is receiving oxygen, monitor the flow of oxygen, the tank pressure, and the flow rate as well as the patient's condition. Do not let the tank run completely empty; if necessary, change to a new tank when the pressure drops to 500 psi.

✎ Do You Understand?

1. A full oxygen tank has a pressure of about _____ pounds per square inch.

2. Which oxygen delivery device typically provides the lowest concentration of oxygen?

   _____

3. True or false: You should frequently oil or grease the threads of the oxygen tank and

---

Skill 8-6   Oxygen Administration

1 Check the equipment, the oxygen labels on the cylinder and regulator, and that the tubing and delivery device are ready.

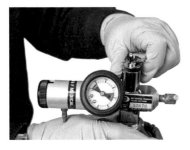

2 Remove any protective seal, point the cylinder opening away from you, and open the main valve for 1 second.

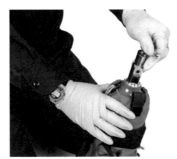

3 Remove any protective seals and attach the regulator to the oxygen cylinder.

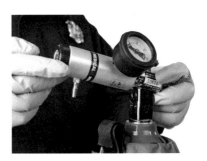

4 Open the main cylinder valve.

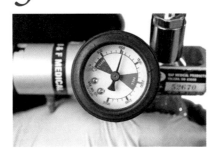

5 Check the pressure regulator gauge.

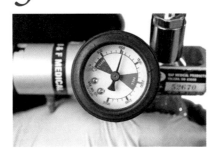

6 Attach the tubing to the flow meter and the oxygen delivery device.

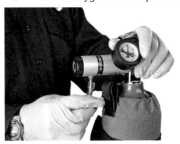

Skill 8-6 **continued**

7 Set the flow meter at the correct oxygen flow rate:
- 1-6 lpm for a nasal cannula
- 10 lpm for a face mask
- 10-15 lpm for a bag mask or nonrebreather mask

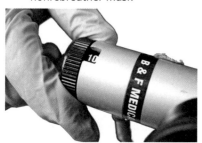

8 Confirm that oxygen is flowing.

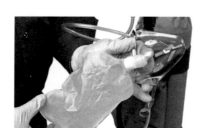

9 Position the delivery device on the patient and continue ventilations (or allow the patient to breathe spontaneously).

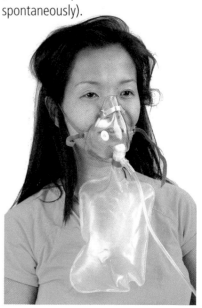

10 Monitor the pressure regulator gauge and be prepared to remove the delivery device and change tanks if the pressure drops below 500 psi. Observe oxygen safety precautions.

regulator to make it easy to connect the equipment.

4. Do you start the flow of oxygen before or after putting the oxygen delivery device on the patient?

_____

Conclusion

Resuscitation adjunctive devices, when available and when you are trained in their use, increase the efficiency of resuscitation techniques and increase the patient's chances for successful full recovery. Never delay care for a patient, however, to get or set up these devices for use.

Key Terms

airways (p. 111)

bag mask (p. 116)

bulb syringe (p. 110)

flow meter (p. 121)

nasal airway (p. 116)

nasal cannula (p. 122)

nasopharyngeal airway (NPA) (p. 116)

nonrebreathing mask (p. 122)

oral airway (p. 114)

oropharyngeal airway (OPA) (p. 114)

oxygen delivery device (p. 121)

oxygen reservoir (p. 120)

pressure regulator (p. 121)

suction (p. 110)

supplemental oxygen (p. 121)

Review Questions

1. In an infant, you should not suction more than how many seconds at a time?
   a. 2
   b. 5
   c. 10
   d. 15

2. To determine the maximum depth of the suction tip's insertion, measure from the
   a. eyebrow to the corner of the mouth.
   b. outside corner of the eye to the earlobe.
   c. nostril to the earlobe.
   d. earlobe to the corner of the mouth.

3. If a patient vomits,
   a. sweep out solids and fluid with your finger before suctioning.
   b. sweep out solids and fluid with your finger after suctioning.
   c. sweep out solids and fluid with your finger during suctioning.
   d. do not use your finger to sweep the mouth; use suction only.

4. To choose the correct size oral airway, measure from the
   a. eyebrow to the corner of the mouth.
   b. outside corner of the eye to the earlobe.
   c. nostril to the earlobe.
   d. earlobe to the corner of the mouth.

5. Use a nasal airway rather than an oral airway in a patient who
   a. is wearing dentures.
   b. needs oxygen.
   c. is responsive.
   d. may have a spinal injury.

6. The bag of a bag mask for use on an infant is
   a. about 1/3 the volume of an adult bag.
   b. about 1/2 the volume of an adult bag.
   c. the same volume as a child bag.
   d. the same volume as an adult bag.

7. The best way to connect oxygen tubing to a bag mask is
   a. to an oxygen reservoir bag.
   b. to the bag you squeeze.
   c. to a portal in the mask.
   d. Oxygen tubing cannot be attached to a bag mask.

8. Give ventilations by squeezing the bag over
   a. 1 second.   c. 3 seconds.
   b. 2 seconds.   d. 4 seconds.

9. Oxygen may be delivered to a patient through
   a. any resuscitation mask.
   b. a resuscitation mask with a special port.
   c. only a nonrebreathing mask.
   d. any face shield.

10. Which oxygen delivery device is best to use for ventilating an unresponsive nonbreathing patient?
    a. Nasal cannula
    b. Resuscitation mask
    c. Nonrebreathing mask with reservoir bag
    d. Bag mask with reservoir bag

Unit 4
Circulation

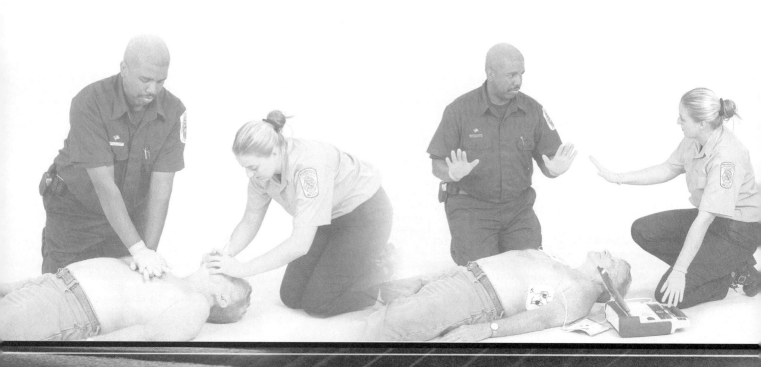

Chapter 9

Cardiac Emergencies and CPR

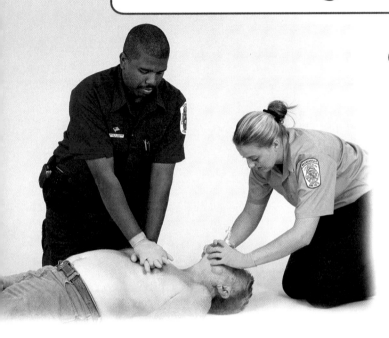

Chapter Preview

- Review of the Circulatory System
- Cardiac Arrest
- Cardiac Chain of Survival
- Call First vs. Call Fast
- Cardiopulmonary Resuscitation (CPR)
- Technique of CPR

You Respond To …

a scene where a businessman in his 40s was seen to collapse suddenly approximately 2 minutes ago. Additional EMS help is on the way. You check his ABCs and find he is not breathing and has no pulse. You know irreversible brain damage will begin within minutes if you do not act quickly.

Introduction

Basic Life Support is needed for a patient whose breathing or heart has stopped. Ventilations are given to oxygenate the blood in someone whose breathing is inadequate or has stopped. If that patient's heart has stopped, as it will soon after breathing stops, chest compressions also are given to circulate blood to vital organs. Ventilation combined with chest compressions is called **cardiopulmonary resuscitation (CPR).** CPR is most commonly given to patients in cardiac arrest as a result of heart attack.

Review of the Circulatory System

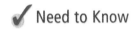 Need to Know

The circulatory system consists of the heart, blood, and blood vessels **(Figure 9-1).**

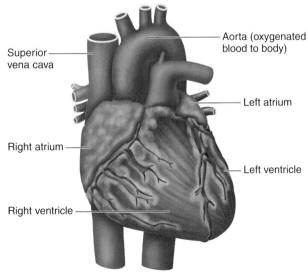

Superior vena cava

Aorta (oxygenated blood to body)

Left atrium

Right atrium

Left ventricle

Right ventricle

Figure 9-1 The heart.

127

Its primary functions are:

☑ Transporting oxygen and nutrients in the blood to all parts of the body

☑ Removing carbon dioxide and other wastes from tissues

Other functions include:

☑ Transporting hormones that regulate other body functions

☑ Helping regulate body temperature

☑ Transporting cells and substances that fight infection

☑ Helping maintain the body's fluid balance

The heart has four chambers: the left and right atria and the left and right ventricles. The ventricles pump the blood through two loops or cycles in the body:

☑ The right ventricle pumps blood to the lungs to pick up oxygen and release carbon dioxide.

☑ The blood returns to the left atrium and then flows into the left ventricle.

☑ The left ventricle pumps the oxygenated blood through the arteries to all areas of the body to release oxygen for use by body cells and pick up carbon dioxide for removal.

☑ The blood returns through the veins to the right atrium, to be pumped again to the lungs.

☑ Within the heart, valves prevent the back flow of blood so that it moves only in one direction through these cycles.

The term *cardiac* refers to the heart. The heart is composed of a unique type of muscle (myocardium) that contracts to make the pumping action. This pumping action, called contractions, is controlled by electrical signals under nervous system control.

The blood flows from the heart to body areas through an extensive network of arteries **(Figure 9-2)**. Arterial blood is oxygenated, bright red, and under pressure. Major arteries include:

☑ Carotid arteries, the major arteries passing through the neck to the head

☑ Femoral arteries, the major arteries to the legs passing through the thigh

☑ Brachial arteries, in the upper arm

☑ Radial arteries, the major artery of the lower arm

With each contraction of the left ventricle, a wave of blood is sent through the arteries, causing

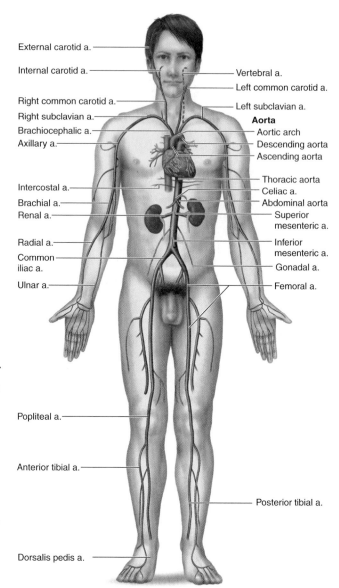

Figure 9-2 Major arteries of the body.

pulsing blood pressure changes in the arteries that can be palpated in certain body locations as the pulse. A pulse can be felt anywhere an artery passes near the skin surface and over a bone:

☑ The carotid pulse can be palpated on either side of the neck.

☑ The femoral pulse can be palpated in the groin area (the crease between the abdomen and the thigh).

☑ The radial pulse can be palpated on the palm side of the wrist proximal to the base of the thumb.

☑ The brachial pulse can be palpated on the inside of the arm between the elbow and the shoulder.

Arteries progressively branch into smaller vessels that eventually reach capillaries:

☑ Capillaries are very small blood vessels connecting arteries with veins throughout the body.

☑ Capillaries have thin walls through which oxygen and carbon dioxide are exchanged with body cells.

From the capillaries, the blood drains back to the heart through an extensive system of veins. Venous blood is dark red, deoxygenated, and under less pressure than arterial blood. Blood flows more evenly through veins, which do not have a pulse. Veins have valves that prevent the backflow of blood.

Arteries are generally deeper in the body than veins and are therefore more protected and less likely to be damaged by injuries.

The heart rate, which can be measured as the pulse, is affected by many factors:

☑ With exercise, fever, or emotional excitement, the heart rate increases to meet the body's greater need for oxygen.

☑ Various injuries and illnesses may either increase or decrease the heart rate.

Emergencies Related to the Circulatory System

The circulatory system's functions are vital for life, health, and well-being.

☑ The most vital function is carrying oxygen to the body's tissues.

☑ Cells begin to die in vital organs, such as the brain, after only a few minutes without oxygen.

☑ Any injury or illness that affects respiration, therefore, also diminishes the ability of the circulatory system to deliver oxygen to the body.

Blood vessel problems may also affect circulatory system functioning:

☑ Bleeding may be so severe that not enough blood is left in circulation to adequately provide the oxygen the body needs.

☑ Arterial bleeding is most severe because the blood may spurt out under pressure, leading to the life-threatening condition of shock within minutes.

☑ Shock occurs when vital body organs are not receiving enough oxygen (Chapter 12).

☑ Bleeding from veins is generally slower but can still be serious or life-threatening if it continues.

☑ Capillary bleeding is generally minor and usually stops by itself as the blood clots.

Problems involving the heart can also affect tissue oxygenation.

☑ Some conditions, such as cardiomyopathy and congestive heart failure, reduce the heart's ability to pump to effectively meet the body's needs.

☑ If the heart muscle does not receive enough oxygenated blood because of blocked cardiac arteries, part of the heart muscle may die (heart attack, or acute myocardial infarction).

The heart may stop (**cardiac arrest**) as a result. Organ damage begins quickly after the heart stops:

☑ Brain damage begins 4 to 6 minutes after the patient suffers cardiac arrest.

☑ Brain damage becomes irreversible in 8 to 10 minutes.

Dysrhythmia, or an abnormal heartbeat, is another type of heart problem that may reduce the heart's pumping effectiveness.

✎ Do You Understand?

1. The two most important functions of the circulatory system are

   _____

   _____

2. Bleeding from _____ is usually the most serious.

3. Irreversible brain damage begins _____ minutes after the heart stops beating.

4. True or false: Injuries and illnesses may either increase or decrease the heart rate.

Cardiac Arrest

 ### Need to Know

Cardiac arrest is determined in a patient by the absence of a pulse. Cardiac arrest may be caused by:

☑ Heart attack or other heart disease

☑ Drowning

☑ Suffocation

☑ Respiratory arrest from any cause

☑ Stroke

☑ Poisoning or drug overdose

☑ Allergic reaction

☑ Diabetic emergency

☑ Prolonged seizures

☑ Electric shock

☑ Trauma and bleeding

CPR is needed for all patients in cardiac arrest. You do not need to know the cause of cardiac arrest before starting CPR.

Cardiac Chain of Survival

■▬ Need to Recognize

To recognize the urgent need for quick actions to save the lives of cardiac arrest patients, the Citizen CPR Foundation created the concept of the **cardiac chain of survival (Figure 9-3).** This chain has four crucial links, and any weak link in the chain lowers the patient's chance for survival.

1. **Early Recognition and Access to EMS.** Recognize that a patient whose heart has stopped needs help immediately! It is also important to recognize the signs and symptoms of a potential life-threatening condition such as a heart attack or a stroke in a responsive person (see Chapter 11). Do not wait until a person becomes unresponsive to start the chain of events needed to keep him or her alive. Ensure additional help is on the way. The patient needs early access to advanced medical care. A citizen who calls 911 has already accessed EMS to get help on the way.

2. **Early CPR.** For a pulseless patient, start CPR immediately. This helps keep the brain and other vital organs supplied with oxygen until an automated external defibrillator (AED) is ready for use. CPR alone seldom resuscitates a patient; defibrillation (Chapter 10) is usually also needed. A citizen with CPR training may already have begun CPR when you arrive. The 911 dispatcher may also direct the citizen to give CPR.

3. **Early Defibrillation.** An AED can help get the heart beating normally again after a cardiac arrest. If not present at the scene, ensure that an AED is on the way.

4. **Early Advanced Care.** The sooner the patient is treated by emergency care professionals with **Advanced Cardiac Life Support (ACLS)** training, the better the chance for the patient's survival. You can help make sure the patient reaches this last link in the chain by acting immediately with the earlier links.

Call First vs. Call Fast

▶ Need to Do

As a general rule, if you are alone with an adult patient, ensure additional EMS personnel have been called first before providing CPR. For a child patient, call fast after providing 5 cycles of CPR (about 2 minutes). Your response depends on the most likely cause of the patient's problem:

♦ Call first for a patient of any age seen to collapse suddenly. These patients are more likely to have a dysrhythmia and to require defibrillation. Calling for help immediately starts the process of getting an AED to the patient sooner.

♦ For unresponsive patients in cardiac arrest because of a likely asphyxial arrest, such as a drowning patient or a child likely to have an airway obstruction, call fast. Give 5 cycles of CPR (about 2 minutes) before stopping to call for help.

✎ Do You Understand?

1. List as many causes of cardiac arrest as you can:

_____ _____ _____

_____ _____ _____

_____ _____ _____

_____ _____ _____

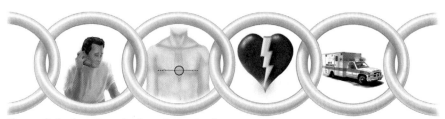

Figure 9-3 Cardiac chain of survival.

2. Fill in the missing links in the cardiac chain of survival:

    1. Early recognition and access

    2. _____

    3. Early defibrillation

    4. _____

3. Generally, if you encounter a pulseless adult when you are alone, you call for help before starting CPR. In what situation should you give an adult 2 minutes of CPR before stopping to call?

_____

Cardiopulmonary Resuscitation (CPR)

✔ Need to Know

CPR helps keep the patient alive by circulating some oxygenated blood to vital organs:

☑ Ventilations move oxygen into the lungs where it is picked up by the blood.

☑ Compressions on the **sternum** (breastbone) increase the pressure inside the chest, resulting in movement of some blood to the brain and other tissues.

The circulation of blood resulting from chest compressions is not nearly as strong as the circulation from a heartbeat, but it can help keep brain and other tissues alive until a normal heart rhythm is restored.

☑ Often an electric shock from an AED or another ACLS medical procedure is needed to restore a heartbeat—and CPR can keep the patient viable until then.

☑ CPR is effective only for a short time.

☑ CPR should be started as soon as possible.

☑ In some instances, the heart may start again spontaneously with CPR.

CPR has clearly been demonstrated to save lives in many circumstances.

☑ With the most common cause of cardiac arrest, a heart attack, CPR and defibrillation within 3 to 5 minutes after the patient collapses can save more than 50% of patients.

☑ Sudden cardiac arrest occurs in more than 900 people with heart disease every day, and CPR followed by AED use can clearly save many thousands of lives every year.

The general technique of CPR involves alternating chest compressions and ventilations. After checking the patient's ABCs and determining that the patient is unresponsive, is not breathing, and has no pulse, start chest compressions. For a patient of any age, these are the general steps of CPR:

1. Find the correct hand position on the lower half of the breastbone midway between the nipples in adults and children **(Figure 9-4).** In infants, the position is just below a line between the nipples.

2. For adults, place the heel of one hand in the correct position; then put your second hand on top of the first and interlock your fingers. For children, depending on their size and your strength, use both hands or the heel of one hand. For infants, use two fingers for one-rescuer CPR.

3. Compress the chest hard and fast at a rate of 100 compressions per minute. Compressions in an adult should be 1 1/2 to 2 inches deep. In an infant or child, compressions should be 1/3 to 1/2 the depth of the chest. Release completely between compressions to let the chest return to its normal height, but do not take your hand(s) from the patient's chest.

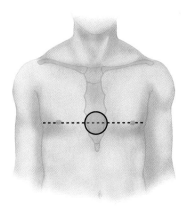
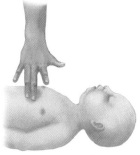

Figure 9-4 Proper hand location for chest compressions.

4. If you are alone, alternate 30 chest compressions and 2 ventilations for patients of all ages. In two-rescuer CPR for an infant or child, alternate 15 compressions (using the chest-encircling method in an infant) and 2 ventilations. For all patients, give each ventilation over 1 second.

5. If supplemental oxygen equipment is present and you are trained in its use, give the patient oxygen during CPR as described in Chapter 8.

Technique of CPR

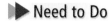 Need to Do

Skill 9-1 gives the sequence of steps of CPR for a patient of any age. Single-rescuer CPR is performed in the same way for all ages—the only differences are the hand placement and the depth of compressions **(Box 9-1)**.

Compressions for Bradycardia in Infants and Children

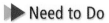 Need to Do

An infant or child being given ventilations may have a pulse but may still have inadequate perfusion.

- If the pulse is less than 60 beats/minute (**bradycardia**) and the infant or child has signs of poor systemic **perfusion** (such as poor skin color), provide CPR with chest compressions.

- Do not wait for the patient to become pulseless if perfusion is poor even with ventilation.

Two-Rescuer CPR for Adults and Children

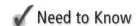 Need to Know

When two rescuers at the scene are trained in CPR, resuscitation performed by both together offers several advantages. Two-rescuer CPR:

BOX 9-1

PROBLEMS WITH CPR TECHNIQUE

It is well known that CPR saves lives and that CPR training is needed to effectively use this procedure. CPR is taught in the classroom using manikins in ideal circumstances rather than real-life situations, which may be very different. It is often difficult to evaluate the effectiveness of CPR given in the field because of the many variables that determine patient outcome.

A recent study, however, demonstrated that CPR, even when given by paramedics, is often ineffective because of poor technique.* This study showed two key problems in the chest compression technique of many of these rescuers. Compressions were not delivered steadily and constantly at all times during the resuscitation efforts. Equally important, more than half of the compressions given were too shallow, resulting in ineffective blood flow. In addition, many rescuers gave compressions at too fast a rate, which does not allow chest pressures to drop sufficiently between compressions to maximize blood flow.

Other studies have also shown that only good-quality CPR improves the patient's chances of survival. The quality depends mostly on giving chest compressions at the correct rate and depth.

More research is likely needed before it is clearly understood why CPR skills seem to deteriorate soon after a rescuer learns or refreshes them, as well as how to correct this problem. The evidence clearly indicates, however, the importance of performing CPR as learned—especially the depth and rate of chest compressions. Perhaps even the knowledge that one is likely to give compressions too shallowly will help rescuers in the future remember to focus on their technique to provide the quality CPR the patient needs to survive.

*From "Quality of Cardiopulmonary Resuscitation During Out-of-Hospital Cardiac Arrest," by Wik, L. et al., JAMA, 293, pp. 299–304. Copyright © 2005 American Medical Association. Reprinted with permission.

Skill 9-1 Single-Rescuer CPR

1 Check the patient's responsiveness, open the airway, and determine that the patient is not breathing adequately.

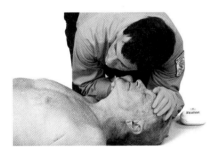

2 Give 2 ventilations, each lasting 1 second. (If the first breath does not go in, reposition the head and try again; if the second breath still does not go in, give choking care).

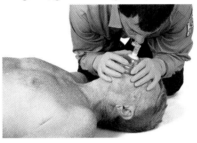

3 Determine the victim has no pulse.

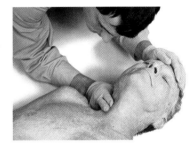

4 Put your hand(s) in the correct position for chest a compressions. Give 30 chest compressions at a rate of 100 per minute. Count aloud for a steady fast rate: "One, two, three...." Then give 2 ventilations.

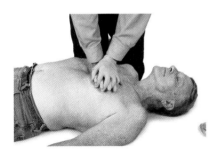

5 Continue cycles of 30 compressions and 2 ventilations.

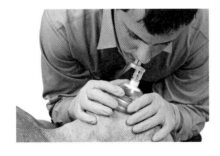

6 Continue CPR until:
- The patient begins to move.
- An AED is brought to the scene and is ready to use.
- Personnel with equal or higher level training arrive and take over.
- You are too exhausted to continue.

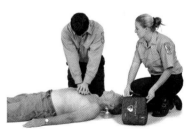

7 a. If the patient starts moving, check for breathing and a pulse. If the patient is breathing adequately and has a pulse, put the patient in the recovery position and monitor breathing.

b. When an AED arrives, start the AED sequence.

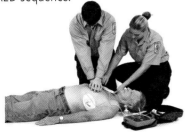

Alert!
Chest Compressions
- Be careful with your hand position for chest compressions. For adults and children, keep your fingers off the patient's chest.
- Do not give compressions over the tip of the breastbone.
- When compressing, keep your elbows straight and keep your hands in contact with the patient's chest at all times.
- Remember to compress the chest hard and fast, but let the chest recoil completely between compressions.
- Minimize the amount of time used giving ventilations between sets of compressions.

☑ Minimizes the time between ventilations and compressions, making CPR more effective

☑ Allows an AED to be set up quickly

☑ Reduces rescuer fatigue

▶▶ Need to Do

The first rescuer, who will be giving ventilations, begins by checking the patient's ABCs while the second rescuer ensures additional help is on the way and moves into position on the opposite side of the patient to give chest compressions. Two-rescuer CPR is performed in the same cycles of 30 compressions and 2 ventilations for an adult, but with 15 compressions and 2 ventilations for an infant or child.

- The first rescuer provides ventilations, and the second rescuer gives the chest compressions at a rate of 100 compressions per minute.

- The second rescuer should count aloud during the compressions and pause after the last compression to let the first rescuer give 2 ventilations.

- The rescuers should switch positions about every 2 minutes (after 5 cycles of 30 compressions and 2 ventilations) to prevent the second rescuer from becoming fatigued and giving ineffective compressions. This change should be done at the end of a full CPR cycle after ventilations are given, and should be accomplished in less than 5 seconds.

- If an AED is present, the first rescuer gives both ventilations and chest compressions while the second rescuer sets up the unit and attaches the pads (see Chapter 10). If the AED unit advises continuing CPR, the rescuers then give CPR together.

- A third rescuer, if present, can give cricoid pressure to help ensure ventilations do not go into the stomach and possibly cause vomiting.

Note: If an advanced airway is placed in the patient for ventilation, chest compressions are given continually, without pauses for ventilations. Ventilation at a rate of 8 to 10 per minute is provided while compressions are ongoing.

Transitioning from One-Rescuer CPR to Two-Rescuer CPR

▶▶ Need to Do

In some situations, a rescuer is already giving CPR when a second rescuer arrives on the scene. The rescuers should coordinate their actions for a smooth transition from one-rescuer CPR to two-rescuer CPR:

1. The second rescuer moves into position on the other side of the patient to prepare to take over chest compressions.

2. The first rescuer completes a cycle of compressions and ventilations.

3. While the first rescuer then pauses to check for a pulse, the second rescuer finds the correct hand position for compressions.

4. When the first rescuer says, "No pulse, continue CPR," the second rescuer begins chest compressions and the first rescuer then gives only ventilations (**Skill 9-2**).

Note: If you are the First Responder who started CPR, the arriving second rescuer may be a rescuer with a higher level of training. In such a case, this rescuer assumes authority for how CPR should best be continued. If this rescuer determines your ventilation or compression technique is inadequate, he or she may ask you to take on the other role—or may take over the CPR alone.

Two-Rescuer CPR for Infants

▶▶ Need to Do

Two-rescuer CPR for an infant uses a different hand position for giving chest compressions:

- The rescuer giving compressions places the thumbs of both hands together in the correct position on the infant's sternum (just below a line between the nipples).

- The fingers of both hands encircle the infant's chest (**Figure 9-5**).

- The chest is compressed with both thumbs while the chest is squeezed with the fingers, as described in **Skill 9-3**.

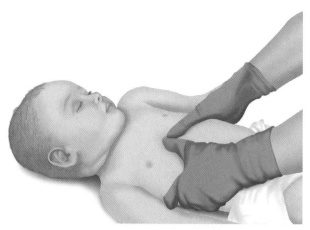

Figure 9-5 Chest-encircling hand position for infant chest compressions in two-rescuer CPR.

Skill 9-2 Two-Rescuer CPR for Adults and Children

1 At the patient's head, Rescuer 1 checks the patient's ABCs. An AED has been summoned. At the patient's side, Rescuer 2 locates the site for chest compressions.

2 Rescuer 1 indicates "No pulse." Rescuer 2 gives 30 compressions for an adult (15 for a child) at rate of 100 per minute, counting aloud for a fast, steady rate, then pauses.

3 Rescuer 1 gives 2 ventilations.

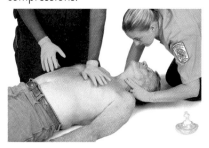

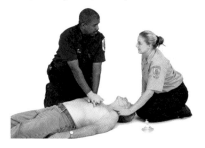

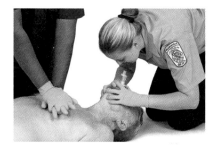

4 Rescuers continue cycles of 30 compressions in an adult (15 in a child) and 2 ventilations for about 2 minutes (or after 5 cycles of compressions and ventilations at a ratio of 30:2) before switching compressor and ventilator roles. The switch should be done quickly (in less than 5 seconds).

5 Rescuers continue CPR until:
• The patient moves.
• An AED is brought to the scene and is ready to use.
• Help arrives and takes over.

6 If the patient starts breathing and has a pulse, put the patient in the recovery position and monitor the ABCs.

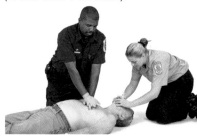

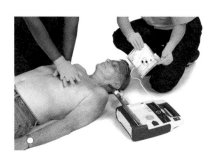

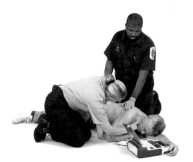

7 If an AED is brought to the scene, start the AED sequence.

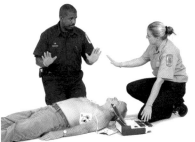

Skill 9-3   Two-Rescuer CPR for Infants

1 At the infant's head, Rescuer 1 checks the ABCs. At the infant's feet, Rescuer 2 locates the site for chest compressions with both thumbs.

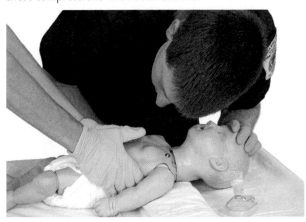

2 If absent, Rescuer 1 says, "No pulse." Rescuer 2 gives 15 chest compressions at a rate of 100 per minute, counting aloud for a fast, steady rate, then pauses.

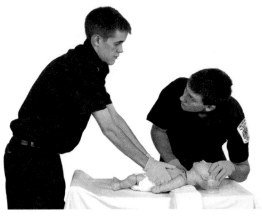

3 Rescuer 1 gives 2 ventilations.

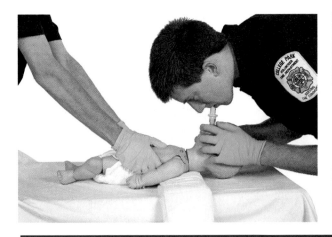

4 Rescuers continue cycles of 15 compressions and 2 ventilations for about 2 minutes before switching compressor and ventilator roles. The switch should be done quickly (in less than 5 seconds). Rescuers continue CPR until:
• The infant has a pulse or is breathing.
• Help arrives and takes over.

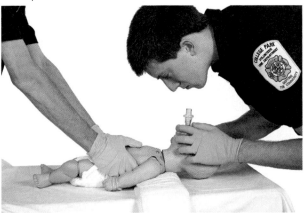

When Not to Perform CPR

◼ Need to Recognize

Generally, BLS skills should be performed on any patient who is not breathing and has no pulse. Exceptions in which it is acceptable to not give CPR to a patient include:

▶ The presence of a Do-Not-Resuscitate (DNR) order

▶ The patient is obviously dead (decapitation; incineration; or clear signs of prolonged death, such as rigor mortis and dependent lividity).

▶ It is not safe to be on the scene and the patient cannot be moved somewhere safe.

Continued

5 If the infant starts breathing, hold the infant in the recovery position and monitor the ABCs.

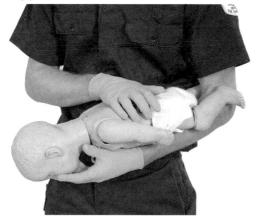

◆ A physician pronounces the patient dead.

✎ Do You Understand?

1. True or false: In most cases, CPR restarts the heart beat to resuscitate the patient.

2. How is the hand position for chest compressions in a child different from in an adult?

   _____

3. What is an exception to the general rule to use a ratio of 30 compressions and 2 ventilations?

   _____

4. Common problems with CPR include compressions that are too shallow and compressions given at too _____ a rate.

5. At what point in CPR do two rescuers switch positions?

   _____

Conclusion

As important as CPR is for saving lives, in most cases, it only serves to keep the patient viable until defibrillation or ACLS begins. Chapter 10 describes how to use an AED along with CPR for patients in cardiac arrest.

Key Terms

Advanced Cardiac Life Support (ACLS) (p. 130)

bradycardia (p. 132)

cardiac arrest (p. 129)

cardiac chain of survival (p. 130)

cardiopulmonary resuscitation (CPR) (p. 127)

perfusion (p. 132)

sternum (p. 131)

Review Questions

1. Oxygenated blood is pumped to the body by the
   a. left ventricle.
   b. right ventricle.
   c. left atrium.
   d. right atrium.

2. The femoral pulse is palpated in the
   a. upper arm.
   b. wrist.
   c. groin area.
   d. neck.

3. How soon may brain damage begin when the heart stops?
   a. 2 minutes
   b. 4 minutes
   c. 8 minutes
   d. 12 minutes

4. The chain of survival link for early recognition includes recognizing
   a. diabetic coma.
   b. anaphylaxis.
   c. internal bleeding.
   d. heart attack.

5. The most urgent reason for ensuring EMS is responding to a patient in cardiac arrest is to
   a. prepare emergency department staff for the incoming patient.
   b. get an AED to the patient as soon as possible.
   c. start two-rescuer CPR as soon as possible.
   d. ensure transport takes place as soon as possible.

6. In infants, the site for chest compressions is
   a. just below the line between the nipples.
   b. just above the line between the nipples.
   c. centered on the line between the nipples.
   d. two finger-widths below the line between the nipples.

7. A single rescuer gives a child chest compressions and ventilations in what ratio?
   a. 15 to 1   c. 30 to 1
   b. 15 to 2   d. 30 to 2

8. When should oxygen, if available, be used to ventilate a patient in cardiac arrest?
   a. For all patients over age 8
   b. For all patients experiencing heart attack
   c. For all trauma patients
   d. For all patients

9. CPR should be given to a child with a pulse with poor perfusion if the pulse is less than _____ beats per minute.
   a. 20   c. 80
   b. 60   d. 100

10. In what situation are ventilations given *simultaneously* with chest compressions?
    a. Whenever three rescuers are present
    b. In all two-rescuer CPR
    c. When the cardiac arrest has lasted longer than 5 minutes
    d. When an advanced airway is in place

Chapter 10

Automated External Defibrillation

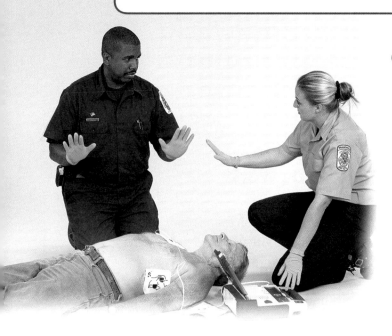

Chapter Preview

- AEDs and Medical Direction
- The Heart's Electrical System
- How AEDs Work
- Using an AED
- AED Alerts
- AEDs for Children
- Special AED Considerations
- AED Problems and Maintenance

You Respond To ...

the scene where a citizen responder is giving CPR to a woman who collapsed suddenly a few minutes previously. You determine that the patient has no pulse. You have an AED with you and are trained to use it. You quickly set it up while the lay provider continues CPR.

Introduction

Not every patient who receives CPR will benefit from an **automated external defibrillator** (**AED**), but many do. In many cases of cardiac arrest, the patient's heart has an abnormal rhythm that does not circulate the blood, and this rhythm can often be corrected with a shock from the AED. Remember the cardiac chain of survival: An AED should be used with any patient who is not responsive, is not breathing, and has no pulse. In many cardiac arrest situations, CPR functions only to keep the patient viable until a shock from the AED restores a normal heart rhythm.

AEDs and Medical Direction

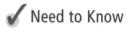 Need to Know

In many areas, the medical director oversees placement and use of the automated external defibrillator (AED). Your course instructor will inform you how to meet the current requirements in your area for using an AED.

Laws regarding AEDs are changing:

☑ After the FDA approved nonprescription AEDs for home use in 2004, AED units that do not require instructor-led training began appearing in homes and other settings.

☑ These devices have been demonstrated for safe use even by lay rescuers who follow the instructions printed on the device and the sound prompts during use.

☑ AEDs have become so simple to use that additional changes in AED regulations may be forthcoming.

The Heart's Electrical System

✔ Need to Know

The heart pumps blood to the lungs to pick up oxygen and pumps oxygenated blood to all parts of the body. The heart's electrical system keeps the four chambers of the heart synchronized and working together:

- ☑ The sinoatrial (SA) and atrioventricular (AV) nodes help organize and control the rhythmic electrical impulses that keep the heart beating properly **(Figure 10-1)**.

- ☑ The heart's normal rhythm is called the **sinus rhythm.**

- ☑ With a heart attack or other heart problems, this rhythmic electrical control may be disrupted, causing an abnormal heart rhythm.

Ventricular Fibrillation

✔ Need to Know

Ventricular fibrillation (VF), sometimes called V-fib, is the most common abnormal heart rhythm that occurs with cardiac arrest. Although we say a patient in VF is in cardiac arrest, the heart is not completely still but is beating abnormally.

- ☑ **Fibrillation** means the ventricles of the heart are quivering instead of beating rhythmically.

- ☑ Blood is not filling the ventricles and is not being pumped to the lungs or body as normal.

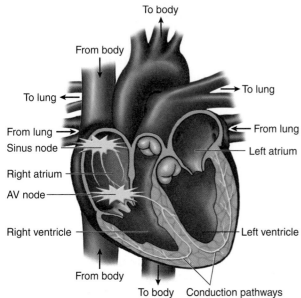

Figure 10-1 The heart's electrical system.

Heart attack is the most common cause of cardiac arrest in adults, so ventricular fibrillation is a common occurrence. Studies show that in approximately half the cases of cardiac arrest, the patient's heart is in fibrillation and therefore would gain from a shock delivered by the AED.

✎ Do You Understand?

1. The normal rhythm of the heart is called the _____ rhythm.

2. True or false: When ventricular defibrillation occurs during a heart attack, the heart is pumping blood too fast through the body.

How AEDs Work

✔ Need to Know

- ☑ The AED automatically checks the patient's heart rhythm by detecting electrical signals in the body picked up by the AED's electrodes.

- ☑ If the patient's heart is in VF, the AED will advise giving an electric shock in an attempt to return the heart to a normal rhythm. This is called **defibrillation,** or stopping the fibrillation of the heart **(Figure 10-2)**.

- ☑ The AED's **electrodes,** or pads, are placed on the patient's chest (or on the front and back of the chest in a small child) as directed by the manufacturer's picture on the pads. The unit then analyzes the patient's heart rhythm.

- ☑ When the unit delivers a shock, electricity travels through the chest to the heart and stops the heart's electrical impulses that are causing the abnormal heart rhythm, often restoring a normal heartbeat.

Contemporary AEDs are easy and simple to use, but they must be used right away. Even when CPR is being given, with every minute that goes by before defibrillation begins, the patient's chances for survival drop by about 10%.

- ☑ AEDs contain a battery or battery pack and are portable.

- ☑ All units have two pads connected to them with cables. The pads are placed on the patient's chest.

- ☑ The unit then analyzes the patient's heart rhythm and advises whether to give a shock.

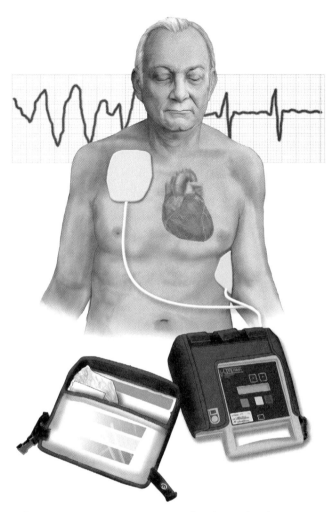

Figure 10-2 An AED gives a shock to the heart.

☑ Some models have a screen that tells you what to do; all models give directions in a clear voice.

☑ AED models vary somewhat in other features, but all work in the same basic way **(Figure 10-3)**.

Using an AED

▶ Need to Do

In any situation in which a patient suddenly collapses or is found unresponsive, be thinking about the possibility of cardiac arrest even as you approach the patient. If someone else is present and you know an AED is available nearby, send that person to get it immediately. It is better to have it right away and not use it than to need it and have to wait for it. The steps for using an AED are simple:

1. Determine the need for the AED (no response, no breathing, no pulse).

2. Start CPR until the AED is set up and ready to use.

3. Attach the AED to the patient.

4. Analyze the patient's rhythm and give a shock when advised.

AED and CPR

▶ Need to Do

As always, first check the patient's ABCs.

▶ If the patient is not breathing and has no pulse, ensure that additional help is on the way and get an AED.

▶ Always use an AED if there is no response, no breathing, and no pulse.

Lay rescuers are taught to use the AED on any nonbreathing adult as soon as the unit is available. When two rescuers are present, one should give CPR while the other sets up the AED. Lay rescuers are taught to give 5 cycles of CPR (2 minutes), without pausing to check for a pulse, for a nonbreathing child found unresponsive (not observed to have collapsed suddenly). For a patient without a pulse, First Responders in out-of-hospital settings should also use the AED as soon as it is ready *except* in the following two situations:

▶ For a pulseless child who was not observed to have collapsed suddenly, provide 5 uninterrupted cycles of CPR (about 2 minutes) before using the AED.

▶ For an adult found pulseless on your arrival, when more than 4-5 minutes have passed since you were called to respond, provide 5 uninterrupted cycles of CPR (about 2 minutes) before using the AED.

Attach the AED to the Patient

▶ Need to Do

▶ Be sure the patient is not in water or in contact with metal. Water or metal conducts electricity that may pose a risk to you or others.

▶ Place the AED at the patient's side, next to the rescuer who will use it. Turn it on, and attach the pads (electrodes) to the patient's chest.

▶ Most AED units have a diagram on the pads or the unit to remind you where to position them **(Figure 10-4)**. Typically, the first pad is placed on the right side, below the collarbone

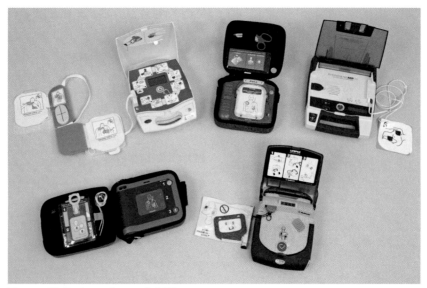

Figure 10-3 A variety of AEDs.

and to the right of the breastbone. The second pad is placed below and to the left of the left nipple and above the lower rib margin.

- Attach the AED pads to the patient only if the patient is unresponsive, is not breathing, and has no pulse.

- Expose the patient's chest, and dry the skin if needed with a towel or dry clothing (heart attack patients are often sweating).

- If the patient has heavy chest hair, quickly shave the pad areas. If a razor is not available, use scissors or trauma shears (which should be kept with the AED) to trim the hair and allow skin contact with the pads. Alternatively, if two sets of pads are available, press one pad to the chest and then remove it, bringing much of the chest hair with it stuck to the pad's adhesive; then position a new pad on the area.

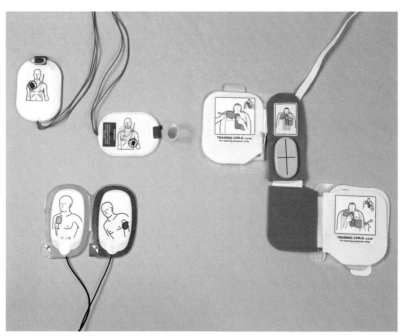

Figure 10-4 AED pads usually include diagrams showing correct pad placement.

◗ Remove the backing from the pads and apply the pads firmly on the patient's chest.

◗ If required with your AED model, plug the pad cables into the main unit.

Analyze and Shock

▶ Need to Do

◗ With the pads in place and the AED unit on, most AED models automatically analyze the patient's heart rhythm.

◗ Do not move or touch the patient while it is analyzing. After it analyzes the heart rhythm, the unit will advise you whether to give a shock or to continue CPR.

◗ If a shock is advised, be sure no one is touching the patient. Look up and down the patient and say, "Everybody clear!" Once everyone is clear, administer the shock (when advised).

◗ After the shock, immediately give CPR for 5 cycles (about 2 minutes). Do not check for a pulse.

◗ Then the AED will analyze again and advise another shock, if needed, or continuing CPR (with the pads left in place).

Different AEDs may use different prompts.

◗ Follow the unit's voice and picture prompts through this process.

◗ Some units can be programmed to administer the shock automatically rather than prompt you to push the shock button; in this case, as always, follow the unit's prompts.

If the patient recovers (moves and is breathing) and spinal injury is not suspected, put an unresponsive, breathing patient in the recovery position and continue to monitor breathing. Keep the AED pads in place as some patients may return to VF and require defibrillation again.

The AED may also say no shock is indicated.

◗ This means the patient's heart will not benefit from defibrillation.

◗ Immediately continue CPR (see **Skill 10-1**).

AED Alerts

▶ Need to Do

◗ Move the patient away from standing water before using the AED and dry the patient's chest well before attaching the electrodes.

◗ Avoid any flammable materials, including oxygen flowing through a mask. Do not use alcohol to wipe the patient's skin.

◗ Do not use the AED when in motion in a vehicle or boat.

◗ Do not use a cell phone or 2-way radio within 6 feet of an AED.

◗ Remember not to touch the patient while the AED is analyzing the rhythm or administering a shock. (Note: Research is underway for the development of new AEDs that can analyze the patient's heart rhythm while CPR is being given.)

✎ Do You Understand?

1. When should you first send for an AED?

_____

2. If you find a child pulseless on your arrival, what should you do first?

_____

3. What is your first action after administering a shock?

_____

4. List at least four precautions to observe when using an AED.

_____ _____

_____ _____

AEDs for Children

✔ Need to Know

Follow the adult guidelines and use adult pads for children over age 8. Although much rarer, sudden cardiac arrest can also occur in younger children from causes such as:

☑ Sudden infant death syndrome (SIDS)

☑ Poisoning

☑ Drowning

☑ A heart problem

▶ Need to Do

In most cases, cardiac arrest in a child is caused by a respiratory problem, not a heart problem, and the child's heart is not in VF.

◗ Give a child 2 minutes of CPR before using the AED unless the child was witnessed to collapse suddenly.

Skill 10-1 **Using an AED**

1 Position the patient away from water and metal. Place the unit at the patient's side and turn it on.

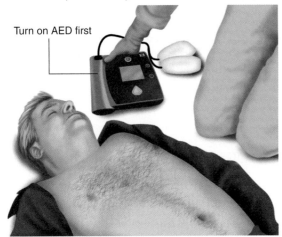

Turn on AED first

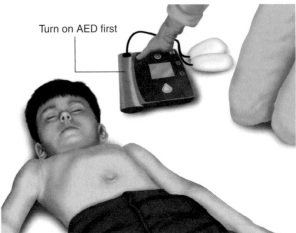

Turn on AED first

2 Expose the patient's chest, and dry or shave the area if necessary.

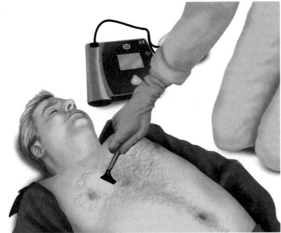

3 Apply pads to the patient's chest. If needed, plug the cables into the unit.

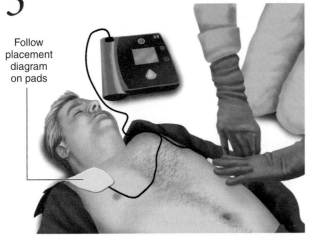

Follow
placement
diagram
on pads

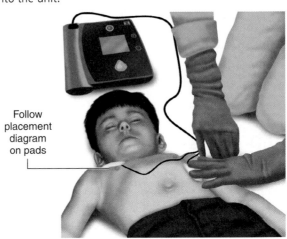

Follow
placement
diagram
on pads

4 Stand clear during the rhythm analysis.

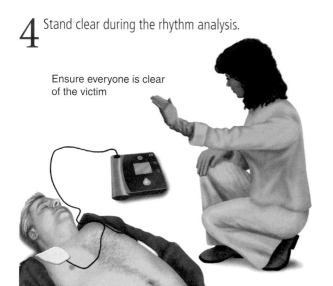

Ensure everyone is clear of the victim

Ensure everyone is clear of the victim

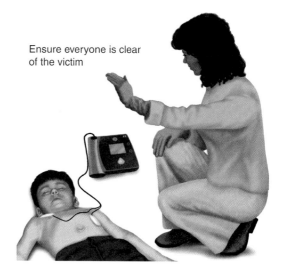

5 Follow prompts from the AED unit to (a) press the shock button or (b) do not shock. Immediately give CPR with the pads remaining in place, starting with chest compressions.

Give shock when indicated

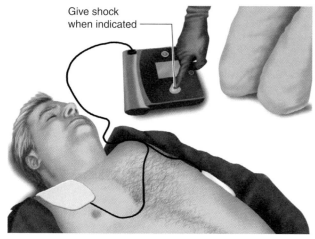

6 Stand clear when the AED prompts to analyze the rhythm again after 5 cycles of CPR (about 2 minutes).

7 Continue steps 5 and 6 until the patient moves or help arrives and takes over.

8 If the patient recovers, put a breathing, unresponsive patient in the recovery position (with pads remaining in place) and continue to monitor the ABCs.

- If the child does not recover, then use the AED as usual.
- This is different from the protocol for adults, in whom cardiac arrest is more likely to be the result of heart attack.

In recent years, the value of defibrillating a young child in sudden cardiac arrest has been recognized, and pediatric AED units and electrode pads are available.

- Use only approved pediatric AED electrode pads, which are smaller than those for adults and produce lower-energy shocks on a child under age 8.

- Usually the pads have a distinctive appearance to prevent confusing adult and pediatric pads, such as pink connectors and teddy bear emblems.
- If pediatric pads are not available, using adult pads is better than not using the AED at all.
- Pediatric pads should not be used for an adult because the lower energy is insufficient to affect the heart rhythm.

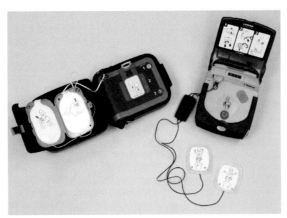

Figure 10-5 Pediatric AED units.

Be sure to follow the device's instructions for pad placement on a small child. The AED shown in **Figure 10-5,** on the right, uses pad placement on the front and back of the child's chest. With small children and infants, it can be difficult to position both pads on the front of the chest, and studies have shown placement on the front and back also delivers an effective shock **(Box 10-1)**.

Currently, AED use on both adults and children from ages 1 to 8 is recommended. AED use for infants is not recommended against, but the evidence is considered "indeterminate" regarding the benefit of AED use for infants versus the risks of incorrectly analyzing rhythm or delivering an inappropriate shock level. There are proponents for infant AED use, however, and AED manufacturers claim they are safe and appropriate when using the correct pediatric pads.

Special AED Considerations

Internal Pacemaker or Defibrillator

▶ Need to Do

When you expose the patient's chest to apply the AED pads, you may see a bulge or lump beneath the patient's skin from an implanted **pacemaker** or defibrillator, often on the upper left side of the chest **(Figure 10-6)**.

- Do not place a pad directly over this area but instead place it at least one or more inches away.

- If the patient's chest or body is jerking, there may be an implanted defibrillator giving

BOX 10-1

CHANGING AED TECHNOLOGY

AEDs were first designed for use on adults and older children and therefore originally had pads that came in one size only and were placed in the typical manner on the upper right and lower left chest. When research showed the benefit of lower-energy shocks for pediatric patients, newer units were developed that used separate pediatric pads, sometimes placed on the front and back of the chest because of the difficulty of placing both pads far enough apart on a child's small chest. At this time, AED technology continues to evolve, with some new units now able to determine characteristics of the patient and adjust the shock level automatically. Other new units now use the same pads for all patients, regardless of size and weight, but have a separate switch on the unit used for pediatric patients. With such advances, separate pediatric pads may eventually become obsolete.

Until December 2005, most AED units used a protocol that advised a series of up to three shocks. Recent studies showed that a single shock immediately followed by CPR was more effective, and this became the recommended protocol. It is anticipated that older AEDs will be reprogrammed to follow this revised protocol, although some older units may retain the outdated settings for a time. Always follow the prompts of the AED unit you are using.

shocks; wait until jerking has ended before applying the pads.

Medication Patches

▶ Need to Do

If the patient has a medication patch or paste on the chest, remove it and wipe the chest before applying the AED pads **(Figure 10-7)**.

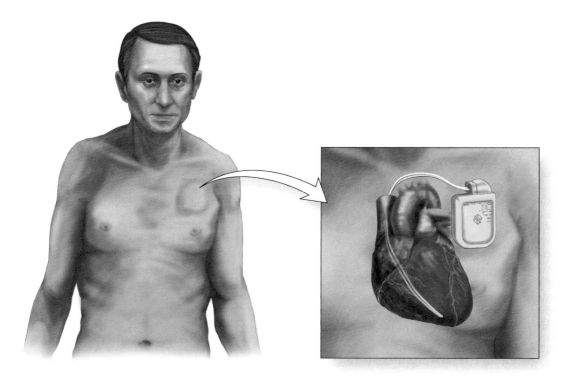

Figure 10-6 Vary AED pad placement if there is an internal device.

AED Problems and Maintenance

▶▶ Need to Do

With regular maintenance, an AED should not have any problems during use.

The AED may prompt you to avoid problems.

- If you get a low-battery prompt, change the battery or battery pack before continuing.

- Another prompt may advise you to prevent moving the patient if the AED detects motion.

- An error message may be given if the electrodes are not firmly in contact with the patient's skin.

AEDs require regular maintenance:

- Check the manual from the manufacturer for periodic scheduled maintenance and testing of the unit.

- The battery or battery pack must be kept charged, and a charged backup battery or battery pack should be available.

- Pads should be sealed and replaced before their expiration dates.

- A daily inspection of the unit helps ensure the AED is always ready for use and all needed supplies are present.

- You may be instructed to inspect the unit at the beginning of your shift.

- Most facilities with an AED use a daily checklist form **(Figure 10-8)**. The checklist should always be adapted for the specific AED model,

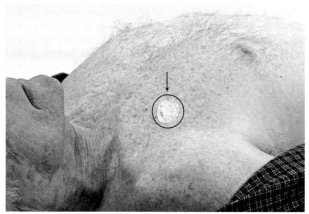

Figure 10-7 Remove medication patches prior to AED pad placement.

AED INSPECTION CHECKLIST

Date: _____ Location: _____ AED Model: _____

Inspected by: _____ Signed: _____

Criteria	ok/no	Corrective action/remarks
AED unit		
verify correctly placed	_____	_____
clean, clear of objects	_____	_____
no cracks or damage to case	_____	_____
cables/connectors present and not expired	_____	_____
fully charged battery in place	_____	_____
charged spare battery present	_____	_____
check status/service light indicator	_____	_____
check absence of service alarm	_____	_____
power on, self-test	_____	_____
Supplies		
Two sealed sets of electrode pads	_____	_____
Verify expiration date on pad packages	_____	_____
Razor	_____	_____
Medical exam gloves	_____	_____
Hand towels	_____	_____
Alcohol wipes	_____	_____
Scissors	_____	_____
Pocket mask or face shield	_____	_____

Figure 10-8 Example of an AED inspection checklist.

including the manufacturer's daily and periodic maintenance guidelines.

◗ Many units come with a self-diagnostic test or simulator device to be used to check that the AED is correctly analyzing rhythms and delivering shocks; this may be part of the daily inspection routine.

Do You Understand?

1. Children at what ages are recommended for use of an AED with pediatric pads? _____
2. True or false: Never use an AED with adult pads on a child.

3. What should you do if a patient has a medication patch on the chest where you want to position an AED pad?

_____

Conclusion

Ventilation, chest compressions, and AED are used together in the treatment of patients in cardiac arrest **(Table 10-1)**. These are crucial skills for First Responders, and they also require periodic refreshing to remain effective. Even if you are now becoming certified in CPR and AED, remember that to continue to use these lifesaving skills in the future, you will eventually need a refresher course.

Table 10-1

Summary of Basic Life Support

Step	Infant (under 1 year)	Child (1-puberty except 1-8 for AED)	Adult
1. Check for responsiveness	Stimulate to check response	"Are you okay"—Tap shoulder	
2. If unresponsive, call for help	Send someone to call; give 2 minutes of care before calling yourself if alone	Send someone to call; give 2 minutes of care before calling yourself if alone (except for known heart problem)	Send someone to call; call immediately if alone (give 2 minutes of care for patients of drowning, poisoning, and other injuries)
3. If unresponsive: Open airway	Head tilt-chin lift (but do not overextend the neck)	Head tilt-chin lift or jaw thrust	
4. Check breathing	Look, listen, feel for breathing		
5. If not breathing: Give 2 ventilations, watch the chest rise	Use a barrier device or cover the mouth, nose, or stoma Each ventilation lasts 1 second		
6. If the chest does not rise with first ventilation: Reposition the airway and try again	Each ventilation lasts 1 second		
7. If the chest still does not rise: Start care for airway obstruction	Start CPR beginning with chest compressions Check the mouth for an object each time ventilations are given		
8. If the chest rises with ventilations: Check for a pulse	Check for a brachial pulse	Check for a carotid or femoral pulse	Check for a carotid pulse
9. If a pulse is present but there is no breathing, give ventilations	1 ventilation every 3-5 seconds		1 ventilation every 5-6 seconds
10. If there is no pulse, give CPR	For compressions, use 2 fingers just below the line between the nipples; compress the chest 1/3 to 1/2 the depth of the chest	For compressions use one or two hands midway between the nipples; compress the chest 1/3 to 1/2 the depth of the chest	For compressions, use both hands, one on top of other, midway between the nipples; compress the chest 1 1/2-2 inches
Chest compressions:	Rate of 100 per minute Cycles of 30 compressions and 2 ventilations (Except 15:2 in 2-rescuer CPR for an infant or a child)		*(continued)*

Table 10-1 continued

Summary of Basic Life Support

Step	Infant (under 1 year)	Child (1-puberty except 1-8 for AED)	Adult
11. Continue to check for breathing and a pulse	Look, listen, and feel for breathing Check pulse		
12. Use AED when available (if no breathing and no pulse)	Not recommended for or against	Use pediatric electrode pads	Use adult AED electrode pads
13. If the patient recovers adequate breathing and a pulse, put the patient in the recovery position	Hold the infant and monitor the ABCs	Lay the patient preferably on the left side, in the recovery position, and monitor the ABCs	

Key Terms

automated external defibrillator (AED) (p. 139)

defibrillation (p. 140)

electrodes (p. 140)

fibrillation (p. 140)

pacemaker (p. 146)

sinus rhythm (p. 140)

ventricular fibrillation (VF) (p. 140)

Review Questions

1. What are the electrodes of an AED?
   a. The pads placed on the patient's chest
   b. Small sensors applied to the patient's neck to check pulse
   c. The wires connected to the AED unit
   d. The screen readouts of the patient's heart rhythm

2. When does the AED deliver a shock to the patient?
   a. Immediately after you position the pads
   b. When you push the shock button after analysis
   c. About 3 seconds after you stop CPR
   d. When the unit determines the patient is dead

3. Use the AED with a patient as soon as you have
   a. determined unresponsiveness.
   b. opened the airway.
   c. determined the patient is not breathing.
   d. determined the patient has no pulse.

4. For an adult found pulseless after more than 5 minutes have passed since the call,

   a. use the AED immediately.

   b. give 2 minutes of CPR before using the AED.

   c. give 5 minutes of CPR before using the AED.

   d. it is too late to use the AED.

5. When do you use an AED immediately with a child?

   a. If the child was pulled from water

   b. If the child was known to be choking before becoming unresponsive

   c. If the child was seen to have collapsed suddenly

   d. If you are the only responder present at the scene

6. On an adult, place the AED pads

   a. in an area of the least chest hair.

   b. as close as possible to the site for chest compressions during CPR.

   c. where the pad diagram indicates they should be placed.

   d. close together, immediately over the heart.

7. Following a shock, for how long should you give CPR before the AED unit again analyzes the patient?

   a. 2 minutes

   b. 3 minutes

   c. 4 minutes

   d. 5 minutes

8. Should an AED be used with an infant under the age of 1 year?

   a. No one should ever use an AED with an infant.

   b. Follow local protocol for AED use with an infant.

   c. Always use an AED with an infant without a pulse.

   d. Use an AED only with an infant known to have a heart problem.

Unit 5

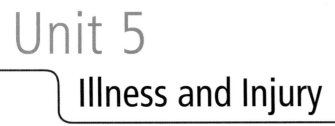

Illness and Injury

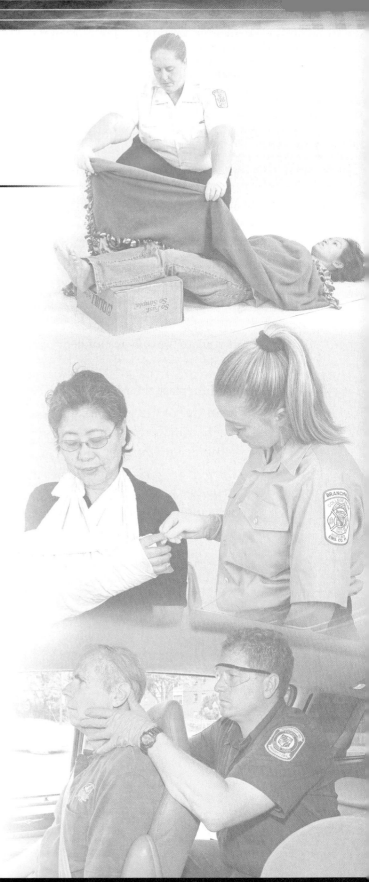

Chapter 11

Medical Emergencies

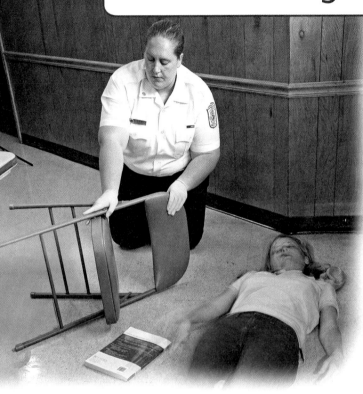

Chapter Preview

- General Medical Complaints
- Heart Attack
- Respiratory Emergencies
- Altered Mental Status
- Fainting
- Stroke
- Seizures
- Cold Emergencies
- Heat Emergencies
- Diabetic Emergencies

- Poisoning
- Inhaled Poisons
- Alcohol and Drug Emergencies
- Bites and Stings
- Allergic Reactions (Anaphylaxis)
- Severe Abdominal Pain
- Behavioral Emergencies

You Respond To ...

a scene where a man is lying on a sofa, obviously ill. His wife says he was fine until a few minutes ago, but then he started "acting funny" and seemed to have trouble breathing. He is responsive but seems confused. He says his head hurts, and you note that he is short of breath and cannot speak a full sentence without stopping to catch his breath.

Introduction

A medical emergency occurs because of illness or a medical problem, rather than trauma. Some medical emergencies develop slowly, whereas others may develop very quickly and become life threatening. It is important to know the signs and symptoms of common medical problems and the appropriate emergency medical care to provide.

General Medical Complaints

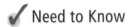 Need to Know

Many different illnesses and medical conditions can occur suddenly and become medical emergencies.

☑ The patient or a family member may call for help for a variety of signs and symptoms.

☑ In some cases you may suspect or know the cause of the problem, but in other cases neither you nor the patient may know the cause of the problem.

☑ The general approach is the same for all sudden illness emergencies, and you do not have to know for sure what the patient's specific illness is before giving the following emergency care.

Need to Recognize

Perform the standard assessment:

1. Size up the scene before beginning emergency medical care.

2. Complete the initial assessment.

3. Perform a physical examination as appropriate.

4. Complete ongoing assessments.

General signs and symptoms of medical emergencies:

▶ Person feels ill, dizzy, confused, or weak

▶ Skin color changes (flushed or pale), sweating

▶ Breathing changes

▶ Nausea, vomiting

Need to Do

Perform standard patient care:

1. Ensure EMS has been activated.

2. Take body substance isolation precautions.

3. Maintain the patient's airway and provide artificial ventilation if needed.

4. Comfort, calm, and reassure the patient while awaiting additional EMS resources.

In addition:

▶ Follow local protocol to administer oxygen if it is available and you are so trained.

▶ Help patient rest and avoid getting chilled or overheated.

▶ Do not give the patient anything to eat or drink.

▶ Watch for changes, and be prepared to give Basic Life Support (BLS).

Heart Attack

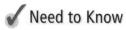 Need to Know

Heart attack, or **acute myocardial infarction (AMI),** involves a sudden reduced blood flow to the heart muscle. It is a medical emergency and

may lead to cardiac arrest. Heart attack can occur at any age but is very rare in children **(Box 11-1)**. Heart attack is caused by a reduced blood flow or blockage in the coronary arteries, which supply the heart muscle with blood, usually as a result of narrowing of the vessels due to **atherosclerosis.**

Need to Recognize

The signs and symptoms of heart attack vary considerably, from vague chest discomfort (which the patient may confuse with heartburn) to crushing pain, with or without other symptoms **(Figure 11-1)**.

▶ The patient may have no signs and symptoms at all before suddenly collapsing.

▶ The patient may have milder symptoms that come and go for two or three days before the heart attack occurs.

▶ Some heart attack symptoms are more common in women. Chest pain or discomfort is still the most common symptom, but women are somewhat more likely to have shortness of breath, jaw or back pain, and nausea and vomiting.

▶ Consider the possibility of heart attack with a wide range of symptoms rather than expecting a clearly defined situation, including a lack of chest pain or discomfort.

▶ Heart attack patients occasionally deny that they are having a heart attack.

Perform the standard assessment:

1. Size up the scene before beginning emergency medical care.

2. Complete the initial assessment.

3. Perform a physical examination as appropriate.

4. Complete ongoing assessments.

BOX 11-1

FACTS ABOUT HEART ATTACK

• About 180,000 people a year in the United States die from heart attacks—many of whom could have been saved by prompt medical treatment.

• Heart attack is more likely in those with a family history of heart attacks.

• One-fifth of heart attack patients do not have chest pain—but often have other symptoms.

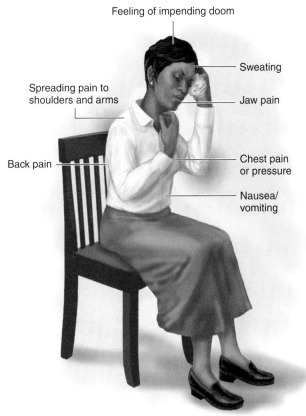

Feeling of impending doom

Sweating

Jaw pain

Spreading pain to shoulders and arms

Chest pain or pressure

Back pain

Nausea/ vomiting

Figure 11-1 Signs and symptoms of a heart attack.

Signs and symptoms of heart attack:

- Complaints of persistent pressure, tightness, ache, or pain in the chest
- Complaints of pain spreading to neck, shoulders, or arms
- Complaints of shortness of breath
- Complaints of dizziness, lightheadedness, a feeling of impending doom
- Pale, moist skin or heavy sweating
- Nausea

Need to Do

Perform standard patient care:

1. Ensure EMS has been activated.
2. Take body substance isolation precautions.
3. Maintain the patient's airway and provide artificial ventilation if needed.
4. Comfort, calm, and reassure the patient while awaiting additional EMS resources.

In addition:

- Help the patient rest in a comfortable position (often sitting). Loosen any tight clothing. Keep the patient from moving.

- Ask the patient if he or she is taking heart medication, and follow local protocol to help the patient with the medication (**Box 11-2**).
- Follow local protocol to allow the patient to take one adult aspirin (unless allergic).
- Follow local protocol to administer oxygen if it is available and you are so trained.
- Stay with the patient, and be reassuring and calming. Be prepared to give care if the patient becomes unresponsive and breathing stops.
- Do not let the patient eat or drink anything.

It is important to act quickly when the patient may be having a heart attack, because deaths from heart attack usually occur within an hour or two after symptoms begin.

Angina

Need to Know

Angina pectoris, usually just called angina, is chest pain caused by heart disease that usually happens after intense activity or exertion. Other factors may trigger the pain of angina, such as stress or exposure to extreme heat or cold.

- ☑ The pain is a sign that the heart muscle is not getting as much oxygen as needed, usually because of narrowed or constricted coronary arteries.
- ☑ The pain may also radiate to the jaw, neck, or left arm or shoulder.
- ☑ The pain usually goes away after a few minutes of rest.
- ☑ Patients usually know when they have angina and may carry medication for it, usually nitroglycerin.

Need to Do

- Help a person with angina take his or her own medication and rest.
- If the pain persists more than 10 minutes or stops and then returns, or if the patient has other heart attack symptoms, give emergency care as for a heart attack.

Respiratory Emergencies

Need to Know

Respiratory distress, or difficulty breathing, can be caused by many different illnesses and injuries. If

BOX 11-2

MEDICATION FOR HEART ATTACK

Aspirin has a clot-preventing benefit, and many healthcare providers advise their patients who are at risk for cardiovascular disease to take one low-dose aspirin daily unless they are allergic or experience side effects. Some benefit has been demonstrated for aspirin during a heart attack, and for patients who do not need to avoid aspirin, one adult aspirin is often recommended to be taken when experiencing heart attack symptoms. Follow your local protocol to allow the patient to take an adult aspirin (325 mg) or four baby aspirin (81 mg).

Nitroglycerin is another medication of benefit for a heart attack patient who has been prescribed this drug. Nitroglycerin increases blood flow through partially restricted arteries. Nitroglycerin is generally prescribed for angina, a condition of pain in the chest caused by narrowed coronary arteries. Forms of nitroglycerin include small tablets dissolved under the tongue; tablets that dissolve in the cheek;

extended-release capsules; oral sprays; and extended-release patches applied to the chest, usually daily **(Figure 11-2)**. Follow local protocol and the patient's prescribed instructions to help with the drug. The patient should be seated because dizziness or fainting may occur. Do not attempt to give the drug if the patient is unresponsive.

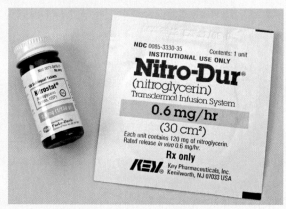

Figure 11-2 Nitroglycerin tablets and patch.

the cause of a patient's breathing problem is not obvious, look for other signs and symptoms that may reveal the problem.

- ☑ Respiratory distress can be a sign of many different injuries and medical emergencies.

- ☑ If you can determine the cause of a patient's breathing difficulty, give emergency care for that problem.

- ☑ Respiratory distress may also result as a sudden emergency in those with a chronic illness such as asthma or chronic obstructive pulmonary disease (COPD).

- ☑ If you do not know the cause of a patient's respiratory distress, give the general emergency care described in a later section.

■ Need to Recognize

Assessing Respiratory Distress

Perform the standard assessment:

1. Size up the scene before beginning emergency medical care.
2. Complete the initial assessment.
3. Perform a physical examination as appropriate.
4. Complete ongoing assessments.

Signs and Symptoms of Respiratory Distress:

- ♦ The patient is gasping or unable to catch his or her breath, and typically cannot speak a full sentence without pausing to breathe.

- Breathing is faster or slower, or deeper or shallower, than normal.
- Breathing involves sounds such as wheezing or gurgling.
- The patient feels dizzy or lightheaded or shows other signs of altered mental status.
- The patient's skin may look pale or ashen and be cool and moist; the lips and nail beds may be bluish.
- Lowered oxygen levels in the blood may make the patient feel dizzy or disoriented. **(Figure 11-3).**
- The patient may be sitting and leaning forward, hands on knees, in the tripod position. **(Figure 11-4).**
- An infant or child may have obviously flaring nostrils and more obvious movements of chest muscles with the effort to breathe.

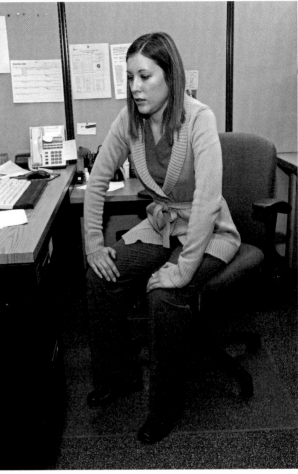

Figure 11-4 The tripod position is commonly assumed by patients in respiratory distress.

Because respiratory distress in an infant or child may rapidly progress to arrest, it is crucial to act quickly when an infant or child is having a problem breathing.

Emergency Care for Respiratory Distress

▶ Need to Do

Perform standard patient care:

1. Ensure EMS has been activated.
2. Take body substance isolation precautions.
3. Maintain the patient's airway and provide artificial ventilation if needed.
4. Comfort, calm, and reassure the patient while awaiting additional EMS resources.

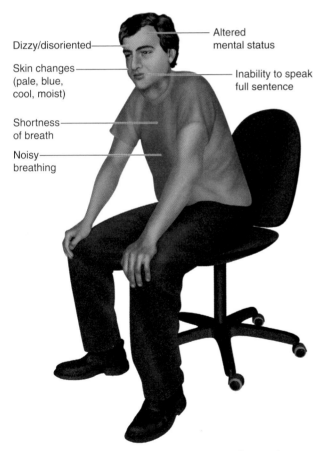

Dizzy/disoriented
Altered mental status
Skin changes (pale, blue, cool, moist)
Inability to speak full sentence
Shortness of breath
Noisy breathing

Figure 11-3 Signs and symptoms of respiratory distress.

In addition:

◆ Help the patient rest in a position of easiest breathing (often sitting up).

◆ Ask the patient about any prescribed medicine he or she may have, and help the patient take it if needed.

◆ Be prepared to give BLS, because respiratory distress may progress to respiratory arrest.

◆ Follow local protocol to administer supplemental oxygen if it is available and you are trained in its use.

Asthma

✓ Need to Know

Asthma is a common problem affecting 1 in 20 adults and 1 in 7 children. Asthma attacks in the United States result in more than 1.5 million emergency department visits a year and more than 5,500 deaths.

☑ Asthma is a chronic disease and cannot be cured.

☑ In an asthma attack, the airways become narrow and the person has difficulty breathing.

☑ Many asthma patients know they have the condition and carry medication, typically an inhaler, for emergency situations.

☑ Untreated, a severe asthma attack can be fatal.

Assessing Asthma

◼ Need to Recognize

Perform the standard assessment:

1. Size up the scene before beginning emergency medical care.

2. Complete the initial assessment.

3. Perform a physical examination as appropriate.

4. Complete ongoing assessments.

In addition:

◆ If a young child away from his or her usual caretakers has trouble breathing, always ask if he or she has medication.

Signs and symptoms of an asthma attack:

◆ Wheezing and difficulty breathing and speaking

◆ Dry, persistent cough

◆ Fear, anxiety

◆ Gray-blue skin

◆ Changing levels of responsiveness

Emergency Care for Asthma Attack

▶ Need to Do

Perform standard patient care:

1. Ensure that EMS has been activated if the patient does not know he or she has asthma (first attack). Local protocol may require activating EMS for all patients with respiratory distress.

2. Take body substance isolation precautions.

3. Maintain the patient's airway and provide artificial ventilation if needed.

4. Comfort, calm, and reassure the patient while awaiting additional EMS resources.

In addition:

◆ Follow local protocol to assist the patient in using his or her medication (usually in an inhaler) when these conditions are met:
  ◦ The patient confirms that it is an asthma attack.
  ◦ The patient identifies the inhaler as his or her asthma medication.
  ◦ The patient cannot self-administer the medication.

◆ Help the patient rest and sit in a position for easiest breathing.

◆ The patient may use the inhaler again if needed.

◆ If the breathing difficulty persists after using the inhaler, activate EMS.

◆ Follow local protocol to give supplemental oxygen if available and you are trained in its use.

◆ Never unnecessarily separate a child from a parent or loved one when providing care.

Helping a Child with an Inhaler

✓ Need to Know

A small child with asthma may need help using an inhaler during an asthma attack (**Figure 11-5**). The medication is usually a **bronchodilator,** a drug that relaxes the muscles of the airway, allowing airway passages to open wider (dilate) to make breathing easier. Use only the child's prescribed inhaler.

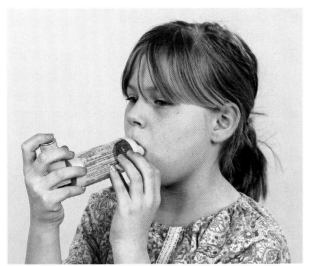

Figure 11-5 Many people with asthma use an inhaler.

Need to Do

The following general instructions may need modification for the specific medication device for a particular child.

1. Shake the inhaler.
2. If a spacer is used, position it on the inhaler. (A spacer is a tube or chamber that fits between the inhaler and the child's mouth.)
3. Have the child breathe out fully through the mouth.
4. With the child's lips around the inhaler mouthpiece or the spacer, have the child inhale slowly and deeply; press the inhaler down to release one spray of medication as the child inhales. (A facemask is generally used for an infant instead of a mouthpiece.)
5. Have the child hold his or her breath for up to 10 seconds if possible and then exhale slowly.
6. Reassess the patient's breathing.

Chronic Obstructive Pulmonary Disease

✔ Need to Know

Chronic obstructive pulmonary disease (COPD) includes **emphysema,** chronic bronchitis, and other conditions. More than 12 million people in the United States have emphysema or chronic bronchitis, leading to more than 124,000 deaths a year. Both of these diseases may cause respiratory distress and breathing emergencies.

▶ Need to Do

Patients with breathing difficulty related to COPD generally have the same signs and symptoms as respiratory distress:

- The emergency care is the same.
- Ask the patient whether he or she has a chronic disease.
- If the patient has a prescribed medication to help with breathing, you may help the person take the medication.

Hyperventilation

Hyperventilation is fast, deep breathing usually caused by anxiety or stress, although it may also be caused by some injuries or illnesses. The rapid breathing causes an imbalance in the body's levels of oxygen and carbon dioxide. Hyperventilation caused by emotional stress usually does not last long or become an emergency.

▦ Need to Recognize

Perform the standard assessment:

1. Size up the scene before beginning emergency medical care.
2. Complete the initial assessment.
3. Perform a physical examination as appropriate.
4. Complete ongoing assessments.

Signs and symptoms of hyperventilation:

- Fast, deep breathing
- Anxiety
- Confusion or dizziness
- Numbness or tingling of the fingers, toes, and lips
- Muscle twitching or cramping

▶ Need to Do

Perform standard patient care:

1. Ensure EMS has been activated.
2. Take body substance isolation precautions.
3. Maintain the patient's airway and provide artificial ventilation if needed.
4. Comfort, calm, and reassure the patient while awaiting additional EMS resources.

In addition:

- Help the person calm down, relax, and breathe more slowly. Breathing slowly along with the patient often helps the patient slow the breathing rate.

- Do not have the person breathe into and out of a bag, which could lower the person's oxygen level too far.
- Rapid breathing may also be caused by injury or sudden illness, so do not assume the patient is simply hyperventilating. Look for other signs of injury or illness, and ask the patient what happened to start the problem.
- If there are other signs or symptoms that suggest injury or illness, or if the patient's breathing does not return to normal in a few minutes, activate EMS.
- A patient who often has this problem should seek medical care, because some medical conditions can cause rapid breathing.

Do You Understand?

1. True or false: With an unknown sudden illness, do not give the patient anything to eat or drink.
2. Check off the common signs and symptoms of heart attack:
   - _____ Skin red and flushed
   - _____ Nausea
   - _____ Tingling in fingers and toes
   - _____ Headache
   - _____ Shortness of breath
   - _____ Pale skin
   - _____ Chest pain or pressure
   - _____ Unusual cheerfulness
   - _____ Sweating
   - _____ Dizziness
3. True or false: You cannot care for a person with difficulty breathing unless you know the specific cause of the problem.
4. What is the best thing a patient with asthma can do when having an asthma attack?

Altered Mental Status

Need to Know

Altered mental status refers to a sudden or gradual change from a person's normal responsiveness and awareness.

- The patient may be confused, disoriented, combative, drowsy, or partially or wholly unresponsive.

- The duration of altered mental status may be brief or prolonged.
- Altered mental status is not a condition but is a sign or symptom that may result from many different injuries and illnesses.
- Altered mental status is often a sign of deteriorating condition.

Following are among the many causes of altered mental status:

- Seizures
- Stroke
- Head injury
- Poisoning, drug use or overdose
- High fever
- Infection
- Diabetic emergencies
- Psychiatric conditions
- Any condition, such as respiratory problems, that causes lowered blood oxygen levels

Need to Recognize

Perform the standard assessment:

1. Size up the scene before beginning emergency medical care.
2. Complete the initial assessment.
3. Perform a physical examination as appropriate.
4. Complete ongoing assessments.

Need to Do

Perform standard patient care:

1. Ensure EMS has been activated.
2. Take body substance isolation precautions.
3. Maintain the patient's airway and provide artificial ventilation if needed.
4. Comfort, calm, and reassure the patient while awaiting additional EMS resources.

In addition:

- Determine the nature of the problem if possible. If the patient is responsive, gather a SAMPLE history.
- Place a patient who becomes unresponsive in the recovery position unless spinal injury is suspected.
- Have suction available.
- Consider the use of an airway adjunct because a patient with altered mental status may not be able to protect the airway.

If the person's altered mental status is due to drug or alcohol use, and the person is acting erratically or potentially violently, the situation may involve a behavioral emergency (see later section). Never assume, however, that a person with an altered mental status is intoxicated or is using drugs, because injuries and sudden illnesses such as a diabetic emergency can produce behavior easily mistaken for intoxication. Even if the person is intoxicated, he or she may still have an injury or illness requiring emergency care.

Fainting

✓ Need to Know

Fainting is caused by a temporary reduced blood flow to the brain.

☑ Fainting commonly occurs in hot weather or after prolonged inactivity.

☑ Fainting may be caused by fright, emotional shock, or a lack of food.

☑ A temporary drop in blood pressure caused by suddenly standing after prolonged sitting or lying down may cause dizziness or fainting, especially in the elderly.

In a young, healthy, nonpregnant adult, fainting is usually not a sign of a more serious problem, unless the person faints often or does not recover quickly. In someone who has heart disease, is pregnant, or is over age 65, fainting may be a sign of a serious problem requiring immediate medical attention.

◼ Need to Recognize

Perform the standard assessment:

1. Size up the scene before beginning emergency medical care.

2. Complete the initial assessment.

3. Perform a physical examination as appropriate.

4. Complete ongoing assessments.

Signs and symptoms of fainting:

▶ Before fainting, the patient may experience dizziness, sweating, nausea, a blurring or dimming of vision, and generalized weakness.

▶ Sudden brief loss of responsiveness and collapse

▶ Pale, cool skin; sweating

▶ Need to Do

Perform standard patient care:

1. Ensure EMS has been activated.

2. Take body substance isolation precautions.

3. Maintain the patient's airway and provide artificial ventilation if needed.

4. Comfort, calm, and reassure the patient while awaiting additional EMS resources.

In addition:

▶ If fainting is anticipated, have the person sit or lie down.

▶ Injury may result if the fainting person falls—try to catch the person and gently lower him or her to the floor.

▶ Unless the patient may have a spinal or leg injury, lay the patient down and raise his or her legs about 12 inches.

▶ Loosen constricting clothing.

▶ Check for possible injuries caused by falling.

▶ Be prepared to provide BLS if needed.

▶ Place a patient who remains unresponsive in the recovery position.

▶ Reassure the patient as he or she recovers.

▶ Do not pour or splash water on the patient's face, which could be aspirated into the lungs.

▶ Do not use ammonia inhalants or similar remedies to arouse the patient.

▶ Activate EMS if the patient does not regain responsiveness soon or faints repeatedly. Always call EMS for all older adults, people with heart disease, and pregnant women.

Stroke

✓ Need to Know

A stroke, also called a **cerebrovascular accident (CVA)** or a brain attack, is an interruption of blood flow to a part of the brain, killing nerve cells and affecting the patient's functioning.

☑ Stroke, like heart attack, may be caused by atherosclerosis. A blood clot may form in a brain artery or may be carried there in the blood and lodge in the artery, obstructing flow to that part of the brain.

☑ Stroke may also result when an artery in the brain ruptures or other factors impede flow.

☑ Some 700,000 people in the United States have a stroke each year, resulting in more than 162,000 deaths.

☑ Strokes are more common in older adults.

It is important to be able to identify the signs and symptoms of stroke because a stroke patient needs medical help immediately to decrease the chance of permanent damage.

Assessing Stroke

■■ Need to Recognize

Perform the standard assessment:

1. Size up the scene before beginning emergency medical care.
2. Complete the initial assessment.
3. Perform a physical examination as appropriate.
4. Complete ongoing assessments.

Signs and symptoms of stroke:

♦ Complaints of sudden, severe headache

♦ Complaints of sudden weakness or numbness in one side of the face, arm, or leg

♦ Dizziness, confusion, difficulty understanding speech

♦ Difficulty speaking or swallowing, vision problems

♦ Unequal pupils

♦ Changing levels of responsiveness or unresponsiveness

♦ Bladder or bowel incontinence

In addition:

♦ When gathering SAMPLE history information from a potential stroke patient, find out when the signs and symptoms first occurred, because the time may affect medical treatment. Ask family members or others present at the scene as well as the patient.

♦ The exact signs and symptoms vary somewhat depending on the exact site in the brain where an artery is blocked.

♦ Be careful not to attribute the patient's signs and symptoms to some other condition because it is important for medical care for stroke to begin as soon as possible.

The Cincinnati Prehospital Stroke Scale

The **Cincinnati Prehospital Stroke Scale (CPSS)** and other screening methods are used widely to

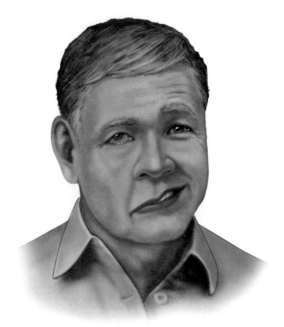

Figure 11-6 The facial droop of a stroke patient.

accurately and quickly identify a potential stroke patient. The CPSS uses three simple assessments:

1. Ask the patient to smile. (Only one side of the face makes a smile; the other side seems to "droop"; **Figure 11-6**).
2. Ask the patient, with eyes closed, to raise both arms out in front of the body. (One arm drifts down lower than the other in front of the body.)
3. Ask the patient to repeat a simple sentence such as: "You can't teach an old dog new tricks." (The patient slurs words, uses the wrong words, or cannot speak.)*

Emergency Care for Stroke

▶ Need to Do

Perform standard patient care:

1. Ensure EMS has been activated.
2. Take body substance isolation precautions.
3. Maintain the patient's airway and provide artificial ventilation if needed.
4. Comfort, calm, and reassure the patient while awaiting additional EMS resources.

In addition:

♦ Relay your stroke assessment to the arriving EMS crew so that they can quickly begin med-

Reprinted from The Annals of Emergency Medicine, 33(4): Kothari RU, Pancioli A, Liu T, Broderick J, Cincinnati Prehospital Stroke Scale, pp. 373-378. © 1999, with permission from The American College of Emergency Physicians.

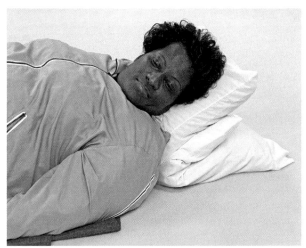

Figure 11-7 Turn a stroke patient's head to the side to allow drool or vomit to drain.

ical care at the scene and plan to transport the patient to the best setting for immediate care.

▶ Monitor the patient and be prepared to give BLS.

▶ Follow local protocol to administer oxygen if you are so trained.

▶ Have the patient lie on his or her back with head and shoulders slightly raised. Loosen a constrictive collar.

▶ If necessary, turn the patient's head to the side to allow drool or vomit to drain **(Figure 11-7).**

▶ Do not let a stroke patient eat or drink anything.

▶ Keep the patient warm and quiet until additional help arrives.

▶ Put an unresponsive patient in the recovery position.

Seizures

✔ Need to Know

Seizures, or convulsions, result from a brain disturbance caused by many different conditions.

☑ The brain's normal electrical activity becomes out of balance, resulting in sudden altered mental status and uncontrolled muscular contractions that cause jerking or shaking of the body.

☑ Seizures are rarely life threatening but are a serious emergency.

☑ Most seizures are caused by **epilepsy.** Epilepsy and seizures affect 2.5 million people of all ages in the United States. Approximately 181,000 new cases of seizures and epilepsy occur each year. About 10% of the U.S. population will experience a seizure in their lifetime.

Other causes include:

☑ Head injuries

☑ Low blood sugar in a person with diabetes

☑ Poisoning, including drugs and alcohol

☑ Electric shock

☑ High fever, especially in infants and young children

☑ Any condition causing low levels of oxygen

☑ Brain tumors

☑ Complications of pregnancy

Seizures follow a wide variety of different patterns, depending in part on the cause. The following are some of the more common types of seizures:

☑ **Complex partial seizures.** The person is conscious but does not interact normally with others and is not in control of movements or speech. They are called "partial" because only part of the brain is involved and typically only part of the body is affected. The person seems dazed and may mumble or wander. This type of seizure is often mistaken for a behavioral problem.

☑ **Absence seizures.** The person seems to stare blankly into space and does not respond to others. The seizure begins and ends abruptly, often lasting only a few seconds.

☑ **Generalized tonic clonic seizures.** Also called convulsions or grand mal seizures, the person loses consciousness and falls. The person is at first stiff (tonic) and then experiences jerking of muscles (clonic phase) throughout the body. Breathing may stop momentarily but restarts spontaneously. After the seizure, the person may be confused or agitated.

☑ **Febrile seizures.** Unrelated to epilepsy, febrile seizures are caused by high fever in infants or young children. The convulsions are similar to those of tonic clonic seizures, and the emergency care is the same, followed by measures to bring down the patient's body temperature.

Assessing Seizures

◼ Need to Recognize

Perform the standard assessment:

1. Size up the scene before beginning emergency medical care.

2. Complete the initial assessment.

3. Perform a physical examination as appropriate.

4. Complete ongoing assessments.

Signs and symptoms:

▶ Minor seizures: staring blankly ahead; slight twitching of lips, head, or arms and legs; other movements such as lip-smacking or chewing

▶ Major seizures: crying out and then becoming unresponsive; body becomes rigid and then shakes in convulsions; the jaw may clench

▶ Fever convulsions in young children: hot, flushed skin; violent muscle twitching; arched back; clenched fists

In addition:

▶ Seizures generally occur suddenly and without warning.

▶ Some patients have an unusual feeling in advance of the seizure called an **aura,** a generalized sensation or a hallucinated sensation involving any of the senses.

▶ Most patients are unresponsive and may vomit during the convulsion.

▶ Bowel or bladder incontinence may occur.

▶ The length of the seizure may be brief (less than 5 minutes) or prolonged.

▶ Patients are typically tired and sleep following the attack.

Emergency Care for Seizures

▶▶ Need to Do

Perform standard patient care:

1. Ensure EMS has been activated.

2. Take body substance isolation precautions.

3. Maintain the patient's airway and if the patient is bluish or breathing inadequately, provide artificial ventilation.

4. Comfort, calm, and reassure the patient while awaiting additional EMS resources.

In addition:

▶ Support the patient; do not worry about determining the cause of the seizure.

▶ Protect the patient from the environment. Move dangerous objects away and put something flat and soft under the head (**Figure 11-8**). Remove eyeglasses.

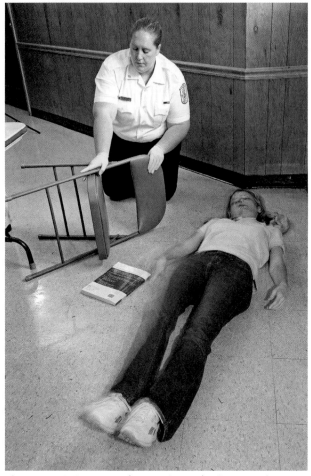

Figure 11-8 Protect the patient during a seizure.

▶ Loosen clothing around the neck to ease breathing.

▶ Never restrain the patient.

▶ Do not put anything in the patient's mouth.

▶ Have suction available; often seizure patients will have significant oral secretions and require suctioning.

▶ Look for a medical identification bracelet or necklace.

▶ Gently turn the person onto one side to help keep the airway clear if vomiting occurs.

▶ Protect the patient's modesty; ask bystanders to leave the area.

▶ For an infant or child with fever convulsions, sponge the body with lukewarm water to help cool the patient.

▶ Someone having a complex partial seizure may wander about; if the person is moving into a hazardous situation, gently guide the person away from danger.

- Keep track of how long the seizure lasts.
- Place an unresponsive patient in the recovery position after convulsions have ended unless there may be a spinal injury.
- Afterwards, the person is likely to be confused or disoriented and drowsy or agitated; be reassuring and help the person rest as needed.
- If the recovering patient seems agitated or angry, stay back but close enough nearby to prevent any dangers.
- Follow your local protocol for administering oxygen if it is available and you are so trained.
- Report your assessment findings to arriving EMS personnel. Observe and describe the seizure to arriving EMS personnel; this information may be important in determining the cause of the seizure.

Seizures in Special Circumstances

Need to Do

A person who has a seizure while in the water is at risk of aspirating water into the lungs or even drowning.

- Since a seizure lasts only a few minutes at most, do not try to move the person from the water but support him or her with the head tilted to keep water out of the person's mouth.
- After the seizure, help the person out of the water.
- If the person is not responsive, check for breathing and give CPR if needed.

Another special circumstance is a seizure that occurs in an airplane, a motor vehicle, or another confined area.

- If there are empty seats around the person, fold back the arm rests so the person can lie on his or her side across the seats with his or her head on a cushion.
- If there is no room to lie down, use pillows to protect the person's head from striking hard objects around the seat.
- Try to lean the person to one side to keep the airway open.

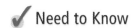 Do You Understand?

1. List at least eight causes of altered mental status.

_____ _____
_____ _____
_____ _____
_____ _____

2. What are the three assessments of the Cincinnati Prehospital Stroke Scale?

1. _____
2. _____
3. _____

3. What should you do for a patient having seizures?

a. Lay the patient facedown on the floor.
b. Ask others to help you hold the patient's head, arms, and legs still.
c. Put something flat and soft under the patient's head.
d. Put something wooden, like a pencil, between the patient's teeth.

Cold Emergencies

Body temperature problems may occur when the body becomes either cold or hot (**Box 11-3**).

Hypothermia

✔ Need to Know

When the body cannot make heat as fast as it loses it in a cold environment, **hypothermia** develops. Hypothermia is a generalized cold emergency in which the body temperature drops below 95°F (35°C).

- ☑ It does not have to be freezing cold for hypothermia to occur.
- ☑ Hypothermia can occur at almost any cool temperature if the body is unprotected, especially if the patient is wet, exposed a long time, or unable to restore body heat because of a medical condition.
- ☑ Because hypothermia alters a person's mental status, an affected patient may not take corrective actions to avoid continued exposure to cold.
- ☑ About 700 people die of hypothermia each year in the United States, about half of them over age 65.

BOX 11-3

BODY TEMPERATURE ISSUES

A fairly constant internal body temperature is necessary for many body functions. The body has several mechanisms to create heat or to lose heat when necessary. In most environments, these mechanisms, along with protective clothing and shelter, work well. With prolonged exposure to environmental temperature extremes, these mechanisms cannot maintain a constant internal temperature, particularly if the patient is injured or in poor health. Infants and the elderly also are more susceptible to temperature extremes.

Mechanisms for Staying Warm

Most of the body's heat is produced by metabolic processes that break down food nutrients to release energy for use by the body. Contraction of muscle tissue also produces heat. Shivering is an involuntary movement of muscles to produce additional heat when the body needs it.

The body also has mechanisms to conserve heat when needed. Much of the body's heat is lost to a cooler environment through the process of radiation. If the body is losing too much heat, blood vessels in the skin contract (**vasoconstriction**) so that less internal heat is brought by the blood to the skin to radiate away from the body.

Mechanisms for Staying Cool

Cold is the absence of heat: the body cannot produce cold when a hot environment or prolonged exertion threatens to raise body temperature. Nor can the body shut down heat-producing processes, because energy production must be continuous. The body must lose internal heat when necessary to prevent overheating. **Vasodilation** opens blood vessels to bring more blood to the skin where it can be radiated from the body.

Sweating is a second mechanism. Sweat evaporates from the skin's surface, cooling the skin by helping dissipate the heat brought to the surface by the blood.

The Body in Temperature Extremes

With extended exposure to temperature extremes, the body's normal heat production, heat conservation, and heat loss mechanisms often cannot maintain a normal body temperature.

With prolonged exposure to cold, especially when wet (water conducts heat away from the body much faster than it radiates into air), not enough heat can be conserved and shivering cannot produce enough heat to keep the body warm. The person develops hypothermia, a potentially life-threatening condition. Organ systems gradually begin to fail, leading eventually to death.

With prolonged exposure to heat, the body eventually cannot lose enough heat to maintain a normal temperature. Profuse sweating frequently leads to dehydration, which reduces blood volume and blood pressure. Even when the environment is not very hot, prolonged sweating caused by physical exertion can lead to dehydration. Without sufficient fluid, the body cannot cool itself adequately. Heatstroke occurs when the body temperature rises; sweating stops as the body attempts to conserve its remaining fluid. Without treatment, organ damage eventually occurs, followed by death.

Hypothermia and heatstroke are the most dangerous temperature injuries. Both develop gradually and worsen with continued exposure, so the signs and symptoms of a developing problem must be recognized early and the condition corrected before it becomes life threatening.

Rick Factors for Cold and Heat Injuries

- **Age:** Young children and the elderly are at greater risk. Young children are at risk because their shivering produces less heat due to their smaller muscle mass. They also have less body fat, making them more likely to lose heat. Older people are at a greater risk because a lower metabolic rate can result in a failure to maintain a normal body temperature, even indoors, when the air temperature falls below 64°F (17.8°C). Older adults are also more likely to have a chronic illness, such as diabetes, that increases the risk for hypothermia.

- **Illness or injury:** Many injuries and chronic health problems, particularly those affecting circulation or the heart, increase one's susceptibility to heat and cold injuries. For example, a patient in shock often produces insufficient body heat, making it important to keep a shock patient warm. The body responds less well to heat and cold in diabetes, infection, burns, head injuries, and other conditions.

- **Mental impairment:** Individuals with cognitive disabilities are generally less likely to take action to prevent hypothermia when exposed to cold.

- **Dehydration:** Not drinking enough fluid makes one more susceptible to both heat and cold emergencies.

- **Body type:** People with little body fat have a greater risk of hypothermia, because body fat slows environmental cooling. People with more body fat have a greater risk of a heat emergency.

- **Activity:** Those who work or exercise outdoors in hot environments are more likely to experience a heat emergency if they do not rest frequently and drink sufficient fluids. People outdoors in extreme cold are at greater risk for hypothermia, especially if not dressed properly or in situations where they may not be able to reach shelter.

- **Drugs and medications:** Many medications and drugs increase the risk for heat and cold injuries. Alcohol dilates blood vessels, making hypothermia more likely. It also reduces body fluid levels, making the person more susceptible

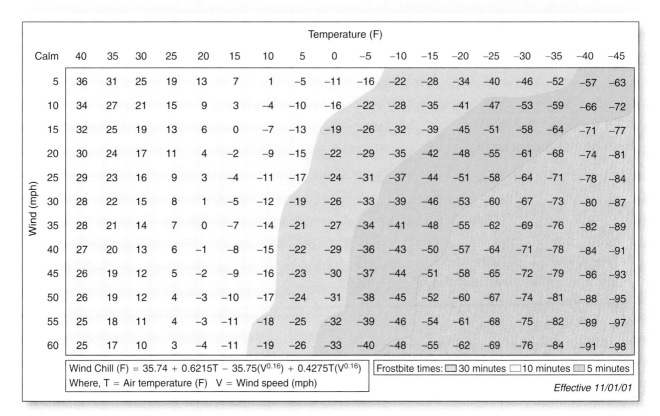

Wind Chill (F) = $35.74 + 0.6215T - 35.75(V^{0.16}) + 0.4275T(V^{0.16})$
Where, T = Air temperature (F)   V = Wind speed (mph)

Frostbite times: ☐ 30 minutes ☐ 10 minutes ☐ 5 minutes

Effective 11/01/01

Figure 11-9 Wind chill. (National Oceanic and Atmospheric Administration)

BOX 11-3 continued

to heatstroke. Alcohol and some other abused drugs can suppress shivering, thereby reducing heat production, and can prevent surface blood vessels from constricting. Many prescription medications also can increase a person's susceptibility to either heat or cold emergencies. As well, alcohol and drugs that affect the user's judgment often lead to the person taking risks or entering situations where a heat or cold emergency is more likely.

- **Environmental variables:** The risk of hypothermia is increased by becoming wet from rain or immersion in water. Wind also increases heat loss through the "wind chill" effect **(Figure 11-9)**. High humidity increases the risk of heat emergencies because sweat evaporates more slowly and provides less cooling effect, as shown in the heat index chart **(Figure 11-10)**.

Temperature (F) versus Relative Humidity (%)

F	90%	80%	70%	60%	50%	40%
80	85	84	82	81	80	79
85	101	96	92	90	86	84
90	121	113	105	99	94	90
95		133	122	113	105	98
100			142	129	118	109
105				146	133	121
110						135

HI	Possible Heat Disorder
80F–90F	Fatigue possible with prolonged exposure and physical activity.
90F–105F	Sunstroke, heat cramps, and heat exhaustion possible.
105F–130F	Sunstroke, heat cramps, and heat exhaustion likely, and heatstroke possible.
130F or greater	Heatstroke highly likely with continued exposure.

Figure 11-10 Heat index. (National Weather Service)

Hypothermia is a progressive problem, as the patient transitions from just feeling cold to mild hypothermia and eventually, unless warmed, to more serious symptoms and possibly to death. This progression may occur gradually, over hours or even days, or very quickly.

Assessing Hypothermia

Need to Recognize

Perform the standard assessment:

1. Size up the scene before beginning emergency medical care.
2. Complete the initial assessment.
3. Perform a physical examination as appropriate.
4. Complete ongoing assessments.

Signs and symptoms of hypothermia:

- The patient is in a cool or cold environment
- Pale, cool skin—even under clothing (check the patient's abdomen under clothing)
- Slow breathing
- Shivering, which may be uncontrollable (but stops in severe hypothermia)
- Decreasing mental status or motor function correlated with the degree of hypothermia
- The patient seems apathetic, confused, or irrational; displays mood changes; may be belligerent
- Lethargy, clumsy movements, drowsiness, dizziness
- Memory disturbances/confusion
- Reduced or a loss of touch or sensation
- The patient is less communicative, experiences speech difficulty
- Poor judgment; the patient may remove clothing
- Stiff or rigid posture, muscular rigidity, complaints of joint/muscle stiffness

Hypothermia may begin gradually, so it is crucial to recognize the first signs and symptoms to take early action:

- Shivering, numbness, lethargy, poor coordination, and slurred speech are early manifestations.
- Patients in early or mild hypothermia often experience the "umbles": mumbles, fumbles, stumbles.

◆ Infants may have bright red skin and little energy.

As body temperature drops, hypothermia progresses and becomes more serious:

◆ Shivering typically stops and the patient may not even feel cold.

◆ Breathing becomes shallow.

◆ Mental status continues to deteriorate.

◆ In severe cases, the patient becomes unresponsive and may stop breathing.

Emergency Care for Hypothermia

▶ Need to Do

Perform standard patient care:

1. Ensure EMS has been activated.

2. Take body substance isolation precautions.

3. Maintain the patient's airway and provide artificial ventilation if needed.

4. Comfort, calm, and reassure the patient while awaiting additional EMS resources.

In addition:

◆ Remove the patient from the cold environment.

◆ Protect the patient from further heat loss: Remove any wet clothing and cover the patient with a blanket.

◆ Have the patient lie down, and handle the patient gently because abrupt movement may cause a dysrhythmia.

◆ Follow local protocol to administer oxygen if it is available and you are so trained.

◆ Do not allow the patient to walk or exert him- or herself.

◆ Do not give the patient anything to eat or drink.

◆ Do not allow the patient to eat or drink stimulants; coffee, tea, or smoking may worsen the condition.

◆ Do not massage the skin or extremities.

◆ Do not immerse a patient with hypothermia in hot water or use direct heat (hot water bottle, heat lamp, heating pad) because rapid warming can cause heart problems.

◆ In an unresponsive patient, assess for a pulse for 30 to 45 seconds before starting CPR.

Localized Cold Injury: Frostbite

✓ Need to Know

Frostbite is the freezing or near-freezing of skin or deeper tissues. Frostbite occurs when the temperature is 32°F (0°C) or colder.

☑ Frostbite usually happens to exposed skin areas on the head or face, hands, or feet.

☑ Wind chill increases the risk of frostbite.

☑ Severe frostbite kills tissue and can result in gangrene, necessitating amputation of the body part.

Assessing Frostbite

■ Need to Recognize

Perform the standard assessment:

1. Size up the scene before beginning emergency medical care.

2. Complete the initial assessment.

3. Perform a physical examination as appropriate.

4. Complete ongoing assessments.

Signs and symptoms of frostbite:

◆ Early or superficial frostbite:
  ◦ Skin blanching: color does not return after palpation
  ◦ Skin remains soft
  ◦ The area is numb or feels tingly or aching when rewarmed

◆ Severe frostbite:
  ◦ Skin looks waxy and white, gray, yellow, or bluish **(Figure 11-11)**
  ◦ The area feels hard
  ◦ Swelling or blisters may be present
  ◦ The affected area may become painless
  ◦ After warming, the area becomes swollen and may blister and appear flushed with areas of purple and blanching, or it may be mottled and cyanotic

Emergency Care for Frostbite

▶ Need to Do

Perform standard patient care:

1. Ensure EMS has been activated.

2. Take body substance isolation precautions.

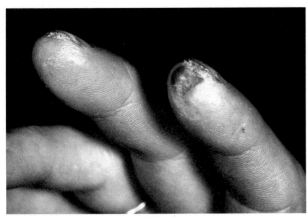
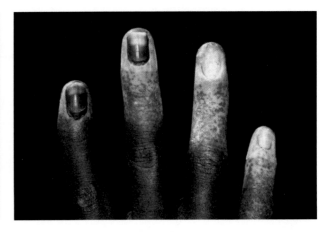

Figure 11-11 Severe frostbite.

3. Maintain the patient's airway and provide artificial ventilation if needed.

4. Comfort, calm, and reassure the patient while awaiting additional EMS resources.

In addition:

- Remove the patient from the cold environment, and remove wet or constrictive clothing.
- Check the patient for hypothermia.
- Protect the cold-injured area from further injury.
- For early or superficial injury:
  - Manually stabilize and cover the extremity.
  - Do not rub or massage the area.
  - Do not allow the area to be exposed to cold again.
- For late or deep cold injury:
  - Remove jewelry and tight clothing.
  - Cover the area with dry clothing or dressings. Put dry gauze or fluffy cloth between frostbitten fingers or toes **(Figure 11-12)**. Protect the area from being touched or rubbed by clothing or objects.
  - Do not:
    Break blisters
    Rub or massage the area
    Apply heat
    Rewarm the area
    Allow the patient to walk on the affected extremity

Remote Location Emergency Care

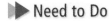 Need to Do

If the frostbitten area is at any risk of being refrozen, it should not be rewarmed, because

warming followed by freezing increases the tissue damage:

- If the extrication, rescue, or transport of a frostbite patient may subject the area to cold again, do not warm it.
- Wait for healthcare or EMS professionals to treat the frostbite.

If help will be delayed, and only if refreezing can be prevented, then severe frostbite can be rewarmed:

- Immerse the area in lukewarm—not hot—water (about 100 to 104°F; 37.8 to 40°C) for at least 20 minutes and up to 45 minutes.
- Never apply a direct heat source to frostbitten skin, such as heat lamp, hot water bottle, or heating pad, because of the risk of additional tissue damage.

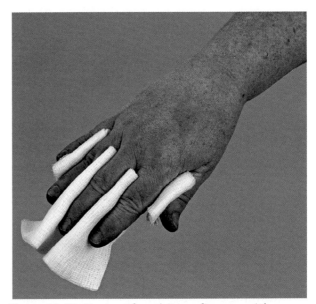

Figure 11-12 Protect frostbitten fingers with gauze or fluffy cloth.

Heat Emergencies

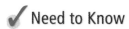 Need to Know

Heat exhaustion develops when the body becomes dehydrated in a hot environment. **Heatstroke,** with a seriously high body temperature, may develop from untreated heat exhaustion.

- ☑ Heatstroke causes a body temperature of 104°F (40°C) or higher and is more severe than heat exhaustion.
- ☑ Altered mental status occurs when heat exhaustion progresses into heatstroke.
- ☑ Heatstroke is a medical emergency and, if untreated, usually causes death.
- ☑ Most heatstroke deaths occur from exposure to a high temperature for a sustained period, including in settings where heat is generated, such as furnace rooms, factories, or vehicles.
- ☑ An average of 400 heat-related deaths a year have occurred in the United States.

Like hypothermia, heat emergencies are progressive:

- ☑ In the mild stage (heat exhaustion), the patient becomes dehydrated and the body is unable to cool itself.
- ☑ If the condition is not corrected, with continuing exposure, the body temperature begins to rise (heatstroke) and more serious symptoms occur, potentially leading to death.
- ☑ Prevention of life-threatening heatstroke depends on recognizing the early signs and symptoms and providing care before the condition becomes more serious.

Assessing Heat Exhaustion

◼◼ Need to Recognize

Perform the standard assessment:

1. Size up the scene before beginning emergency medical care.
2. Complete the initial assessment.
3. Perform a physical examination as appropriate.
4. Complete ongoing assessments.

Signs and symptoms of heat exhaustion:

- ◗ Sweating, pale or ashen moist skin (often cool)
- ◗ Thirst
- ◗ Fatigue, weakness, exhaustion
- ◗ Muscle cramps
- ◗ Later signs and symptoms:
  - ◦ Headache, dizziness, fainting
  - ◦ Nausea, vomiting
  - ◦ Fast, shallow breathing
  - ◦ Rapid heart rate

Emergency Care for Heat Exhaustion

▶ Need to Do

Perform standard patient care:

1. Ensure EMS has been activated.
2. Take body substance isolation precautions.
3. Maintain the patient's airway and provide artificial ventilation if needed.
4. Comfort, calm, and reassure the patient while awaiting additional EMS resources.

In addition:

- ◗ Move the patient from the heat to rest in a cool place. Loosen or remove unnecessary clothing.
- ◗ As long as the patient does not have altered mental status, give a sports drink or water to drink, but not liquids containing caffeine or alcohol (follow local protocol).
- ◗ Raise the legs 8 to 12 inches.
- ◗ Cool the patient with one of these methods **(Figure 11-13)**:
  - ◦ Put wet cloths on the forehead and body.
  - ◦ Sponge the skin with cool water.
  - ◦ Spray the skin with water from a spray bottle and then fan the area.
- ◗ Do not give a heat exhaustion or heatstroke patient salt tablets. If the patient is awake and alert, give a sports drink or water instead.
- ◗ If the patient is lethargic, nauseous, or vomiting, do not give any liquids.
- ◗ Seek medical care if the patient's condition worsens or does not improve within 30 minutes.
- ◗ Seek urgent medical attention if the patient has a heart condition or high blood pressure.

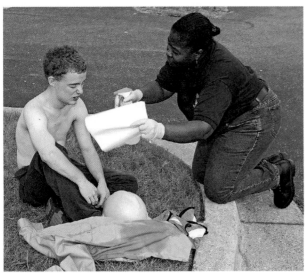

Figure 11-13 Cool a patient in heat exhaustion such as by spraying water and fanning.

Assessing Heatstroke

◼️ Need to Recognize

Perform the standard assessment:

1. Size up the scene before beginning emergency medical care.
2. Complete the initial assessment.
3. Perform a physical examination as appropriate.
4. Complete ongoing assessments.

◗ In heatstroke, the patient's skin is flushed and feels very hot to the touch. In heat exhaustion, the skin may be pale or ashen and clammy.

◗ In heatstroke, the patient becomes very confused and irrational and may become unresponsive or have convulsions. In heat exhaustion, the patient is dizzy or tired or may be irritable or have a headache.

Signs and symptoms of heatstroke:

◗ Skin that is flushed, dry, and hot to the touch; sweating usually has stopped

◗ Fast breathing

◗ Headache, dizziness, extreme confusion

◗ Irrational behavior

◗ Possible convulsions or unresponsiveness

Emergency Care for Heatstroke

▶ Need to Do

Perform standard patient care:

1. Ensure EMS has been activated.
2. Take body substance isolation precautions.
3. Maintain the patient's airway and provide artificial ventilation if needed.
4. Comfort, calm, and reassure the patient while awaiting additional EMS resources.

In addition:

◗ Move the patient to a cool place.

◗ Remove outer clothing.

◗ Cool the patient quickly with any means at hand, such as one of these methods **(Figure 11-14)**:

  ◦ Spray the skin with water from a spray bottle and then fan the area.
  ◦ Wrap the patient in a wet sheet and keep it wet.
  ◦ Sponge the patient with cold water.
  ◦ Put ice bags or cold packs beside the neck, armpits, and the femoral pressure point area near the groin.
  ◦ Partly submerge the patient in cool water and splash the skin (do not immerse fully in cold water).

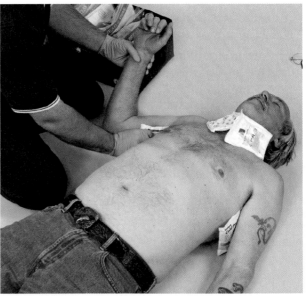

Figure 11-14 Cool a heatstroke patient by any means at hand, such as icepacks at the neck and armpits.

- Follow local protocol to administer oxygen if it is available and you are so trained.

- Keep cooling until the patient's temperature drops to about 101°F (38.3°C).

- Do not apply rubbing alcohol to the patient's skin.

- The patient should not take pain relievers or salt tablets.

- Do not give any beverage containing caffeine or alcohol.

- If the patient is nauseous, vomiting, or experiencing diminished mental status, do not give liquids.

- Monitor the patient and provide care as needed.

- Put an unresponsive patient in the recovery position and monitor breathing and vital signs.

- Protect a patient having convulsions from injury.

Diabetic Emergencies

✓ Need to Know

Diabetes is a group of related diseases in which blood sugar (**glucose**) levels are not well regulated by the body:

- ☑ The hormone **insulin,** produced in the pancreas, is needed for body cells to be able to use glucose.

- ☑ When insulin levels are too low, glucose levels rise too high. The problem results if the body is not producing enough insulin or if the body does not use the insulin well, a condition called *insulin resistance.*

- ☑ Currently, more than 18 million people in the United States have diabetes, 5 million of whom have not been diagnosed.

In a person with diabetes, the blood sugar level may become either too low or too high as a result of many interacting factors. Low blood sugar, called **hypoglycemia,** may result if a person:

- ☑ Takes too much insulin

- ☑ Does not eat enough of the right foods

- ☑ Uses blood sugar too fast through exercise or emotional stress

High blood sugar, called **hyperglycemia,** may result if a person:

- ☑ Takes too little insulin

- ☑ Eats too much high-sugar food

- ☑ Is not active

Untreated hypoglycemia or hyperglycemia can progress to a medical emergency without treatment. Hypoglycemia may cause abrupt or quickly developing altered mental status (drowsiness, disorientation) and a generalized feeling of sickness **(Figure 11-15).** Hyperglycemia may also cause altered mental status but occurs less commonly and develops more slowly.

- ☑ When taking the SAMPLE history of any patient who suddenly feels ill, ask about diabetes or other medical conditions, and look for a medical alert ID.

- ☑ If the patient is responsive and alert, he or she may know from experience whether the problem is hypoglycemia or hyperglycemia.

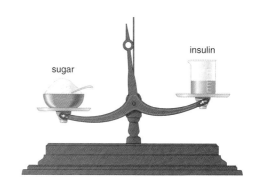

Hypoglycemia
- Sudden dizziness
- Shakiness
- Mood change
- Headache
- Confusion
- Pale skin
- Sweating
- Hunger

Hyperglycemia
- Frequent urination
- Drowsiness
- Dry mouth
- Thirst
- Shortness of breath
- Deep, rapid breathing
- Nausea/vomiting
- Fruity-smelling breath

Figure 11-15 Signs and symptoms of diabetic emergencies.

Assessing Diabetic Emergencies

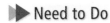 Need to Recognize

Perform the standard assessment:

1. Size up the scene before beginning emergency medical care.

2. Complete the initial assessment.

3. Perform a physical examination as appropriate.

4. Complete ongoing assessments.

Signs and symptoms of hypoglycemia:

♦ Sudden dizziness, shakiness, or mood change (even combativeness)

♦ Headache, confusion, difficulty paying attention

♦ Pale skin, sweating

♦ Hunger

♦ Clumsy, jerky movements

♦ Possible seizure

♦ The patient may appear to be intoxicated (slurred words, staggering gait, confusion, etc.)

Signs and symptoms of hyperglycemia:

♦ Frequent urination

♦ Drowsiness

♦ Dry mouth, thirst

♦ Shortness of breath, deep rapid breathing

♦ Breath that smells fruity

♦ Nausea, vomiting

♦ Eventual unresponsiveness

Emergency Care for Diabetic Emergencies

▶ Need to Do

Perform standard patient care:

1. Ensure EMS has been activated.

2. Take body substance isolation precautions.

3. Maintain the patient's airway and provide artificial ventilation if needed.

4. Comfort, calm, and reassure the patient while awaiting additional EMS resources.

In addition:

♦ Talk to the patient and confirm he or she has diabetes; look for a medical alert ID.

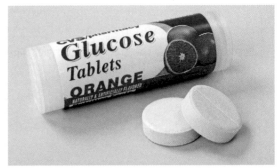

Figure 11-16 Diabetics often carry glucose tablets in case of low blood sugar.

♦ *For hypoglycemia:* Ensure the patient can maintain an open airway (for example, if the patient can speak), and follow local protocol to give the patient sugar: glucose gel or paste, 3 glucose tablets, 1/2 cup fruit juice, 1 or 2 sugar packets (but not non-sugar sweetener packets), or 5 to 6 pieces of hard candy **(Figure 11-16)**. If the patient still feels ill or has signs and symptoms after 15 minutes, give more sugar.

♦ If you cannot judge whether the patient has hypoglycemia or hyperglycemia, give sugar as for low blood sugar (following local protocol). If it happens that the patient has hyperglycemia, this additional sugar will not worsen the patient's condition, but it could solve the problem if the patient has low blood sugar.

♦ Follow local protocol to administer oxygen if it is available and you are so trained.

♦ If a diabetic patient becomes unresponsive, do not try to inject insulin or put food or fluids in the patient's mouth.

♦ If a patient becomes unresponsive or continues to have significant signs and symptoms, ensure EMS has been activated and monitor breathing.

♦ Put an unresponsive patient in the recovery position and monitor breathing and vital signs.

Glucose Paste for Hypoglycemia

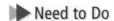 Need to Do

Some First Responders may have and be trained to use oral glucose paste or gel, which may be administered to a diabetic patient with signs and symptoms of hypoglycemia. The gel or paste form is generally safer for a patient with mild altered mental status who can still swallow and is not snoring or gagging. It is typically available in small, single-dose tubes **(Figure 11-17)**.

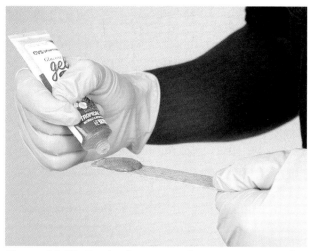

Figure 11-17 Oral glucose gel or paste may be given, following local protocol, to a diabetic patient experiencing hypoglycemia.

1. Squeeze a small amount of paste onto a tongue depressor.

2. Carefully spread the paste between the cheek and gums of the patient, where it will be quickly absorbed.

3. Continue to administer small doses until all of the tube has been used (or follow local protocol for the dose to administer).

Do You Understand?

1. You are called to a scene where a man who was working outside in the cold has just been brought inside. His movements are clumsy and he seems confused. One of your first actions should be to

   a. give him a warm drink.

   b. have him take off his outer clothes and sit close to a heater.

   c. send him to a hot shower.

   d. remove his damp clothing and warm him with a blanket.

2. List at least four ways to cool down a patient experiencing heatstroke.

   _____ _____

   _____ _____

3. You respond to a patient whose coworkers called 911 because she seemed suddenly ill. She is sitting at a table staring into space. When you ask her if she is okay, she does not seem to understand what you are saying. She

looks ill, her skin is pale, and she is sweating even though the room is not warm. Her coworkers tell you that she is diabetic and that she might have skipped lunch today. You cannot be sure whether she has low or high blood sugar. What should you do?

Poisoning

Swallowed Poisons

✔ Need to Know

Most cases of poisoning involve swallowed substances. Depending on the type and amount of poison, the effects may begin almost immediately or may be delayed.

☑ Emergency care is most effective if given as soon as possible after the poison is swallowed. In some cases, the effects can be prevented or minimized by acting quickly.

☑ Poisoning is like sudden illness in that often there is no visible injury and you may not know immediately what happened.

☑ The patient may be unresponsive or, even if responsive, may be confused and disoriented and unable to tell you what happened.

Assessing Swallowed Poisoning

■■ Need to Recognize

Perform the standard assessment:

1. Size up the scene before beginning emergency medical care.

2. Complete the initial assessment.

3. Perform a physical examination as appropriate.

4. Complete ongoing assessments.

In addition:

▶ Look for any sign that the patient may be poisoned. Look for containers nearby or any clue that the person was using a substance or product.

▶ Ask others at the scene if anyone saw anything or knows what the person was doing when the problem occurred.

▶ If the patient is responsive and identifies a substance to which he or she was exposed, try to learn how much the person may have swallowed and how long ago.

The specific signs and symptoms of poisons depend on the particular substance and many other factors, although many poisons cause similar general effects:

- A general appearance of not looking well
- Abdominal pain or cramps
- Nausea and vomiting, diarrhea
- Altered mental status; the patient may become unresponsive
- Burns, stains, or odors around the patient's mouth
- Dilated or constricted pupils
- An abnormal breathing pattern

Emergency Care for Swallowed Poison

▶ Need to Do

Perform standard patient care:

1. Ensure EMS has been activated.
2. Take body substance isolation precautions.
3. Maintain the patient's airway and provide artificial ventilation if needed.
4. Comfort, calm, and reassure the patient while awaiting additional EMS resources.

In addition:

- Be aware that the condition of a poisoning patient may change rapidly.
- Emergency care depends on the patient's condition.
- Follow local protocol to administer oxygen if it is available and you are so trained.
- For an unresponsive patient:
  - Ensure EMS has been activated.
  - Check breathing and provide BLS if needed.
  - Put a breathing, unresponsive patient in the recovery position, because of the risk of vomiting.
  - Continue to monitor breathing and vital signs.
- For a responsive patient:
  - If the mouth or lips are burned by a corrosive chemical, rinse the mouth with cold water (without swallowing).
  - Follow local protocol to call the Poison Control Center (PCC) or medical direction and follow their instructions (Box 11-4).
  - Do not give any substance to eat or drink unless instructed by the PCC or medical direction.

BOX 11-4

POISON CONTROL CENTERS

A system of **Poison Control Centers (PCC)** exists throughout the United States to provide information and treatment recommendations for all types of poisonings. All can be reached through one number 24 hours a day: 1-800-222-1222. Your call will be routed to the regional PCC in your area. The PCC usually has more accurate and up-to-date information than many healthcare providers. Personnel staffing each PCC have information about all known poisons and can advise what emergency care to give in a specific poisoning case. Follow your local protocol for situations in which you may call the PCC rather than calling medical direction or waiting for arriving EMS personnel.

The American Association of Poison Control Centers (AAPCC) also provides much valuable information about how to prevent poisonings and information about specific poisons (http://www.aapcc.org).

- Do not follow instructions on household product labels because they may be incorrect.
- Depending on the poison, you may be directed to take any of the various actions:
  - Some poisons may be diluted by having the patient drink water or milk.
  - With some poisons, the patient may benefit from drinking a solution of activated charcoal, which absorbs some types of poison (Figure 11-18). Follow local protocol and the instructions of the PCC to administer activated charcoal.

Inhaled Poisons

✓ Need to Know

Various gases and fumes may be present in both home and work settings.

☑ Products such as paints, thinners, and many chemicals give off toxic fumes.

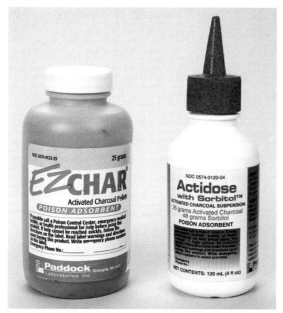

Figure 11-18 The Poison Control Center may advise giving activated charcoal in some cases of poisoning.

☑ Inhaled poisons also include gases that may escape from pipelines or tanks being transported.

☑ Whenever you smell gas or have other evidence of a leak, stay away from the scene and let a specially trained hazardous materials team manage the situation.

   Carbon monoxide is especially dangerous because it is invisible, odorless, and tasteless—and lethal.

☑ This gas results in more fatal unintentional poisonings in the United States than any other poison.

☑ Carbon monoxide may be present from motor vehicle or boat exhaust, a faulty furnace, a kerosene heater, industrial equipment, a poorly vented fireplace or wood stove, or fire.

Assessing Inhaled Poisoning

■ Need to Recognize

Perform the standard assessment:

1. Size up the scene before beginning emergency medical care. Do not enter the scene without protection if the inhaled poison may still be in the air.

2. Complete the initial assessment.

3. Perform a physical examination as appropriate.

4. Complete ongoing assessments.

Signs and symptoms of inhaled poison:

◗ Breathing difficulty

◗ Headache

◗ Dizziness, lightheadedness, confusion, weakness

◗ Nausea, vomiting

◗ Chest pain

◗ Convulsions

◗ Changing levels of responsiveness

Emergency Care for Inhaled Poisoning

▶ Need to Do

Perform standard patient care:

1. Ensure EMS has been activated.

2. Take body substance isolation precautions.

3. Maintain the patient's airway and provide artificial ventilation if needed.

4. Comfort, calm, and reassure the patient while awaiting additional EMS resources.

In addition:

◗ Immediately move the patient into fresh air.

◗ Monitor the patient's breathing and vital signs, and give BLS as needed.

◗ Put an unresponsive patient in the recovery position.

◗ Loosen tight clothing around the neck or chest.

Alcohol and Drug Emergencies

✓ Need to Know

Excessive alcohol consumption causes problems that may lead to a medical emergency. In some cases, someone who behaves as if intoxicated may not be under the influence of alcohol or a drug but may be experiencing a problem such as a diabetic emergency that causes altered mental status.

☑ Drinking a large amount of alcohol in a short time can cause alcohol poisoning, which may result in unresponsiveness, seizures, or death.

☑ Alcohol has depressant effects on the respiratory system and can cause an overdose similar to that of depressant drugs.

Illicit drugs and prescription drugs used for non-medical purposes cause a wide variety of effects, depending on the type and amount of drug used.

☑ You do not need to know the type of drug taken to provide emergency care.

☑ Consider the possibility of drug abuse or overdose whenever a patient's behavior or signs and symptoms cannot otherwise be explained.

An accidental overdose of a prescription medication may similarly result in a wide range of behaviors and symptoms, depending on the drug.

Assessing Alcohol and Drug Emergencies

◼ Need to Recognize

Perform the standard assessment:

1. Size up the scene before beginning emergency medical care.
2. Complete the initial assessment.
3. Perform a physical examination as appropriate.
4. Complete ongoing assessments.

In addition:

▶ Question the patient and others present at the scene about the drug or substance used, the amount used, and when it was used. Give this information to arriving EMS personnel.

▶ Assess the patient for injuries or illness. Do not assume alcohol or a drug is the factor, or the only factor, involved.

Signs and symptoms of alcohol poisoning:

▶ Smell of alcohol about the person
▶ Flushed, moist face
▶ Vomiting
▶ Slurred speech, staggering
▶ Fast heart rate
▶ Impaired judgment and motor skills
▶ Agitated or combative behavior
▶ Changing levels of responsiveness, coma

Signs and symptoms of drug abuse or overdose:

▶ Signs and symptoms similar to alcohol poisoning
▶ Dilated or constricted pupils of the eye

▶ Stumbling, clumsiness, drowsiness, incoherent speech
▶ Difficulty breathing (very slow or fast)
▶ Changing levels of responsiveness
▶ Unusual or erratic behavior
▶ Agitated or combative behavior
▶ The presence of drug paraphernalia (e.g., needles and syringes; eye droppers; burnt spoons; straws or rolled-up dollar bills used for snorting, pipes; glass bulbs; razor blades; paper or plastic bags reeking of inhalants; or bottles of pills, powder, or liquid)

Emergency Care for Alcohol and Drug Emergencies

▶ Need to Do

Perform standard patient care:

1. Ensure EMS has been activated.
2. Take body substance isolation precautions.
3. Maintain the patient's airway and provide artificial ventilation if needed.
4. Comfort, calm, and reassure the patient while awaiting additional EMS resources.

In addition:

▶ For a responsive patient:
  ○ Stay with the patient and protect from injury (take away car keys).
  ○ Do not let the patient lie down on his or her back.
  ○ Care for any injuries.
  ○ For a responsive patient known to have taken a drug or other substance, follow local protocol to call the PCC and follow their instructions.

▶ For an unresponsive patient:
  ○ Position the patient in the recovery position (preferably on left side to reduce the risk of vomiting); be prepared for vomiting.
  ○ Monitor the patient's breathing and provide BLS if necessary.
  ○ In a cold environment, an intoxicated patient is likely to experience hypothermia because dilated peripheral blood vessels allow the body's heat to escape more easily. Take steps to keep the patient warm.

- For an injured intoxicated patient:
  - Do not rely on the patient's perception of an injury to guide your care, because alcohol may keep the patient from feeling pain.
  - Give emergency care as you would if the patient were unresponsive, based on your assessment of the signs of injury or illness rather than reported symptoms.
  - If the mechanism of injury suggests the patient could have a spinal injury, do not move the patient but keep the head aligned with the body.
- Put an unresponsive patient in the recovery position (preferably on left side to reduce the risk of vomiting). Monitor breathing, and give BLS as needed.
- Provide care for any condition that occurs (e.g., seizures, shock, cardiac arrest).
- Keep the patient from harming him- or herself or others.
- Do not try to induce vomiting, which may cause further harm and is unlikely to help the patient.
- Alcohol and some drugs make some people hostile and violent. Stay a distance away and call law enforcement if violence threatens.
- When illegal drugs are involved, this is also a crime scene (see Chapter 3).

Alcohol Withdrawal

✓ Need to Know

Someone who drinks heavily for a long time may develop a physical dependence on alcohol. Withdrawal from alcohol dependence may cause **delirium tremens** ("the DTs"), an altered mental status characterized by confusion, disorientation, agitation, and altered perception such as hallucinations or illusions. Other signs and symptoms include hand trembling, head shaking, nausea, vomiting, and seizures.

Give the same emergency care as for an intoxicated patient, including the use of the recovery position for an unresponsive patient and monitoring breathing.

Bites and Stings

✓ Need to Know

The bites and stings of some snakes, spiders, insects, and marine life can result in a medical emergency caused by either an injected venom or a severe allergic reaction to the bite or sting. The bites and stings from the following are poisonous:

- ☑ Snakes
  - Rattlesnakes
  - Copperheads
  - Water moccasins (cottonmouths)
  - Coral snakes
- ☑ Spiders
  - Black widow
  - Brown recluse
- ☑ Some scorpion species
- ☑ Portuguese man-of-war and some jellyfish

Stings from bees, wasps, and other insects can cause life-threatening allergic reactions, called anaphylaxis, in patients with severe allergies to them.

Assessing Bites and Stings

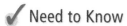 Need to Recognize

Perform the standard assessment:

1. Size up the scene before beginning emergency medical care.
2. Complete the initial assessment.
3. Perform a physical examination as appropriate.
4. Complete ongoing assessments.

In addition:

- Check the scene and try to identify the biting or stinging creature, but do not attempt to capture it.
- Check the patient's skin for signs of a bite or sting.

General signs and symptoms of many bites and stings:

- Pain or burning sensation at the site
- Redness and swelling at the site
- Depending on the species:
  - Difficulty breathing
  - Numbness or muscle paralysis
  - Nausea and vomiting
  - Blurred vision
  - Drowsiness or confusion, weakness
  - Signs of shock
- Possible allergic reaction

Emergency Care for Bites and Stings

▶▶ **Need to Do**

Perform standard patient care:

1. Ensure EMS has been activated.

2. Take body substance isolation precautions.

3. Maintain the patient's airway and provide artificial ventilation if needed.

4. Comfort, calm, and reassure the patient while awaiting additional EMS resources.

In addition:

♦ Have the patient lie down and stay calm. (Do not move the patient unless absolutely necessary.)

♦ Wash the wound with soap and water.

♦ Remove jewelry or tight clothing before swelling begins.

♦ Do not put a tourniquet on the patient.

♦ Do not cut the wound open to try to drain or suck out the venom.

♦ Remove the stinger and venom sac from the skin by scraping it away gently with a piece of plastic (not a knife blade); grasping it with your fingers may result in additional venom being squeezed into the skin.

♦ Observe the patient for any signs or symptoms of allergic reaction (difficulty breathing, swelling in other areas, anxiety, nausea or vomiting) and treat for shock.

♦ If the patient knows he or she is allergic to bee or wasp stings and has an **EpiPen**® or other emergency medication, follow local protocol to assist the patient with the medication.

♦ Place an unresponsive patient in the recovery position, monitor breathing and vital signs, and give BLS as needed.

Allergic Reactions (Anaphylaxis)

✔ **Need to Know**

Anaphylaxis, or anaphylactic shock, is a severe allergic reaction following exposure to a substance.

☑ The patient's airway may swell, making breathing difficult or impossible.

☑ The signs and symptoms of anaphylactic shock may begin within minutes, even seconds, of the patient's contact with the allergen.

☑ As a general rule, the more quickly the reaction occurs, the more serious it is likely to be.

The most common causes of anaphylaxis are:

☑ Certain drugs (such as penicillins or sulfa)

☑ Certain foods (such as peanuts, shellfish, eggs)

☑ Insect stings and bites (such as bees or wasps)

Assessing Anaphylaxis

■■ **Need to Recognize**

Perform the standard assessment:

1. Size up the scene before beginning emergency medical care.

2. Complete the initial assessment.

3. Perform a physical examination as appropriate.

4. Complete ongoing assessments.

In addition:

♦ In the SAMPLE history, always ask about allergies and recent things they ate or drank.

♦ With patients with a known severe allergy, ask whether they have emergency medication with them.

Signs and symptoms of anaphylaxis:

♦ Early signs and symptoms:
   ◦ Skin flushing, itching or burning, and rash
   ◦ Swelling of the face and neck, puffy eyes
   ◦ Sneezing, watery eyes and nose
   ◦ Coughing or a feeling of a tickle or lump in the throat that does not go away
   ◦ Nausea, vomiting

♦ Developing signs and symptoms:
   ◦ Anxiety, agitation
   ◦ A feeling that the throat is closing and the chest is becoming tight
   ◦ Rapid, weak pulse
   ◦ Difficulty breathing
   ◦ Coughing, wheezing, or hoarseness
   ◦ Altered mental status
   ◦ Severe headache
   ◦ Weakness or dizziness
   ◦ Pale or ashen skin or cyanosis (bluish color of the lips and nail beds)

Emergency Care for Anaphylaxis

▶▶ **Need to Do**

Perform standard patient care:

1. Ensure EMS has been activated.

2. Take body substance isolation precautions.

3. Maintain the patient's airway and provide artificial ventilation if needed.

4. Comfort, calm, and reassure the patient while awaiting additional EMS resources.

In addition:

- Follow local protocol to administer oxygen if it is available and you are so trained.

- Help the patient into a position for easiest breathing.

- Follow local protocol to help a responsive patient use his or her emergency epinephrine kit **(Box 11-5)**.

- Put a breathing, unresponsive patient (if no suspected spinal injury) in the recovery position, monitor breathing and vital signs, and be prepared to give BLS.

Do You Understand?

1. Check off the common signs and symptoms of a swallowed poison.

_____ Nausea	_____ Red lips
_____ Uncontrolled shaking	_____ Vomiting
_____ Dizziness	_____ Unresponsiveness
_____ Drowsiness	_____ Hyperactivity

2. Check off appropriate actions to take for a person with a drug or medication overdose:

_____ Position an unresponsive patient on the back with legs raised (shock position).

_____ Call the Poison Control Center or medical direction for a responsive patient.

BOX 11-5

EMERGENCY EPINEPHRINE KITS

Some patients with severe allergy carry an emergency epinephrine kit such as an EpiPen®, EpiPen Jr.® (for children), or Anakit®. This medication usually will stop the anaphylactic reaction. Ask a patient about this and, if allowed by local protocol and if needed, help the patient open and use the kit.

The EpiPen® is removed from its case and the cap is removed. The tip is pressed firmly against the outer thigh, causing the medica-

tion to be injected. The tip is held in place 5 to 10 seconds. Then the injector is removed and disposed of properly in a biohazard container. The injection site is massaged for a few seconds. The effects of the emergency epinephrine generally last 15 minutes. You may observe the patient experiencing the side effects of epinephrine: fast heartbeat, breathing difficulty, nausea and vomiting, dizziness or nervousness, and headache.

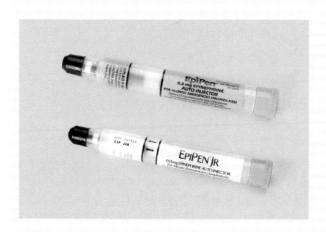

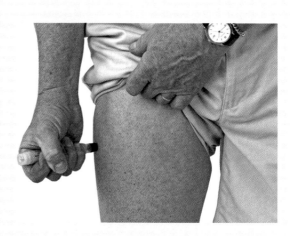

_____ Allow a responsive patient to lie in any position he or she chooses.

_____ Check for injuries that may require emergency care.

_____ Induce vomiting if the person is responsive.

_____ Base emergency care for an injury on the patient's reported level of pain.

_____ Try to find out what the person took.

3. The major risk for a patient in anaphylaxis is

   a. swelling around the eyes.

   b. heart attack.

   c. internal bleeding.

   d. breathing problems.

Severe Abdominal Pain

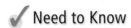 Need to Know

Abdominal injuries are described in Chapter 13. Sudden severe abdominal pain, called an **acute abdomen,** may also result from a medical condition that becomes a serious medical emergency. Many medical problems can cause such pain, but it is not necessary to determine the cause.

Assessing Severe Abdominal Pain

▪ Need to Recognize

Perform the standard assessment:

1. Size up the scene before beginning emergency medical care.

2. Complete the initial assessment.

3. Perform a physical examination as appropriate.

4. Complete ongoing assessments.

In addition:

♦ In the SAMPLE history, gather detailed information about the nature and location of the pain and give this information to arriving EMS personnel.

Emergency care is needed for severe abdominal pain in these situations:

In adults:

♦ Sudden, severe, intolerable pain, or pain that causes awakening from sleep

♦ Pain that begins in the general area of central abdomen and later moves to the lower right

♦ Pain accompanied by fever, sweating, black or bloody stool, or blood in the urine

♦ Pain in pregnancy or accompanying abnormal vaginal bleeding

♦ Pain accompanied by dry mouth, dizziness on standing, or decreased urination

♦ Pain accompanied by difficulty breathing

♦ Pain accompanied by vomiting blood or a greenish-brown fluid

In young children:

♦ Pain that occurs suddenly, stops, and then returns without warning

♦ Pain accompanied by red or purple, jelly-like stool; or with blood or mucus in the stool

♦ Pain accompanied by greenish-brown vomit

♦ Pain with a swollen abdomen that feels hard

♦ Pain with a hard lump in the lower abdomen or groin area

Emergency Care for Severe Abdominal Pain

▶ Need to Do

Perform standard patient care:

1. Ensure EMS has been activated.

2. Take body substance isolation precautions.

3. Maintain the patient's airway and provide artificial ventilation if needed.

4. Comfort, calm, and reassure the patient while awaiting additional EMS resources.

In addition:

♦ Follow local protocol to administer oxygen if available and you are so trained.

♦ Allow the patient to assume the position of greatest comfort.

♦ Be prepared for vomiting.

♦ Do not give the patient anything to eat or drink.

Behavioral Emergencies

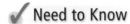 Need to Know

The process of giving emergency care is sometimes complicated by the patient's behavior. Many injuries and medical emergencies may cause altered mental status, which can lead to a patient behaving in unusual or unpredictable ways. Behavior is the manner in which a person acts in any way, including physical and mental activities.

- ☑ Injury and illness often cause emotional responses that may affect how emergency care must be given.
- ☑ Other patients may have emotional problems such as panic reactions, anxiety, or depression that also must be addressed.

Behavioral emergencies involve situations in which the patient's behavior, whether caused by the injury or illness or by personality or mental health factors, results in or complicates an emergency situation. In addition, the patient may manifest self-destructive behavior such as becoming suicidal or may be a danger to others with threatening behavior or violence.

Common causes of altered behavior include:

- ☑ Situational stresses
- ☑ Illness or injury
- ☑ Low blood sugar
- ☑ Low oxygen levels
- ☑ Inadequate blood flow to the brain
- ☑ Head trauma
- ☑ Environmental temperature extremes
- ☑ Poisoning; mind-altering substances, including alcohol and drugs
- ☑ Seizures
- ☑ Stroke
- ☑ High fever
- ☑ Psychiatric problems

Assessing Behavioral Emergencies

◼ Need to Recognize

Perform the standard assessment:

1. Size up the scene before beginning emergency medical care.
2. Complete the initial assessment.
3. Perform a physical examination as appropriate.
4. Complete ongoing assessments.

In addition:

- ◆ Assess the patient's mental status by observing:
  - ○ Appearance
  - ○ Actions
  - ○ Speech
  - ○ Orientation for time, person, and place

- ◆ Assess the potential for violence:
  - ○ Check the scene for potential weapons.
  - ○ In the history, ask family members and bystanders about any known history of aggression or combativeness.
  - ○ Observe the patient's posture: whether he or she stands or sits in a position that threatens self or others (e.g., may have clenched fists, be holding lethal objects, or have tense muscles).
  - ○ Observe what the patient says and how: whether he or she is yelling or verbally threatens harm to self or others, or seems to be hallucinating or yelling at someone not present.
  - ○ Consider the warning signs for suicide **(Box 11-6).**
  - ○ Observe the patient's physical activity: watch for movement toward you and quick irregular movements.
  - ○ Observe the patient's emotional mood, such as being uncontrollably angry, or kicking or throwing things.

BOX 11-6

SUICIDE RISK FACTORS AND WARNING SIGNS

Risk Factors
- Mental disorders, including depression
- History of substance abuse
- Feelings of hopelessness
- Recent emotional crisis or painful illness
- Impulsive or aggressive tendencies
- Past attempts at suicide

Warning Signs
- Talking about suicide (it is a myth that people who talk about it rarely do it)
- Comments about feeling hopeless or worthless
- Taking risks that could cause death, such as driving too fast
- Loss of interest in one's past activities
- Suddenly and unexpectedly seeming calm or happy after being sad

Emergency Care for Behavioral Emergencies

▶ Need to Do

Perform standard patient care:

1. Ensure EMS has been activated.

2. Take body substance isolation precautions.

3. Maintain the patient's airway and provide artificial ventilation if needed.

4. Comfort, calm, and reassure the patient while awaiting additional EMS resources.

In addition:

▸ Do not leave the patient alone.

▸ Consider the need for law enforcement personnel. Be prepared to leave the scene if necessary to maintain personal safety, because such emergencies are frequently unsafe.

▸ Give any medications or drugs you find to arriving EMS resources.

▸ Do not assume the patient is intoxicated, using drugs, or otherwise impaired, because the patient's behavior may result from a medical condition. Even if you smell alcohol on the patient's breath, do not assume a problem is due only to intoxication.

▸ Make a special effort to calm and reassure the patient:
   - Identify yourself and let the patient know you are there to help.
   - Ask for the patient's name, and use it when speaking to him or her.
   - Inform the patient what you are about to do.
   - Ask questions in a calm, reassuring voice.
   - In cultures where it is acceptable, make good eye contact, and stay at the patient's eye level.
   - Without being judgmental, allow the patient to tell what happened and what is troubling him or her.
   - Show you are listening by rephrasing or repeating part of what the patient says.
   - Acknowledge the patient's feelings and restate that you are there to help.
   - Maintain a comfortable distance, and avoid unnecessary physical contact. Do not make quick moves.
   - Respond honestly to patient's questions; do not lie to the patient.
   - Do not threaten, challenge, or argue with disturbed patients.
   - Do not "play along" with visual or auditory hallucinations, but do not challenge them.
   - Involve trusted family members or friends in care activities.
   - Be prepared to stay at the scene for a long time. Always remain with the patient.
   - Call for additional help if needed.

Restraining Patients

✔ Need to Know

A patient is restrained only if he or she is a danger to self or others. Most First Responders do not restrain patients. Restrain a patient only if you have been trained to do so and this is part of your local protocol, which may require first contacting medical direction and/or law enforcement.

☑ Before using a **restraint,** have police present, if possible. Work with responding EMS personnel.

☑ When restraining a patient, avoid unreasonable force. Use only as much force as needed to keep the patient from injuring himself or others.

☑ You may also use reasonable force to defend yourself or others against an attack by an emotionally disturbed patient.

☑ Realize that after a period of combativeness and aggression, some apparently calm patients may cause sudden, unexpected injury to self or others.

☑ Avoid acts or physical force that may cause injury to the patient.

Reasonable force also depends on the circumstances, including the:

☑ Patient's size, strength, and gender

☑ Patient's abnormal behavior

☑ Patient's mental state

☑ Method of restraint

Legal Considerations

✔ Need to Know

Patients in behavioral emergencies are more likely to threaten or make false accusations about responders' actions, including accusations of sexual misconduct. To protect yourself while providing emergency care:

☑ Document the patient's abnormal behavior.

☑ Ensure others are present as witnesses.

☑ When possible, have same-sex responders provide care.

Emotionally disturbed patients often resist treatment.

☑ Attempt to get the patient's consent, witnessed by others. Consent reduces the risk of later legal actions.

☑ If the patient threatens to harm him- or herself, and you, or others, have a reasonable belief that this may occur, you can provide care against the patient's will if it is safe to do so.

☑ The assistance of law enforcement personnel is usually required.

 Do You Understand?

1. True or false: For a patient experiencing severe abdominal pain, follow local protocol to administer oxygen if it is available and you are so trained.

2. True or false: People who talk about suicide rarely do it.

3. List at least four factors that affect whether the force used to restrain a patient is reasonable:

_____   _____

_____   _____

Conclusion

First Responders frequently encounter patients experiencing medical emergencies. Although medical emergencies may result from many different conditions, you do not have to identify the patient's specific illness before giving emergency care. The general approach is the same for all sudden illness emergencies. Always ensure EMS has been activated, and provide supportive care and Basic Life Support if needed.

Key Terms

acute abdomen (p. 182)

acute myocardial infarction (AMI) (p. 154)

altered mental status (p. 160)

anaphylaxis (p. 180)

angina pectoris (p. 155)

asthma (p. 158)

atherosclerosis (p. 154)

aura (p. 164)

behavioral emergency (p. 183)

bronchodilator (p. 158)

cerebrovascular accident (CVA) (p. 161)

chronic obstructive pulmonary disease (COPD) (p. 159)

Cincinnati Prehospital Stroke Scale (CPSS) (p. 162)

delirium tremens (p. 179)

diabetes (p. 173)

emphysema (p. 159)

epilepsy (p. 163)

EpiPen® (p. 180)

frostbite (p. 169)

glucose (p. 173)

heat exhaustion (p. 171)

heatstroke (p. 171)

hyperglycemia (p. 173)

hyperventilation (p. 159)

hypoglycemia (p. 173)

hypothermia (p. 165)

insulin (p. 173)

nitroglycerin (p. 156)

Poison Control Centers (PCC) (p. 176)

restraint (p. 184)

vasoconstriction (p. 166)

vasodilation (p. 166)

Review Questions

1. The signs and symptoms of heart attack include chest pain,
   a. fever, and flushed skin.
   b. headache, and inability to raise both arms.
   c. sweating, and shortness of breath.
   d. difficulty speaking or swallowing, and vision problems.

2. Low oxygen blood levels caused by respiratory distress may cause
   a. heavy sweating.
   b. dizziness or disorientation.
   c. a reddish coloration of the skin.
   d. hyperactivity.

3. Altered mental status may result from any injury that causes
   a. reduced oxygen levels.
   b. increased oxygen levels.
   c. a faster heartbeat.
   d. fluid loss.

4. A responsive stroke patient should be positioned
   a. lying on the weak side.
   b. lying on the strong side.
   c. on the back with the head and shoulders slightly raised.
   d. on the stomach with the head turned to one side.

5. Following a seizure, the patient typically is
   a. hyperexcitable.
   b. feverish.
   c. comatose.
   d. confused.

6. Emergency care for frostbite includes
   a. rapid rewarming using a heat lamp or heating pad.
   b. protecting the area from rubbing or constricting jewelry.
   c. vigorously rubbing the area.
   d. running hot water over the affected area for 10 minutes.

7. The late signs and symptoms of heat exhaustion include
   a. headache, dizziness, and fainting.
   b. constipation or diarrhea.
   c. extreme excitability.
   d. cool, tingling fingers or toes.

8. Exposure to carbon monoxide may cause
   a. bleeding at the mucous membranes.
   b. dizziness.
   c. dark stains around the mouth.
   d. hyperexcitability.

9. Emergency care for a patient experiencing anaphylaxis includes
   a. cooling the patient's body with ice packs.
   b. giving the patient an aspirin as quickly as possible.
   c. positioning the patient for easiest breathing.
   d. using pressure points on the arms and legs.

10. True or false: Making eye contact with a patient who is irrational, delusional, or potentially violent will likely upset the person and make the situation worse.

Chapter 12

Bleeding and Shock

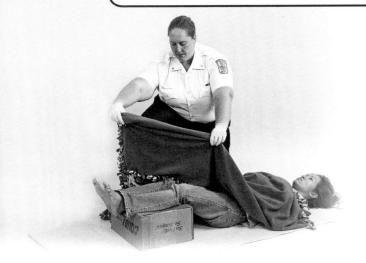

Chapter Preview

- External Bleeding
- Internal Bleeding
- Shock

You Respond To ...

a scene where a woman has cut her wrist on a piece of glass in the kitchen. She is trying to stop the bleeding with her hand, but a pool of blood has formed on the floor. The blood is pulsing out of the wound and running down her arm. She looks pale.

Introduction

External or internal bleeding is commonly present in trauma patients. It is important to act quickly to control bleeding to prevent the patient from going into shock, a life-threatening condition in which vital organs are not receiving enough oxygen.

External Bleeding

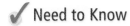 Need to Know

Anatomy and Physiology Review

- ☑ **Arteries** carry oxygenated blood from the heart to all parts of the body.
- ☑ **Veins** carry deoxygenated blood back from the body to the heart.

- ☑ The **capillaries** are the smallest blood vessels, are located between the arteries and veins, and are the site of exchange of nutrients, oxygen, and carbon dioxide between blood and tissue cells.
- ☑ **Perfusion** refers to the adequate flow of blood to body tissues.
- ☑ The **pulmonary** artery carries deoxygenated blood to the lungs for oxygenation, and the pulmonary veins carry oxygenated blood from the lungs back to the heart to be pumped to all parts of the body.

Bleeding

- ☑ Remember the risk of infectious disease from contact with the patient's blood or body fluids. Follow the standard precautions outlined in Chapter 2.
- ☑ The body's normal response to bleeding is constriction of blood vessels and **clotting** of the blood. However, a serious injury may prevent effective clotting.
- ☑ Uncontrolled bleeding leading to significant blood loss will cause shock and possibly death.
- ☑ Bleeding may be external or internal; either can result in severe blood loss.

Types of External Bleeding

Arterial Bleeding

- ☑ The blood spurts from the wound.
- ☑ The blood is bright red (oxygen rich) **(Figure 12-1)**.
- ☑ Arterial bleeding is the most difficult to control because of the pressure at which arteries bleed.
- ☑ Significant blood loss may occur very quickly.
- ☑ As the patient's blood pressure drops, the spurting may also diminish.

Venous Bleeding

- ☑ The blood flows as a steady stream.
- ☑ The blood is dark (oxygen poor).
- ☑ Although bleeding from a vein can be serious, it is usually easier to control because of the lower venous pressure.

Capillary Bleeding

- ☑ Blood oozes from a capillary.
- ☑ The blood is dark red.
- ☑ The bleeding often clots spontaneously.

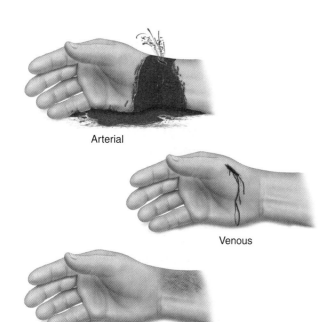

Arterial

Venous

Capillary

Figure 12-1 Arterial, venous, and capillary bleeding.

Assessing External Bleeding

▇▇ Need to Recognize

Perform the standard assessment:

1. Size up the scene before beginning emergency medical care.
2. Complete the initial assessment.
3. Perform a physical examination as appropriate.
4. Complete ongoing assessments.

In addition:

- ♦ Estimate the severity of a patient's blood loss, based on the patient's signs and symptoms and your general impression of the amount of blood loss. Do not, however, delay patient care to make an assessment of the blood loss.
- ♦ In addition, in cases of severe bleeding, assess the patient for shock (see later section in this chapter).

Controlling External Bleeding

▶ Need to Do

Perform standard patient care:

1. Ensure that EMS has been activated.
2. Take body substance isolation precautions.
3. Maintain the patient's airway, provide oxygen (if it is available and you are trained to do so), and be prepared to provide artificial ventilation if needed.
4. Comfort, calm, and reassure the patient while awaiting additional EMS resources.
5. Limit patient movement.

In addition:

- ♦ Control the bleeding as quickly as possible. If the patient is bleeding in several sites, arterial bleeding has the highest priority **(Skill 12-1)**.
- ♦ Apply sterile gauze and apply direct pressure on the point of bleeding. For a small wound, you may use the flat part of your fingers. With a larger wound, use your palm. Direct pressure is usually sufficient to control bleeding. Apply pressure as long as it is needed.
- ♦ With large gaping wounds, apply dressings and direct pressure with the full hand as needed.

Skill 12- Controlling External Bleeding

1 Wearing medical exam gloves, apply pressure directly on the point of bleeding.

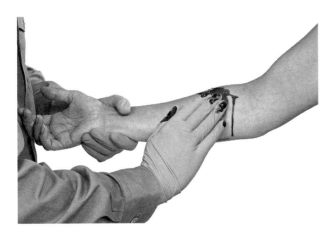

2 With large gaping wounds, apply sterile gauze and apply direct pressure with the full hand if needed to control bleeding.

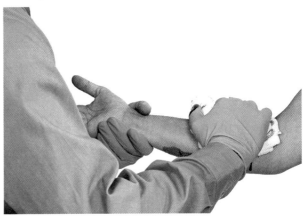

3 If bleeding soaks through the dressing, do not remove it but add another dressing on top and continue to maintain direct pressure.

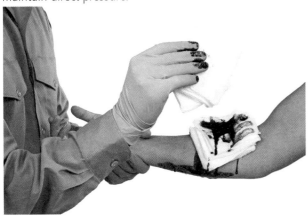

4 With bleeding in an extremity, apply a bandage over a bulky dressing to maintain pressure on the wound.

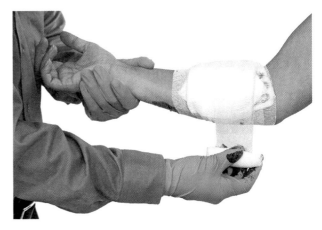

◆ If bleeding soaks through the dressing, do not remove it but add another dressing on top and continue to maintain direct pressure. Removing a dressing would interrupt the clotting process.

◆ With bleeding in an extremity, apply a bandage over a bulky dressing to maintain pressure on the wound. Using a **pressure dressing** made of roller gauze frees you to give other patient care. Check the pulse below the wound to ensure the bandage does not cut off circulation.

◆ Continually monitor the controlled bleeding to identify recurring bleeding.

Note: A **tourniquet** is used only rarely and as an extreme last resort to control bleeding because the arm or leg will likely have to be amputated. This is a "life or limb" decision. If necessary, use a wide band just above the wound and tighten it only enough to stop the bleeding. Record the time of application. Once applied, a tourniquet should not be loosened or removed. Do not cover the tourniquet and ensure that other personnel are aware of it.

Do You Understand?

1. True or false: The first thing to do with any bleeding wound is wash it and apply antibiotic ointment.

2. Number the steps for bleeding control in the correct order:

   _____ Put direct pressure on the wound

   _____ Put on medical exam gloves

   _____ Apply a pressure dressing

Internal Bleeding

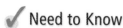 Need to Know

☑ **Internal bleeding** commonly occurs with blunt trauma. Suspect internal bleeding based on the mechanism of injury.

☑ Injured or damaged internal blood vessels may bleed extensively, though the bleeding is concealed. Severe internal bleeding causes shock and is life threatening.

☑ Painful, swollen, and deformed injured extremities may also be involved in serious internal blood loss.

☑ You cannot control internal bleeding. Treat the patient for shock and give supportive care until additional EMS resources arrive.

Assessing Internal Bleeding

 Need to Recognize

Perform the standard assessment:

1. Size up the scene before beginning emergency medical care.

2. Complete the initial assessment.

3. Perform a physical examination as appropriate.

4. Complete ongoing assessments.

Signs and symptoms of internal bleeding:

◆ Discolored, tender, swollen or hard skin tissue, or rigid abdomen

◆ Absence of distal pulse (with internal bleeding in an extremity)

◆ Increased respiratory and pulse rates

◆ Pale, cool, moist skin (or ashen-colored skin in a dark-skinned person)

◆ Nausea and vomiting

◆ Thirst

◆ Mental status changes

◆ Bleeding from body orifices

Emergency Care for Internal Bleeding

▶ Need to Do

Perform standard patient care:

1. Ensure EMS has been activated.

2. Take body substance isolation precautions.

3. Maintain the patient's airway and provide artificial ventilation if needed.

4. Comfort, calm, and reassure the patient while awaiting additional EMS resources.

In addition:

◆ Manage any external bleeding.

◆ Keep the patient in a position of comfort.

- Keep the patient warm.
- Limit the movement of a deformed extremity to reduce bleeding,
- Treat the patient for shock (see next section).
- Administer high-flow oxygen if it is available and you are trained to do so.

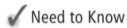 Do You Understand?

1. Describe the skin characteristics of a patient with severe internal bleeding:

_____

2. Put a check mark next to the possible signs and symptoms of internal bleeding:
   _____ Mental status changes
   _____ Feverish, blotchy red skin
   _____ Vomiting or coughing up blood
   _____ Blood in the urine
   _____ Tender, swollen, or rigid abdomen
   _____ Bruising
   _____ Pale, cool, moist clammy skin

3. What is the most important thing you can do for a patient with internal bleeding?

_____

Shock

✓ Need to Know

☑ **Shock,** or **hypoperfusion,** is a condition resulting from the inadequate delivery of oxygenated blood to body tissues.

☑ Shock may result from any condition involving:
   ◦ Failure of the heart to provide oxygenated blood (pump failure)
   ◦ Abnormal dilation of the vessels (pipe failure)
   ◦ Blood volume loss **(Figure 12-2)**

☑ Shock develops as a progressive process and may occur slowly or quickly. The body attempts to **compensate** for reduced perfusion by increasing the heart and breathing rates. With continued reduced perfusion, the body can no longer compensate and vital organs may soon fail.

☑ Definitive treatment for shock is critical. It is a priority to transport the patient for treatment as soon as possible.

☑ Consider the possibility of shock in any serious injury or illness. Shock most commonly results from blood loss but may also result from:
   ◦ Severe burns
   ◦ Heart failure
   ◦ Heart attack
   ◦ Head or spinal injuries
   ◦ Chest injuries
   ◦ Allergic reactions
   ◦ Dehydration (such as with heatstroke or severe vomiting or diarrhea)
   ◦ Electrocution
   ◦ Serious infections
   ◦ Extreme emotional reactions

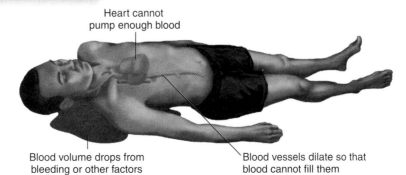

Figure 12-2 Shock may develop from disruption of the heart, blood volume, or blood vessels.

Assessing Shock

▬◀ Need to Recognize

Perform the standard assessment:

1. Size up the scene before beginning emergency medical care.
2. Complete the initial assessment.
3. Perform a physical examination as appropriate.
4. Complete ongoing assessments.

Signs and symptoms of shock:

- Restlessness, anxiety
- Extreme thirst
- Rapid, weak pulse
- Rapid, shallow respirations
- Mental status changes
- Pale, cool, moist skin (or ashen-colored skin in a dark-skinned person)
- Decreased blood pressure (a late sign)

Emergency Care for Shock

▶▶ Need to Do

Perform standard patient care:

1. Ensure EMS has been activated.
2. Take body substance isolation precautions.
3. Maintain the patient's airway and provide artificial ventilation if needed.
4. Comfort, calm, and reassure the patient while awaiting additional EMS resources.

In addition:

- Prevent further blood loss.
- Position the patient lying on the back with the legs raised 8 to 12 inches (unless there is a head, spinal, leg, or pelvis injury—assess for such injuries before raising the legs) **(Figure 12-3)**.
- Keep the patient warm: Attempt to maintain a normal body temperature. If available, put a blanket under the patient as well.
- Do not give the patient anything to eat or drink.
- Provide care for specific injuries.
- Administer high-flow oxygen if it is available and you are trained to do so.
- Continue to monitor the patient's breathing and vital signs every 5 minutes. Be prepared to maintain an open airway in case of vomiting.

✎ Do You Understand?

1. True or false: Because a patient in shock is thirsty and may be dehydrated, offer clear fluids to drink.

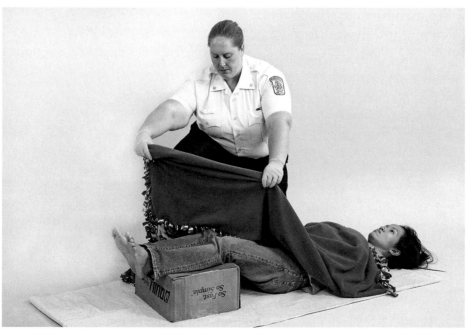

Figure 12-3 The shock position.

2. True or false: A spinal injury can cause shock.

3. You are successful in stopping the bleeding in a patient, but she is pale and seems "out of it" when you ask her what happened. She had lost a significant amount of blood even before you arrived.

   What other signs and symptoms are you likely to observe if she is going into shock?

   a. Vomiting, diarrhea, red blotchy face

   b. Nausea, thirst, clammy skin

   c. Incontinence, hives, swollen legs

   d. Headache, painful abdomen, coughing

4. Which of these actions should you always take first for a patient in shock caused by external bleeding?
   a. Stop the bleeding
   b. Raise the legs
   c. Loosen constricting clothing
   d. Cover the patient with a blanket

Conclusion

Always check for external bleeding during the initial assessment and consider the possibility of internal bleeding in any patient with a serious injury or blunt trauma. Similarly, be alert for the signs and symptoms of shock in any patient with a serious injury or illness. It is important to recognize shock early in its development so that the patient reaches definitive care before the body can no longer compensate.

Key Terms

arteries (p. 187)
capillaries (p. 187)
clotting (p. 187)
compensate (p. 191)
hypoperfusion (p. 191)
internal bleeding (p. 190)
perfusion (p. 187)
pressure dressing (p. 190)
pulmonary (p. 187)
shock (p. 191)
tourniquet (p. 190)
veins (p. 187)

Review Questions

1. The body attempts to slow or stop bleeding from a damaged blood vessel by
   a. contracting skeletal muscles.
   b. blood clotting.
   c. producing more red blood cells.
   d. stopping the heart beat.

2. Which type of bleeding is usually most serious?
   a. Arterial
   b. Venous
   c. Capillary
   d. All bleeding is equally serious.

3. What do you do if blood soaks through the pressure dressing?
   a. Ignore the blood but maintain the pressure.
   b. Put a new dressing on top of the first and maintain pressure.
   c. Replace the bloody dressing with a new dressing and maintain pressure.
   d. Apply a tourniquet on top of the dressing.

4. A pressure dressing is applied
   a. around the extremity from the joint above the wound to the joint below the wound, to apply equal pressure to the whole area.
   b. above the wound to cut off the blood flow.
   c. on the wound to control bleeding.
   d. both above and below the wound to control blood flow and bleeding.

5. Internal bleeding into the abdomen may result in the abdomen feeling
   a. rigid.
   b. hot.
   c. pulsing.
   d. soft and squishy.

6. Severe internal bleeding may cause the
   a. patient to feel thirsty.
   b. patient's skin to be cool and clammy.
   c. patient to be confused.
   d. All of the above.

7. Which is fundamental to the definition of shock?
   a. Not enough oxygen reaching vital organs
   b. Too much waste building up in the urine
   c. The heart beat stopping
   d. An abdominal injury

8. The signs and symptoms of shock may include
   a. confusion.
   b. rapid, shallow breathing.
   c. pale, bluish, or ashen skin.
   d. All of the above.

9. Which is important in the treatment of shock?
   a. Giving the patient water to drink to replace lost fluids
   b. Keeping the patient warm
   c. Keeping the patient moving to prevent becoming unresponsive
   d. Applying ice to the injury

Chapter 13

Soft-Tissue Injuries

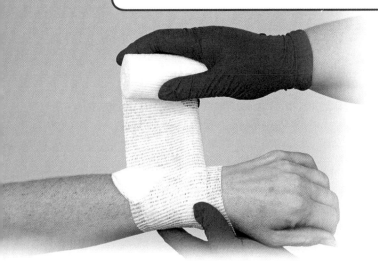

Chapter Preview

- Types of Soft-Tissue Injuries
- General Principle of Wound Care
- Dressing and Bandaging Wounds
- Specific Soft-Tissue Injuries
- Wounds in Specific Body Areas
- Burns

You Respond To …

an industrial scene where a woman has been injured by a boiler explosion. After you check that the scene is safe, you approach and determine that she is unresponsive. As you open her airway and check breathing, you note multiple bleeding soft-tissue injuries caused by the explosion, including a jagged piece of metal impaled in her arm. In addition, her face and hands have apparently been burned by steam or boiling water.

Introduction

Awound is an injury to the skin and sometimes other deeper soft tissues, commonly occurring in trauma and burn patients. In an **open wound,** the skin is torn or cut open, often leading to bleeding. Muscle and other soft tissues beneath the skin may be injured. Different types of soft-tissue injuries require different emergency care, but all open wounds have a risk of becoming infected by pathogens. In addition to controlling bleeding, First Responders should know how to care for different types of soft-tissue injuries and how to apply dressings and bandages.

Types of Soft-Tissue Injuries

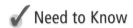 Need to Know

Different mechanisms of injury cause different types of damage to soft tissues. With open wounds, the type and amount of bleeding caused by an injury depend on the type of wound, its location, and depth. Different types of wounds also have different implications for emergency care.

☑ **Closed wounds** are soft-tissue injuries without a break in the skin, such as a bruise (**contusion**) caused by blunt impact. Discoloration and swelling are caused by internal bleeding in the skin and underlying tissue. Internal bleeding caused by damage to organs is described in Chapter 12; musculoskeletal injuries also may be present with open or closed wounds (Chapter 14).

☑ **Abrasions** occur when the top layers of skin are scraped off by shearing forces **(Figure 13-1)**. Abrasions are often painful but not serious injuries because underlying tissues are not usually injured. Bleeding is usually limited to capillary bleeding that typically stops soon by

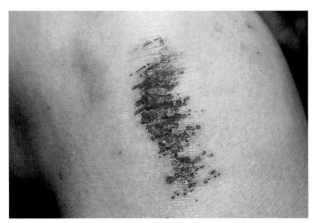

Figure 13-1 Abrasion.

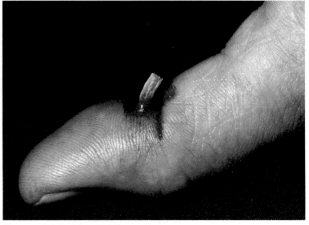

Figure 13-3 Puncture.

itself. Foreign material may be present in the wound, which can cause infection.

☑ **Lacerations,** or cuts, frequently penetrate the skin and may also damage underlying tissue **(Figure 13-2).** Lacerations are either smooth cuts with straight edges (incisions), such as caused by a knife or other sharp object, or jagged cuts with rough edges. Depending on the depth and location of the cut, lacerations may cause heavy bleeding. A laceration through a major artery may cause life-threatening bleeding.

☑ **Punctures** of the skin, also called penetrating wounds, are caused by a sharp, pointed object penetrating into the skin and possibly deeper tissues **(Figure 13-3).** Although there may be little or no external bleeding, internal bleeding may be severe. The wound may penetrate through the body part, such as with a gunshot wound, causing both entrance and exit wounds. Puncture wounds are more likely to trap foreign material in the body, increasing the risk of infection.

☑ **Avulsions** are areas of skin or other soft tissue torn partially from the body, like a flap **(Figure 13-4).** A whole soft-tissue structure, like the ear, may be avulsed, or an area of skin such as in a degloving injury.

☑ **Amputations** are the complete cutting or tearing off of all or part of an extremity: a finger or toe, hand or foot, arm or leg. This wound is often called a traumatic amputation to differentiate from an amputation performed surgically. Depending on the nature of the wound and the time that passes before the patient reaches the hospital, the amputated part may be reattached.

☑ **Burns** are damage caused to skin and other tissue by heat, chemicals, or electricity.

General Principles of Wound Care

Controlling any serious bleeding after the initial assessment is always a priority when caring for a

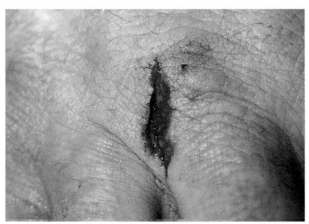

Figure 13-2 Laceration.

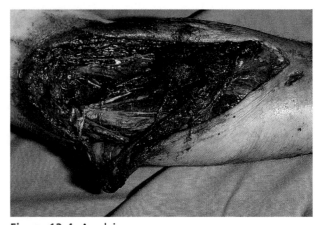

Figure 13-4 Avulsion.

patient with an open wound. Significant bleeding may occur, for example, by an arm breaking through a plate glass window or a leg wound caused by a power saw.

With less serious bleeding, first complete the patient assessment and standard patient care. Then care for the wound.

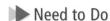 Need to Recognize

Perform the standard assessment:

1. Size up the scene before beginning emergency medical care.

2. Complete the initial assessment.

3. Perform a physical examination as appropriate.

4. Complete ongoing assessments.

In addition:

- Expose the wound completely by cutting away clothing and positioning the patient for a clear view.

Emergency Care for Soft-Tissue Injuries

▶ Need to Do

Perform standard patient care:

1. Ensure that EMS has been activated.

2. Take body substance isolation precautions.

3. Maintain the patient's airway and provide artificial ventilation if needed.

4. Comfort, calm, and reassure the patient while awaiting additional EMS resources.

In addition:

- Consider whether wound care will require BSI precautions in addition to wearing medical exam gloves. Use eye protection, a gown, and other precautions as needed. Wash your hands well after providing care.

- Control bleeding by covering the wound with sterile gauze and applying direct pressure.

- With minor wounds only, such as an abrasion caused by scraping the skin against pavement, resulting in a dirty shallow wound, **irrigate** the wound under running water to flush out any debris and clean the area to prevent infection. Let clean tap water run over the wound for at least 5 minutes or until there appears to be no foreign matter in the wound (**Figure 13-5**). Never delay or interrupt efforts to stop

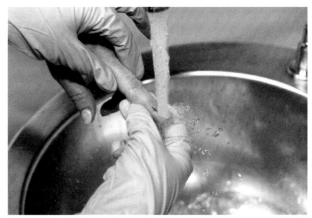

Figure 13-5 Irrigate a shallow wound with running water to help clean it.

bleeding to clean a wound. Then pat the area dry and apply a sterile dressing and bandage.

- Prevent further contamination of the wound with the appropriate dressing and bandage.

- Even with a minor wound, if stitches may be needed or if the patient does not have a current **tetanus** vaccination, ensure the patient receives medical attention.

- Do not let the patient put alcohol, hydrogen peroxide, or iodine on the wound. Alcohol and hydrogen peroxide may damage tissue, and many people have allergic reactions to iodine.

- Avoid breathing or blowing on the wound, because this may transmit pathogens.

- Do not attempt to remove clothing stuck to a wound; cut around the clothing and leave it in place for healthcare providers to manage later.

- Do not scrub a wound, because this can cause further tissue damage.

Dressing and Bandaging Wounds

Dressings

✓ Need to Know

Dressings are put on wounds to help stop bleeding, prevent infection, and protect the wound while healing. Common types of dressings include (**Figure 13-6**):

- ☑ Gauze squares of various sizes (such as 2x2 or 4x4 squares)

- ☑ Roller gauze

- ☑ Nonstick pad dressings

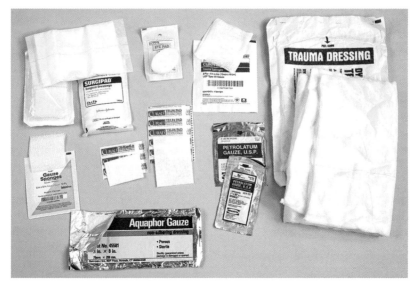

Figure 13-6 A variety of dressings.

☑ Adhesive strips such as Band-Aids® and other dressings combined with a bandage

☑ Bulky dressings, also called **trauma dressings,** are used for large wounds or to stabilize an object impaled in a wound.

☑ **Occlusive dressings** create an airtight seal over certain types of wounds.

If a sterile dressing is not available, use a clean cloth as a dressing; nonfluffy cloth works best because it is less likely to stick to the wound.

☑ Look for a clean towel, handkerchief, or other material.

☑ Avoid using cotton balls or cotton cloth if possible, because cotton fibers tend to stick to wounds.

☑ To improvise bulky dressings, use sanitary pads if available. Although they are not sterile, they are generally individually wrapped and very clean.

☑ Bulky dressings can also be made of towels, baby diapers, or many layers of gauze.

☑ A ring dressing can be made for around an area on which direct pressure should not be used **(Box 13-1).**

Applying Dressings

▶▶ Need to Do

1. Wash hands and put on medical exam gloves.
2. Choose a dressing larger than the wound. Do not touch the part of the dressing that will contact the wound.

3. Carefully lay the dressing on the wound (do not slide it on from the side). Cover the whole wound **(Figure 13-7).**
4. If blood seeps through, do not remove the dressing but add more dressings on top of it.
5. Apply direct pressure if needed to control bleeding (Chapter 12). Apply a bandage to hold the dressing in place and maintain pressure.

Bandages

✓ Need to Know

Bandages are used for covering a dressing, keeping the dressing on a wound, and maintaining pressure to control bleeding **(Box 13-2).**

☑ Only dressings touch the wound, so bandages should be clean but may not necessarily be sterile.

☑ Bandages are also used to support or immobilize an injury to bones, joints, or muscles, and to reduce swelling (Chapter 14).

Different types of bandages are available for different uses **(Figure 13-8):**

☑ Adhesive compresses or strips for small wounds that combine a dressing with an adhesive bandage

☑ Adhesive tape rolls (cloth, plastic, paper)

☑ Tubular bandages for fingers or toes

☑ Elastic bandages

☑ Self-adhering roller bandages

BOX 13-1

RING DRESSING

Direct pressure should not be put over the entire surface of certain wounds, such as a skull fracture, a fractured bone protruding from a wound, or an object impaled in a wound. In these cases, bleeding is controlled with pressure around the object or fracture. A dressing made into a ring shape is appropriate for controlling bleeding and dressing such wounds. Make a ring dressing from a long strip of gauze or other material:

1. Make a circular wrap the right size to surround the area.
2. With the remainder of the strip or an additional strip, wrap it around the circular wrap to give the ring more bulk.
3. Position the ring around the wound and apply pressure as needed.

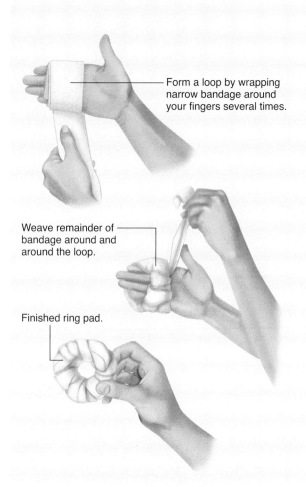

Form a loop by wrapping narrow bandage around your fingers several times.

Weave remainder of bandage around and around the loop.

Finished ring pad.

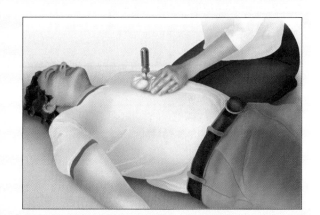

☑ Gauze roller bandages
☑ Triangular bandages (or folded square cloths)
☑ Any cloth or other material improvised to meet the purposes of bandaging

🖊 Do You Understand?

1. How long should a minor wound be irrigated with running water before dressing and bandaging?

   _____ minutes

2. In what situation should you not clean a wound before applying a dressing and bandage?

   _____

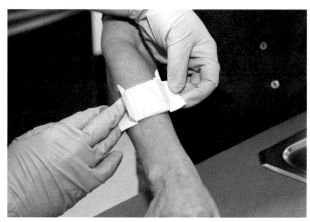

Figure 13-7 Cover the wound with a sterile dressing and apply a bandage.

BOX 13-2

GUIDELINES FOR BANDAGING

1 To put pressure on a wound to stop bleeding or to prevent swelling of an injury, apply the bandage firmly—but not so tightly that it cuts off circulation. Never encircle the neck with a bandage. With a bandage around a limb, check the fingers or toes for color, warmth, and sensation (normal touch, not tingling) to make sure circulation is not cut off. If there are signs of reduced circulation, unwrap the bandage and reapply it less tightly. Do not use elastic bandages for dressings on wounds; these are intended for muscle and joint injuries.

2 Do not cover fingers or toes unless they are injured Keep them exposed so they can be checked for adequate circulation.

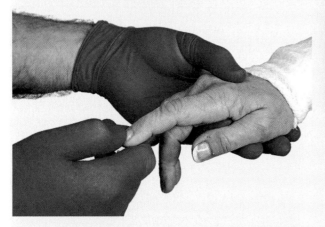

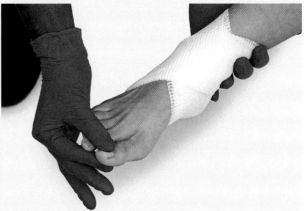

3 Because swelling continues after many injuries, keep checking the tightness of the bandage. Swelling may make a loose bandage tight enough to cut off circulation.

4 With a bandaged wound, be sure the bandage is secure enough that the dressing will not move and expose the wound to possible contamination.

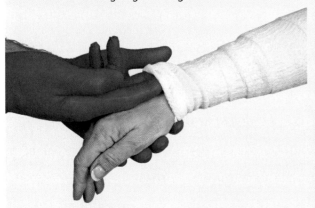

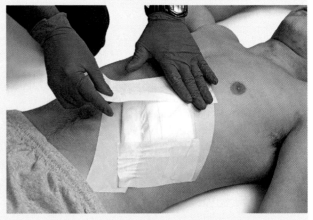

5 With elastic and roller bandages, anchor the first end and tie, tape, pin, or clip the ending section in place. Loose ends could get caught on something and pull the bandage loose or disrupt the wound.

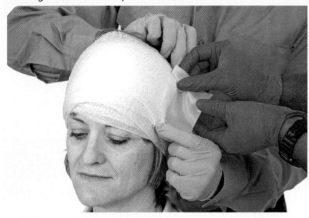

6 Use a non-elastic roller bandage to make a pressure bandage around a limb to control bleeding and protect the wound.

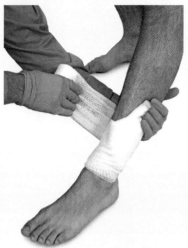

7 An elastic roller bandage is used to support a joint and prevent swelling. At the wrist or ankle, a figure-eight wrap is used.

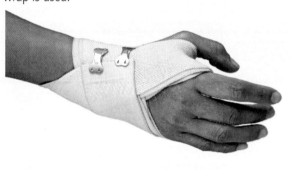

8 Wrap a bandage from the bottom of the limb upward to help prevent cutting off circulation (Skill 13-1).

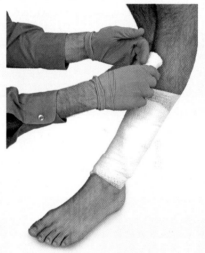

9 Avoid bending a joint once it has been bandaged, because movement may loosen the dressing or cut off circulation. Bandage the joint in the position in which it will be kept.

10 Even with a small wound, use a wide bandage with evenly distributed pressure to avoid a narrow band of pressure around an extremity.

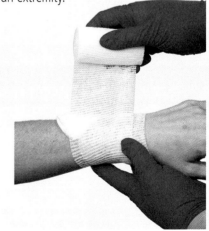

Skill 13-1 Applying a Roller Bandage

1 Anchor the starting end of the bandage.

2 Turn the bandage diagonally across top of foot and around ankle.

3 Continue with overlapping figure-eight turns.

4 Fasten the end of the bandage with clips, tape, or safety pins.

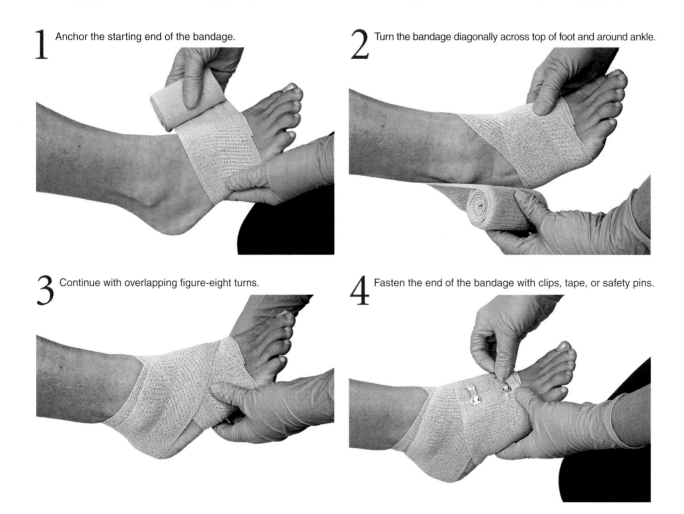

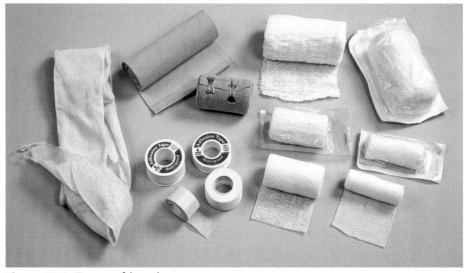

Figure 13-8 Types of bandages.

3. True or false: When bandaging a dressing over a wound that is not bleeding, make the bandage loose enough so that it can be slid to one side later to change the dressing.

4. True or false: An elastic roller bandage makes a good pressure bandage to control bleeding.

Specific Soft-Tissue Injuries

Certain types of wounds require special considerations.

Puncture Wounds

▶ Need to Do

Puncture wounds may involve deeper injuries you cannot see. If a puncturing object may have penetrated the body, such as with a gunshot, check also for an exit wound. In general, puncture wounds carry a greater risk of infection because often there is less external bleeding and therefore germs may not be flushed out. In such injuries, often the significant bleeding is internal.

1. Follow general principles of wound care.

2. Remove any small objects or dirt but not larger impaled objects.

3. With small punctures, gently press on wound edges to promote bleeding to flush out pathogens.

4. Do not put any medication inside or over the puncture wound.

5. Irrigate the wound well with running water directed at the puncture site.

6. Dress the wound and seek medical attention.

Impaled Objects

▶ Need to Do

Removing an object from a wound could cause more injury and bleeding, because often the object seals the wound or damaged blood vessels.

▸ Leave the object in place (unless it would interfere with airway management or chest compressions) and dress the wound around it **(Figure 13-9).** Use bulky dressings (trauma dressings) to stabilize the object and keep it from moving.

▸ Adhesive tape may not stick well enough to hold bulky dressings in place because of blood or sweat on the skin; use a roller ban-

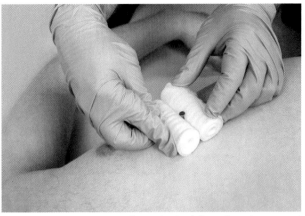

Figure 13-9 Leave an impaled object in place and use bulky dressings to keep it from moving.

dage or strips of cloth to tie the bandage in place around the impaled object.

1. Follow general principles of wound care.

2. Control bleeding with direct pressure at the sides of the object.

3. Dress the wound around the object.

4. Pad the object in place with large dressings or folded cloths.

5. Support the object while bandaging it in place.

6. Keep the patient still and seek medical attention.

Avulsions and Amputations

▶ Need to Do

▸ An avulsion is a piece of skin or other soft tissue torn partially from the body, like a flap. Try to move the skin or tissue back into its normal position unless the wound is contaminated, and then control bleeding and provide wound care.

▸ If the avulsed tissue is completely separated from the body, care for it the same as for an amputated part.

In an amputation, a part has been severed from the body. Bleeding may be massive or limited. Follow general principles of wound care first, then recover and care for the amputated part, which surgeons may be able to reattach:

1. Wrap the severed part in a dry sterile dressing or clean cloth. Do not wash it.

2. Place the part in a plastic bag and seal it.

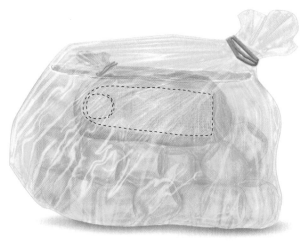

Figure 13-10 Keep an amputated part cold but not directly touching ice.

3. Place the sealed bag in another bag or container with ice and water. Do not let the part touch water or ice directly, and do not bury it in ice or use dry ice **(Figure 13-10).**

4. Make sure the severed part is given to the responding EMS crew or taken with the patient to the emergency department.

Bites

✓ Need to Know

Animal bites can be serious for three reasons:

- ☑ Bleeding and tissue damage can be serious.
- ☑ Bacteria are usually present in animals' mouths, increasing the risk of wound infection.
- ☑ The bite of any animal, even a house pet, carries the risk of **rabies.**

▶ Need to Do

1. Follow general principles of wound care.
2. Clean the wound with soap and water. Run water over the wound for at least 5 minutes (except when bleeding severely).
3. Control bleeding.
4. Cover the wound with a sterile dressing and bandage.
5. Ensure the patient sees a healthcare provider as soon as possible.
6. Do not try to catch any animal that may have rabies.

7. All animal bites should be reported to local animal control officers or law enforcement personnel. State law generally requires specific procedures to be followed when rabies is a risk.

Wounds in Specific Body Areas

Penetrating Chest Wounds

Impaled Object in Chest

Removing an impaled object from the chest could cause additional bleeding, injury, and breathing problems.

▶ Need to Do

1. Follow general principles of wound care.
2. Keep the patient still, seated, or lying down.
3. Use bulky dressings or cloth to stabilize the object.
4. Bandage the area around the object.
5. Monitor the patient's breathing and vital signs. Treat the patient for shock.

Sucking Chest Wound

✓ Need to Know

A **sucking chest wound** is an open wound in the chest caused by a penetrating injury that lets air move in and out of the chest during breathing.

- ☑ During inhalation, air is sucked in through the wound.
- ☑ During exhalation, air is forced out through the wound.
- ☑ You may hear a gurgling or sucking sound and may see air bubbles in the blood around the wound.
- ☑ A sucking chest wound can be life threatening because breathing can be affected.
- ☑ A special dressing is used that prevents air from being sucked into the chest, allowing more normal breathing, while allowing air to escape from the wound, to prevent a buildup of pressure in the chest.

▶ Need to Do

1. Follow general principles of wound care.
2. Put a thin, sterile dressing over the wound.

On inspiration, dressing seals wound, preventing air entry.

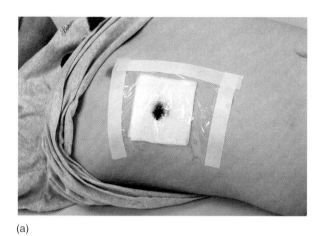

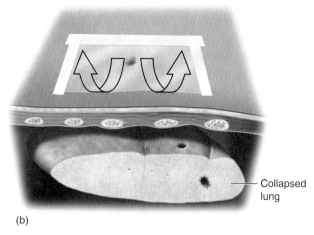

Collapsed
lung

(a)   (b)

Figure 13-11 Occlusive bandage for a sucking chest wound. (a) Tape only three sides to let air escape from a sucking chest wound. (b) When patient breathes in, the dressing seals the wound and prevents air entry.

3. Cover the dressing with an occlusive dressing (or improvise with a plastic wrap or bag) to make an air-tight seal. As the patient exhales, tape it in place on three sides, leaving one side untaped to let exhaled air escape **(Figure 13-11).**

4. If an occlusive dressing is not available, cover the wound with your gloved hand during inhalation to prevent air from entering the chest.

5. Unless a spinal injury is suspected, position the patient lying down inclined toward the injured side or in a position for easiest breathing.

6. If patient's breathing becomes more difficult, remove the occlusive dressing to let air escape; then reapply it.

7. Monitor the patient's breathing until help arrives. Treat the patient for shock.

Closed Chest Injuries

✓ Need to Know

Common chest injuries involving the lungs include pneumothorax and hemothorax, which may occur with either open or closed injuries.

☑ In a **pneumothorax,** air escapes from an injured lung into the thoracic cavity—the space inside the chest around the lungs—causing collapse of some or all of the lung and resulting in respiratory distress.

☑ In a **hemothorax,** blood from internal bleeding accumulates in the thoracic cavity, compressing the lung and causing respiratory distress and possibly shock.

■ Need to Recognize

That the skin is not broken in a closed chest injury does not mean that there is not serious underlying damage. Organ damage or internal bleeding can be serious. Consider the possibility of a pneumothorax or hemothorax, even without outward signs of injury, with any trauma to the chest. Signs and symptoms of a pneumothorax or hemothorax may include:

▶ Little or no external evidence of injury

▶ Signs and symptoms of shock

▶ Respiratory distress

▶ Need to Do

Perform standard patient care:

1. Ensure that EMS has been activated.

2. Take body substance isolation precautions.

3. Maintain the patient's airway and provide artificial ventilation if needed.

4. Comfort, calm, and reassure the patient while awaiting additional EMS resources.

In addition:

▶ Help a responsive victim find the position that is most comfortable and allows for easiest breathing.

▶ Treat for respiratory distress (see Chapter 7).

▶ Follow local protocol to administer supplemental oxygen if it is available and you are so trained.

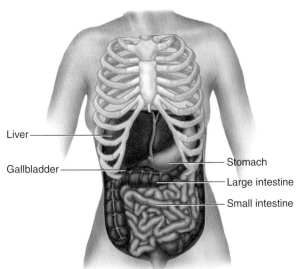

Figure 13-12 Abdominal organs have little protection from injury.

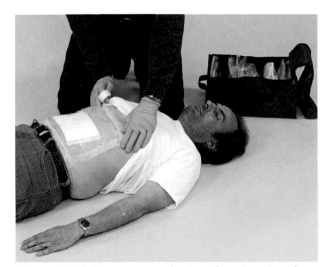

Figure 13-14 Tape an occlusive dressing in place over an open abdominal wound.

Open Abdominal Wounds

✓ Need to Know

Injury may cause internal and/or external bleeding, because large blood vessels are present within the abdomen along with many organs.

- ☑ The abdominal cavity is not protected from injury as the chest is by the ribs **(Figure 13-12)**.
- ☑ Internal organs may be damaged, and organs may protrude from an open wound (**evisceration**) **(Figure 13-13)**.
- ☑ This is a serious emergency because organs can be further damaged by drying out, bleeding from associated blood vessels, or infection.

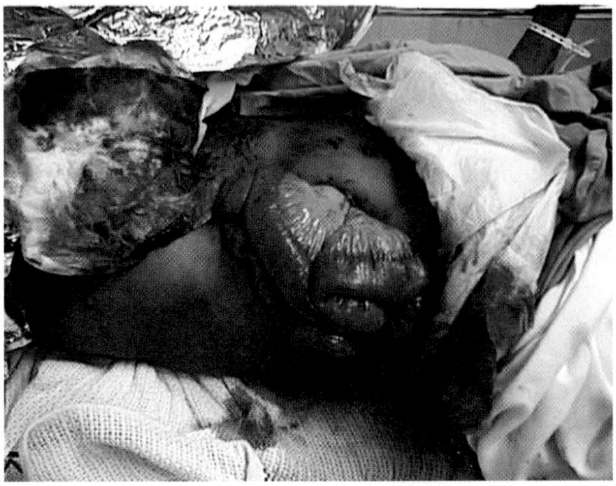

Figure 13-13 Open abdominal wound.

▶ Need to Do

1. Follow general principles of wound care.
2. Position the patient on his or her back and loosen any tight clothing. Allow the patient to bend knees slightly if this eases the pain.
3. Do not push protruding organs back inside the abdomen or apply direct pressure on the wound. Cover the wound and exposed organs with a dry, non-adherent dressing or a sterile, moist dressing. Do not pack the wound with dressings.
4. Cover the dressing with a large, occlusive dressing or plastic wrap, taped loosely in place **(Figure 13-14)**. Then cover the area with a blanket or towel to help maintain warmth.
5. Monitor the patient's breathing and vital signs. Treat the patient for shock.

Genital Injuries

Genital injuries are rare because of their protected location. Injuries may occur from blunt trauma, an impact that creates a wound, or sexual abuse. Provide privacy for a patient when caring for a wound in the genital area.

▶ Need to Do

1. Follow general principles of wound care.
2. Use direct pressure with a sterile dressing or sanitary pad to control external bleeding. Then use a large triangular bandage applied like a diaper to secure the dressings in place **(Figure 13-15)**.

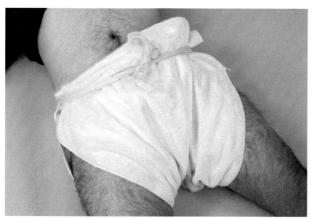

Figure 13-15 Apply a triangular bandage like a diaper to secure dressings in the genital area.

3. For injured testicles, provide support with a towel between the legs like a diaper. For a closed injury caused by blunt trauma, a cold pack may help reduce pain.

4. For vaginal bleeding, have the woman press a sanitary pad or clean folded towel to the area to control bleeding.

5. In the case of rape or sexual abuse, preserve evidence for law enforcement personnel.

Do You Understand?

1. Which type of wound is most likely to become infected?

   a. Abrasion

   b. Laceration

   c. Puncture

   d. Avulsion

2. List three reasons why an animal bite may be serious.

   _____

   _____

   _____

3. True or false: An amputated part should be kept cold but not put in direct contact with ice.

4. Describe the type of dressing put on a sucking chest wound.

   _____

5. True or false: A goal of emergency care for an open abdominal wound with eviscerated organs is to prevent the organs from drying out.

Head and Face Injuries

Soft-tissue injuries of the head or face may require special care. With any significant injury to the head, the patient may also have a neck or spinal injury (see Chapter 15). If you suspect a spinal injury, be careful not to move the patient's head.

Scalp Wound

▶▶ Need to Do

First confirm the following signs of a skull fracture are *not* present (Chapter 15):

- A deformed area of the skull
- A depressed or spongy area in the skull
- Blood or fluid from the ears or nose
- Eyelids swollen shut or becoming discolored (bruising)
- Bruising under eyes (raccoon eyes)
- Bruising behind the ears (Battle's sign)
- Unequal pupils
- An object impaled in the skull

If there are no signs of a skull fracture and the wound is restricted to the scalp, apply a dressing and use direct pressure as usual to control bleeding **(Skill 13-2).** Follow general principles of wound care. *Never wrap a bandage around the neck because of the risk of impeding breathing if the injury causes swelling.*

Neck Injuries

Closed injuries of the neck may cause bruising, swelling, difficulty speaking, and possible airway obstruction by swollen tissues. Minor open neck wounds are treated like other wounds. Significant open neck wounds are a medical emergency because profuse bleeding can occur if arteries in the neck are injured or severed.

▶▶ Need to Do

1. Follow general principles of wound care.

2. Put pressure on the bleeding wound immediately with a gloved hand.

3. Place an occlusive dressing over the whole wound and tape it down on all sides to prevent air from being sucked into the artery. Apply pressure on top of the dressing to control bleeding.

Skill 13-2 Scalp Wound Without Suspected Skull Fracture

1 Replace any skin flaps and cover the wound with a sterile dressing. Use direct pressure as needed to control bleeding.

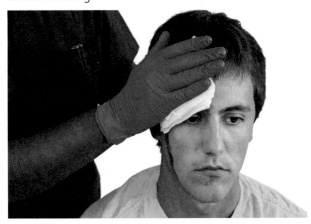

2 Put a roller bandage around the patient's head to secure the dressing, depending on the location and size of the wound.

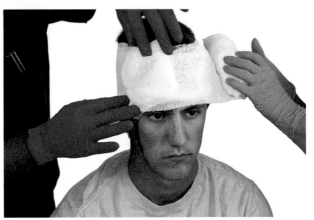

4. When bleeding is controlled, apply a pressure dressing over the occlusive dressing. Do not encircle the neck with a bandage. Apply pressure only to control bleeding, being careful not to obstruct the airway or compress other blood vessels in the neck.

Eye Injuries

✔ Need to Know

Eye injuries are serious because vision may be affected. Eye injuries include blows to the eye, impaled objects in the eye, dirt or small particles in the eye, and chemicals or other substances splashed into the eye.

☑ When caring for an eye injury, avoid putting pressure directly on the eyeball because it is easily injured.

☑ With most eye injuries, movement of the eye will continue to worsen the injury. Bandaging or otherwise covering an injured eye discourages the patient from moving it. Because the eyes move together (sympathetic movement), the unaffected eye must also be covered. Having both eyes covered or bandaged is often frightening, especially to an injured patient. Explain what you are doing and why before covering the good eye.

▉ Need to Recognize

With any significant injury to the eye, assess the patient's vision by checking what the patient can see. The eyelids and other tissue may soon swell and make later assessment of vision difficult, so this early assessment is helpful for EMS personnel who will provide patient care.

▶ Need to Do

For a blow to the eye:

1. Follow general principles of wound care.

2. If the eye is bleeding or leaking fluid, the patient needs emergency medical care immediately.

3. Put a cold pack over the eye for up to 15 minutes to ease pain and reduce swelling, but do not put pressure on the eye **(Figure 13-16)**. If the patient is wearing a contact lens, do not try to remove it.

4. Cover both eyes because movement of the uninjured one causes movement of the injured one.

For a large object embedded in the eye:

1. Follow general principles of wound care.

2. Do not remove the object. Stabilize it in place with dressings or bulky cloth **(Figure 13-17)**.

Skill 13-2 **continued**

3 Use a triangular bandage if needed because of the wound's location or larger size.

a. Start by folding the bandage along the edge.

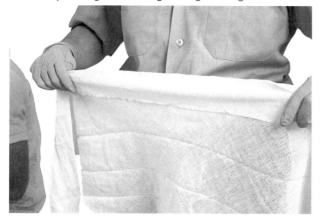

b. Position the bandage and tie the ends behind the head.

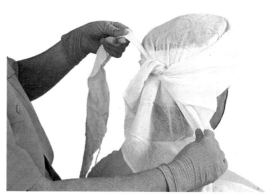

c. Bring the ends around to the front of the head and tie or pin them in place. Then tuck the point in back under the knot.

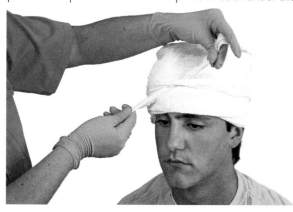

Be careful not to put any pressure on the eye from the object. With a large impaled object or one that may move, use a paper cup or something similar to stabilize the object and keep it from moving in the eye.

3. Cover both eyes because movement of the uninjured one causes movement of the injured one.

For dirt or a small particle in the eye:

1. Follow general principles of wound care.
2. Do not let the patient rub the eye with his or her hands, which could cause scratching of the eye or other soft tissue.

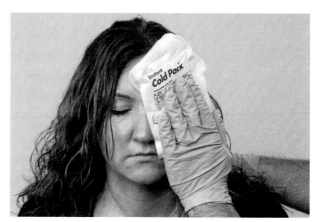

Figure 13-16 For a blow to the eye, hold a cold pack on the eye.

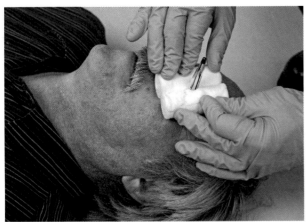

Figure 13-17 Stabilize an object impaled in the eyeball.

3. Wait a minute to see if the patient's tears flush out the object. If not, try these methods:

◆ Gently pull the upper eyelid out and down over the lower eyelid. This allows the lower lashes to catch a particle caught under the upper eyelid.

◆ If the particle remains, gently flush the eye with water from a medicine dropper or water glass. Have the patient tilt the head so that the affected eye is lower than the other so that water does not flow into the unaffected eye. Flush from the corner nearer the nose. Ask the patient to hold the eyelids open with his or her fingers, if needed, and to look in all directions and blink during the flushing.

◆ If the particle remains and is visible, carefully try to brush it out gently with a wet sterile dressing. Lift the upper eyelid and swab its underside if you see the particle **(Figure 13-18).**

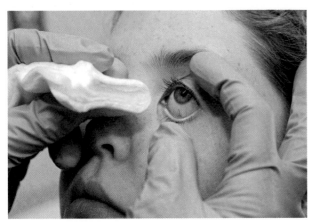

Figure 13-18 Carefully remove a particle from the eyelid.

◆ If the particle still remains or the patient has any vision problems or pain, cover the eye with a sterile dressing. Also cover the uninjured eye to prevent movement of the injured one.

For a chemical or substance splashed in the eye:

1. Follow general principles of wound care.

2. Rinse the eye with running water for at least 20 minutes.

3. Have the patient position his or her head with the affected eye lower than the other so that water does not flow into the unaffected eye.

4. Follow local protocol to consult the Poison Control Center for additional treatment guidance.

Ear Injuries

▶ Need to Do

◆ Bleeding or clear fluid (cerebrospinal fluid) from within the ear can be a sign of a serious head injury. Do not use direct pressure to try to stop fluid from coming out the ear.

◆ Do not try to remove a foreign object from the ear with any tool or object. Never insert tweezers, a pin, or cotton swab into the ear in an attempt to remove an object. Only if the foreign object is clearly visible and easily grasped with your fingers is it safe to remove an object, but do not remove an impaled object.

◆ Occasionally an insect may crawl into the ear when a person is sleeping. If you see or know an insect is in the ear, gently pour lukewarm water into the ear to try to float it out.

With bleeding from the external ear, control the bleeding with direct pressure and dress the wound.

1. Follow general principles of wound care.

2. Help the patient sit up, tilting the affected ear lower to let blood or other fluid drain.

3. Cover the ear with a loose sterile dressing, but do not apply pressure. Do not plug the ear closed to try to stop bleeding.

Nose Injuries

✓ Need to Know

☑ Injury to the nose can cause heavy bleeding.

☑ Bleeding that runs from the back of the nose down the throat is more serious and needs immediate medical attention. Do not tilt the patient's head backward but keep the patient positioned to allow blood to drain out the mouth so that the airway is not threatened.

Need to Do

1. Follow general principles of wound care.
2. Have the patient sit and tilt his or her head slightly forward with the mouth open. Do not try to remove any object you see in the nose. Do not tilt the patient's head backward.
3. Pinch, or have the patient pinch, the nostrils together just below the bridge of the nose for 10 minutes **(Figure 13-19).** Ask the patient to breathe through the mouth and not speak, swallow, cough, or sniff.
4. After 10 minutes, release the pressure slowly. Pinch the nostrils again for another 10 minutes if bleeding continues.
5. With an unresponsive patient or a patient who cannot sit leaning forward, position the patient on one side with the head turned to allow drainage from the nose and mouth while you pinch the nostrils closed. Do not try to pack the nostrils with a dressing in an effort to control the bleeding.

Cheek Injuries

Need to Do

1. Follow general principles of wound care.
2. If an object is impaled in the cheek, check inside the mouth to see if the object has pen-

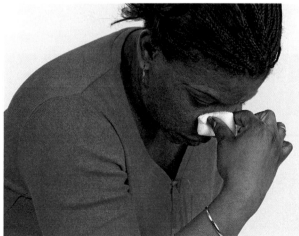

Figure 13-19 For nosebleed, have the patient hold nostrils pinched together.

etrated through. If you can see both sides of the object and can remove it safely, do so. This is the one exception to the rule about not removing an impaled object, because the object may pose a risk to the airway or interfere with ventilation when needed. Gently pull the object out, in the direction from which it penetrated the cheek, taking care with a sharp object not to cut the cheek further.

3. Place a dressing inside the mouth between the cheek wound and the teeth, with the end of the dressing outside the mouth for easy removal if needed. Watch that this dressing does not come out of position and block the airway.
4. Apply another dressing to the outside of the wound, applying pressure as needed to control bleeding.
5. Position an unresponsive patient with the head turned to the side so that blood and other fluid will run out of the mouth.

Teeth and Mouth Injuries

Injuries to the mouth may cause bleeding and may knock out a tooth. Bleeding is controlled with direct pressure on a dressing over the wound. The priority is always to ensure the airway is open and that blood can drain from the mouth until bleeding is controlled.

Need to Do

For bleeding in the mouth:

1. Follow general principles of wound care.
2. Have the patient sit with his or her head tilted forward to let blood drain out.
3. **For a wound penetrating the lip:** Put a rolled dressing between the lip and the gum. Hold a second dressing against the outside lip.
4. **For a bleeding tongue:** Put a dressing on the wound and apply pressure.
5. Do not repeatedly rinse the mouth (this may prevent clotting).
6. Do not let patient swallow blood, which may cause vomiting.

For a tooth knocked out:

1. Follow general principles of wound care.
2. Have the patient sit with his or her head tilted forward to let blood drain out.

3. To control bleeding, fold or roll gauze into a pad and place it over the tooth socket. Have the patient bite down to put pressure on the area.

4. Save the tooth, which may be replanted if the patient sees a dentist soon. Touching only the tooth's crown, rinse it in water only if it is dirty (but do not scrub it or remove attached tissue fragments). Put it in a container of milk, use a commercial tooth saver kit, or wrap it in moist gauze.

5. The tooth should be transported with the patient.

Do You Understand?

1. When is a ring bandage used for a scalp wound?

   _____

2. How long should you flush the eye with running water for a chemical splash?

   _____ minutes

3. Emergency care for ear injuries includes (check all that may apply):

   _____ Removing any objects using tweezers

   _____ Flushing the ear with water to wash out any blood

   _____ Covering the ear with a loose sterile dressing

   _____ Using direct pressure to stop the flow of any clear fluid

4. Describe the one exception to the general rule for not removing objects impaled in a wound.

   _____

Burns

Burns are a major cause of death and injury. Burns of the skin or deeper tissues may be caused by the sun, heat, chemicals, or electricity.

Heat Burns

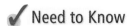 Need to Know

Heat burns may be caused by flames or contact with steam or any hot object. If the patient's clothing is on fire, use a blanket or water to put out any flames or have the patient roll on the ground. Even when the fire is out, the skin will keep burning if it is still hot, so cool the burn area with water immediately, except with very severe burns.

Assessing a Burn

Need to Recognize

Perform the standard assessment:

1. Size up the scene before beginning emergency medical care.

2. Complete the initial assessment.

3. Perform a physical examination as appropriate.

4. Complete ongoing assessments.

In addition, burn assessment involves consideration of several factors:

- Depth of the burn
- Size of the burn
- Specific body areas burned
- Patient's age and health status

Burns are often classified according to their depth into or through the skin:

- **Superficial burns** (also called **first-degree burns**) damage only the skin's outer layer, the epidermis, like a sunburn. The skin is red, typically dry, and painful **(Figure 13-20)**. These are usually minor burns except when covering an extensive area.

- **Partial-thickness burns** (also called **second-degree burns**) damage the skin's deeper layer, the dermis. The skin is red, may look mottled, and is very painful **(Figure 13-21)**. Blisters are often present and may be weeping clear fluid. Partial-thickness burns often require medical attention.

- **Full-thickness burns** (also called **third-degree burns**) damage the skin all the way through the subcutaneous layer and may burn muscle or other tissues. The skin is charred or blackened or may look white and leathery **(Figure 13-22)**.

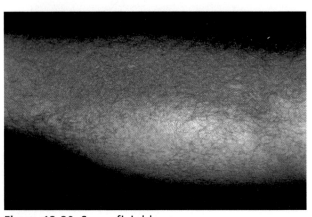

Figure 13-20 Superficial burn.

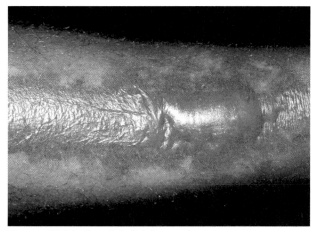

Figure 13-21 Partial-thickness burn.

Pain is not present where the skin has burned through but is likely in adjacent areas. These burns are medical emergencies.

Often a patient with serious burns has a mix of different burn classifications. One area may have a full-thickness burn, while nearby areas have superficial or partial-thickness burns. Care for the most severely burned area first.

In addition to burn depth, the size of the burned area is often assessed. A common method to estimate the body surface area of a burn is the **rule of nines.** In this system, the adult body is divided into a number of areas with percentages based on increments of 9%. As shown in **Figure 13-23**, the percentages are different for a small child.

◗ Each arm is 9% (front or back alone is 4.5%).

◗ Each leg is 18% (front or back alone is 9%).

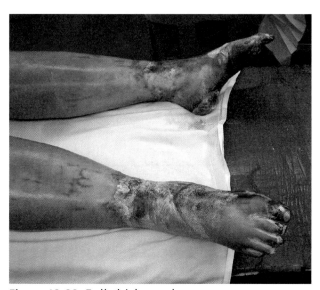

Figure 13-22 Full-thickness burn.

Rule of Nines

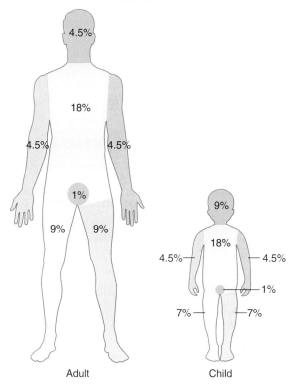

Figure 13-23 The rule of nines for calculating body surface area burned.

◗ The front of the torso is 18% (9% for abdomen and 9% for chest).

◗ The back of the torso is 18% (9% for lower back and buttocks, 9% for upper back).

◗ The head is 9% (face or back of head alone is 4.5%).

◗ The genital region is 1%.

Any full-thickness burn larger than a 50-cent piece or a partial-thickness burn more than 10% of the body in an adult (5% in a child or older adult) is an emergency. A superficial burn over more than 50% of the body may also be an emergency.

Consider also the location of the burn on the body:

◗ Partial- or full-thickness burns on the face, genitals, or hands or feet are considered emergencies and require immediate medical care.

◗ Circumferential burns that wrap around an extremity or a finger or toe should also receive immediate medical attention.

◗ Burns around the nose and mouth may affect breathing and are medical emergencies.

Consider also the patient's age and health:

- A burn in a child under age 5 or an adult over age 55 is more serious than in a younger adult.
- Many **chronic** health disorders also make burns more serious.

Emergency Care for Heat Burns

▶▶ Need to Do

Emergency care for heat burns is based on three general principles of burn care:

- Stop the burning and cool the area with cold water, except for a large burn (over 20% of body surface area, or 10% in a child), because of the risk of hypothermia and shock. Cool as long as the patient feels pain. Be sure the water stays cool by continually adding fresh water.
- Protect the burned area from additional trauma and pathogens.
- Provide supportive care.

Perform standard patient care:

1. Ensure EMS has been activated.
2. Take body substance isolation precautions.
3. Maintain the patient's airway and provide artificial ventilation if needed.
4. Comfort, calm, and reassure the patient while awaiting additional EMS resources.

In addition:

- Follow general principles of wound care.
- Stop the burning by removing the heat source and any smoldering clothing.
- Cool the burn with cold water except for large, full-thickness burns.
- Remove constricting clothing and jewelry before the area swells. If clothing sticks to the burn, do not pull it from the burn but cut around it.
- Treat for shock: Have the patient lie down, elevate the legs, and maintain normal body temperature.
- Carefully cover the burn with a nonstick dressing or a sheet over a larger area.
- If the patient may have inhaled smoke or fumes, watch for airway problems and provide airway and breathing support as needed.
- Follow local protocol to administer oxygen if it is available and you are so trained.

- Do not apply any cream or ointment on the burn, and do not break blisters.
- Do not give the patient anything to drink.
- Monitor the patient's breathing and be ready to give BLS if needed.
- With a child, a large burn may result in greater fluid and heat loss. Keep the environment warm when possible. Depending on the nature of the burn, consider the possibility of child abuse.

Smoke Inhalation

✓ Need to Know

Any patient in the vicinity of a fire could have airway or lung injuries from inhaling smoke or other fumes or even hot air.

- ☑ The lining of the airway may swell and make breathing difficult.
- ☑ The lungs may be damaged, affecting the ability of the body to receive enough oxygen through normal breathing.
- ☑ Carbon monoxide poisoning may also have occurred (see Chapter 11).

■■ Need to Recognize

Perform the standard assessment:

1. Size up the scene before beginning emergency medical care.
2. Complete the initial assessment.
3. Perform a physical examination as appropriate.
4. Complete ongoing assessments.

Signs and symptoms of smoke inhalation:

- Coughing, wheezing, hoarse voice
- Possible burned area or blackening on face or chest
- Difficulty breathing

▶▶ Need to Do

Perform standard patient care:

1. Ensure EMS has been activated.
2. Take body substance isolation precautions.
3. Maintain the patient's airway and provide artificial ventilation if needed.
4. Comfort, calm, and reassure the patient while awaiting additional EMS resources.

In addition:

- Get the patient to fresh air, or fresh air to the patient. Follow local protocol to administer oxygen if it is available and you are so trained.
- Help the patient into a position for easy breathing (often semi-reclining).
- Put an unresponsive patient in the recovery position.
- Monitor the airway and breathing, and be ready to give BLS if needed.

Chemical Burns

✔ Need to Know

Many strong chemicals found in workplaces and the home can burn the skin on contact.

- ☑ Sometimes the burn develops slowly and in some cases the patient may not be aware of the burn for up to 24 hours.
- ☑ Acids and alkalis, liquids and solids can all cause serious chemical burns **(Figure 13-24)**.
- ☑ The chemical reaction can continue as long as the substance is on the skin, so you must remove it immediately.

Assessing Chemical Burns

◼ Need to Recognize

Perform the standard assessment:

1. Size up the scene before beginning emergency medical care.
2. Complete the initial assessment.
3. Perform a physical examination as appropriate.
4. Complete ongoing assessments.

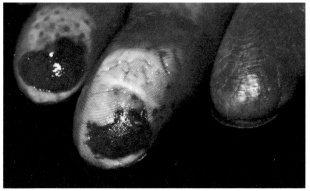

Figure 13-24 A chemical burn.

Signs and symptoms of chemical burns:

- Pain or a burning sensation
- Chemical on the patient's skin or clothing
- Spilled substance on or around an unresponsive patient
- Smell of fumes in the air

Emergency Care for Chemical Burns

▶ Need to Do

Perform standard patient care:

1. Ensure EMS has been activated.
2. Take body substance isolation precautions.
3. Maintain the patient's airway and provide artificial ventilation if needed.
4. Comfort, calm, and reassure the patient while awaiting additional EMS resources.

In addition:

- Wear medical exam gloves and eye protection if appropriate.
- With a dry chemical, first brush it off the patient's skin with a cloth, piece of cardboard or paper, spare article of clothing, or any other available item. Take care not to contaminate skin that has not been in contact with the chemical **(Figure 13-25)**.
- Move the patient or ventilate the area, because of the risk of fumes in a confined area.
- Wash off the area as quickly as possible with running water for at least 30 minutes. Use a sink, hose, or even a shower to flush the whole area of contact **(Figure 13-26)**.
- Do not try to neutralize an acid by applying an alkaline substance, or vice versa, because of the risk of further damage caused by the chemical reaction.
- Remove clothing and jewelry from the burn area while flushing with water.
- Put a dry, nonstick dressing over the burn.
- With a chemical splashed in the eye, flush immediately with running water and continue for at least 20 minutes. Have the patient remove a contact lens. Tilt the patient's head so that the water runs away from the face and not into the other eye. After flushing, have the patient hold a dressing over the eye until he or she receives medical care.

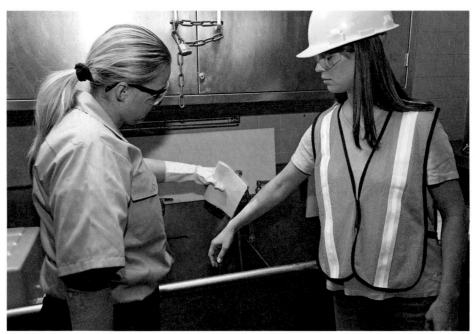

Figure 13-25 Brush a dry chemical from the skin before flushing with water.

Electrical Burns and Shocks

✔ Need to Know

An electrical burn or shock can occur whenever any part of the body comes in contact with electricity. Typical injuries occur with electricity from faulty appliances or power cords or when an appliance comes into contact with water. Two possible injuries may occur from electricity:

- ☑ External burns caused by the heat of electricity
- ☑ Electrical injuries caused by electricity flowing through the body

High-voltage electricity flowing through the body can cause significant injuries to many differ-

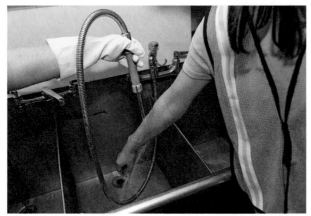

Figure 13-26 Flush the skin after a chemical burn for at least 30 minutes.

ent tissues. Heart damage may cause heart rhythm irregularities that threaten the patient's circulation or cause the heart to stop.

Assessing Electrical Burns

◼ Need to Recognize

Perform the standard assessment:

1. Size up the scene before beginning emergency medical care.

2. Complete the initial assessment.

3. Perform a physical examination as appropriate.

4. Complete ongoing assessments.

Signs and symptoms of electrical injury:

- A source of electricity near the patient: bare wires, power cords, an electrical device

- External burns where the electricity entered and left the body, called **entrance** and **exit wounds (Figure 13-27)**

- Unresponsiveness, seizures, or changing levels of responsiveness

- Breathing abnormalities

- A weak or irregular pulse

Electrical burns can cause massive internal injuries, even when the external burn may look minor.

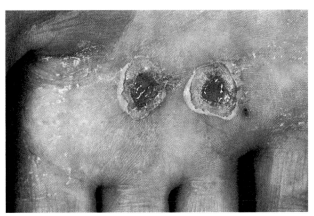

Figure 13-27 An electrical burn.

Emergency Care for Electrical Burns

▶ Need to Do

Perform standard patient care:

1. Ensure EMS has been activated.
2. Take body substance isolation precautions.
3. Maintain the patient's airway and provide artificial ventilation if needed.
4. Comfort, calm, and reassure the patient while awaiting additional EMS resources.

In addition:

- Do not touch the patient until you know the area is safe. Unplug or turn off the power. Do not approach the scene of a downed power line.
- Care for the burn: Stop the burning, cool the area, remove clothing and jewelry, and cover the burn.
- Treat for shock by having the patient lie down, elevating the legs, and maintaining normal body temperature.
- Keep an unresponsive patient in the recovery position and monitor breathing and vital signs. Be prepared to give BLS if needed.
- Assume a patient who experienced a lightning strike or high-voltage shock may have a spinal injury and stabilize the head and neck.

Do You Understand?

1. List four factors that determine the severity of a burn:

   _____   _____

   _____   _____

2. True or false: For a patient with a partial-thickness burn, you should break skin blisters and cover the area with a burn ointment to promote faster healing.

3. Do not use cold water to cool a burn larger than ____% of body surface area.

4. List at least three signs and symptoms that may indicate the patient inhaled smoke.

   _____

   _____

   _____

5. Which is the first action you should take for a patient with a chemical splashed in the eye?

   a. Have the patient keep the eye closed and let tears wash out the chemical.
   b. Apply a bandage and let arriving EMTs treat the eye.
   c. Flush the eye with running water.
   d. Apply a mixture of baking soda and water to the eye.

Conclusion

Soft-tissue injuries are among the most common injuries requiring emergency care. Control bleeding and dress and bandage the wound to help prevent infection. Specific types of wounds, and injuries in certain areas of the body, require additional specific care. When significant traumatic forces are involved, soft-tissue injuries are often accompanied by injuries to muscles and bones, as discussed in the next chapter.

Key Terms

abrasion (p. 195)

amputation (p. 196)

avulsion (p. 196)

burn (p. 196)

chronic (p. 214)

closed wound (p. 195)

contusion (p. 195)

entrance wound (p. 216)

evisceration (p. 206)

exit wound (p. 216)

first-degree burn (p. 212)

full-thickness burn (p. 212)

hemothorax (p. 205)

irrigate (p. 197)

laceration (p. 196)

occlusive dressing (p. 198)

open wound (p. 195)

partial-thickness burn (p. 212)

pneumothorax (p. 205)

puncture (p. 196)

rabies (p. 204)

rule of nines (p. 213)

second-degree burn (p. 212)

sucking chest wound (p. 204)

superficial burn (p. 212)

tetanus (p. 197)

third-degree burn (p. 212)

trauma dressing (p. 198)

Review Questions

1. What is the first priority for a severely bleeding wound?
   a. Transporting the patient
   b. Controlling the bleeding
   c. Preventing infection
   d. Irrigating the wound

2. What is the best way to clean a minor wound?
   a. Soak it in alcohol.
   b. Apply iodine to it.
   c. Irrigate it with water.
   d. Wipe it with a sterile dressing.

3. How would you best care for a traumatically amputated finger?
   a. Wash it under running water and put it in a glass or jar of ice water.
   b. Wrap it in a dressing, place it inside a plastic bag, and put the bag on ice.
   c. Keep it dry and at body temperature (held against the patient's body).
   d. Put it in a plastic bag and place the bag in the freezer.

4. What kind of bandage is most appropriate for an open abdominal wound?
   a. Elastic roller bandage
   b. Adhesive tape
   c. Triangular bandage
   d. Occlusive bandage

5. The bandage over a sucking chest wound is taped in such a way to allow
   a. air to enter the wound.
   b. air to exit the wound.
   c. water to irrigate the wound.
   d. bleeding to be unimpeded.

6. For a painful blow to the eye,
   a. flush constantly with warm water for up to 30 minutes.
   b. have patient sit in a dark room with both eyes covered for 30 minutes.
   c. put a cold pack over the eye for up to 15 minutes.
   d. give the patient aspirin or ibuprofen.

7. Care for a nosebleed includes
   a. having the patient "blow" the nose into a handkerchief to clear out blood.
   b. packing the nose with sterile gauze.
   c. having the patient tilt the head back while sucking on ice chips.
   d. pinching the nostrils closed for up to 10 minutes.

8. The purpose of putting a dressing over a burn is to
   a. protect the area.
   b. squeeze the fluid from blisters.
   c. keep the area moist for 24 hours.
   d. prevent swelling.

9. Using icy water to cool a burn covering 25% of the body could result in
   a. hypothermia and shock.
   b. shock and cardiac arrest.
   c. hypothermia and severe bleeding.
   d. electrolyte imbalances and infection.

10. Emergency care for a dry chemical burn includes
   a. neutralizing an acid burn with an alkaline substance.
   b. neutralizing an alkaline burn with an acidic substance.
   c. brushing off the chemical and then flushing the skin with water.
   d. tightly taping a dressing over the burn.

Injuries to Muscles and Bones

Chapter Preview

- Musculoskeletal System Review
- Mechanisms of Injury to Musculoskeletal System
- Types of Musculoskeletal Injuries
- Assessment of Musculoskeletal Injuries
- Emergency Care of Musculoskeletal Injuries
- Splinting

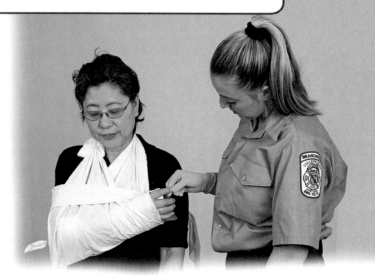

You Respond To ...

a farm where a man has been injured by a heavy piece of equipment that fell on his leg. He is lying on the ground and is responsive and breathing. Blood has soaked through his pants leg above the knee. His upper leg looks oddly angled. He is in significant pain.

Introduction

Trauma patients often have considerable injuries to the musculoskeletal system. With significant mechanisms of injury, bones may fracture and joints may be injured, resulting in pain, disability, and potentially life-threatening injuries with severe bleeding. This chapter covers musculoskeletal injuries to the extremities, ribcage, and pelvis. Injuries to the skull and spine are discussed in Chapter 15.

Musculoskeletal System Review

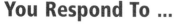 Need to Know

The musculoskeletal system includes the body's bones and muscles along with other structures that join bones at joints **(Figure 14-1)**. The musculoskeletal system's primary functions are the following:

- ☑ The skeletal system provides shape and support for the body as a whole.
- ☑ The muscles acting on bones allow for movement.
- ☑ Groups of bones protect vital internal organs:
  - Ribs protect the heart and lungs.
  - The skull protects the brain.
  - Vertebrae protect the spinal cord.
  - Pelvic bones protect the bladder and other organs.

There are three different types of muscles:

- ☑ Skeletal muscles attach to bones to create body movements and also produce heat **(Figure 14-2)**. These voluntary muscles are under a person's control and provide for movement.
- ☑ Smooth muscles, such as in the esophagus and blood vessels, are involuntary.

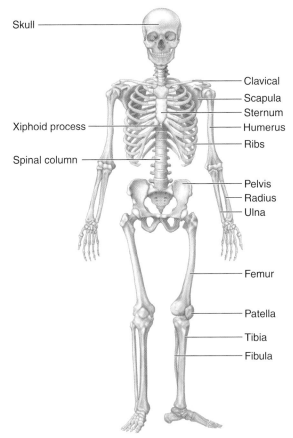

Figure 14-1 The skeletal system.

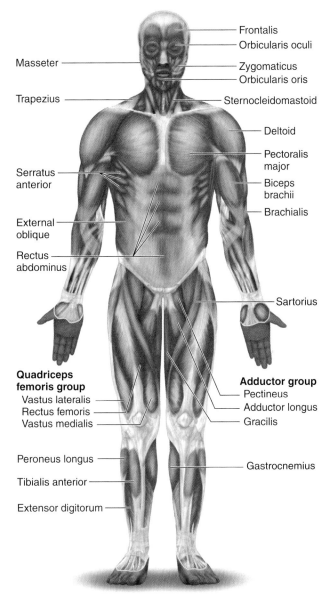

Figure 14-2 Major muscles of the body.

☑ Cardiac muscle is also involuntary.

☑ All muscle activity is controlled by the nervous system.

In addition:

☑ **Tendons** are fibrous tissues that connect muscles to bones.

☑ **Ligaments** are tough bands of tissue that join bones together at joints.

Mechanisms of Injury to Musculoskeletal System

✓ Need to Know

Different types of forces may result in musculoskeletal injuries (**Figure 14-3**).

☑ *Direct force* is a force applied directly to the body, such as being struck by a falling object, the impact of falling on a hard surface, or the impact of the chest against the steering wheel in a vehicle crash.

☑ *Indirect force* is a mechanism of injury in which the force is transferred from its original site in the body along an extremity to impact another point, such as when one falls on an outstretched arm and the force is transferred up the arm and causes dislocation of the shoulder joint.

☑ *Twisting forces* are involved when one part of the body is forced to move in an unnatural direction while the rest of the body remains still, or when the body moves but one part is held stationary. For example, one's foot may be caught in debris when the body falls forward, or a skier's leg may be twisted sideways when one ski is forced sideways while the body moves forward.

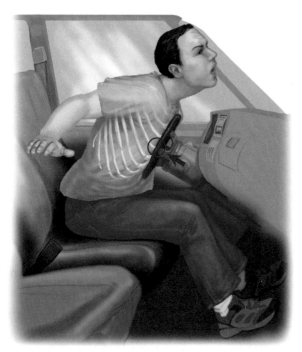

Direct forces often injure that impacted area of the body; the larger the force, the more likely is a serious injury such as a fracture or damage to internal organs.

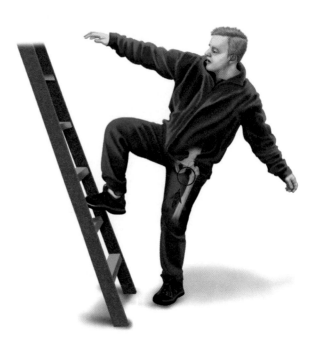

An **indirect force** may also be transferred up or down an extremity, as when falling on one leg. Similarly, falling on an outstretched arm may cause dislocation of shoulder bones.

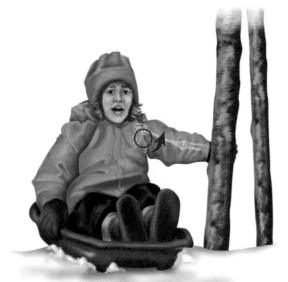

Twisting forces occur when the body moves in one direction but a force keeps some part of an extremity from moving with the rest of the body. Twisting forces may cause fractures or dislocations of bones at joints.

Figure 14-3 Common mechanisms of musculoskeletal injury.

◼▦ Need to Recognize

Consider the type and strength of forces involved when assessing a patient's injury.

◗ The greater the force, the more severe the injury is likely to be and to involve a fracture or joint dislocation.

◗ Many other factors are also involved, such as the patient's age and health status, so do not assume there are no significant injuries with smaller forces. A patient with **osteoporosis** (brittle bones associated with age), for example, may have a severe fracture from a simple fall or other trauma.

Types of Musculoskeletal Injuries

✓ Need to Know

Musculoskeletal trauma may result in either **open** or **closed injuries,** depending on whether there is a break in the skin. Open injuries increase the risk for infection, but even closed injuries may be severe and involve profuse internal bleeding.

Musculoskeletal injuries may also be classified as fractures, joint injuries (dislocations and sprains), and muscle injuries. First Responders are not responsible for determining the type of injury.

☑ **Fractures.** A fracture is a broken bone. The bone may be completely broken with the pieces separated or still together, or it may only be cracked **(Figure 14-4)**. With a closed fracture, the skin is not broken. Internal bleeding may occur. With an open fracture there is an open wound at the fracture site, and the bone end may protrude through the wound **(Figure 14-5)**. An open fracture can be more serious because there is a greater chance of infection and more serious bleeding.

☑ **Dislocations.** In a dislocation, one or more of the bones at the joint are displaced from their normal position when the ligaments that normally hold the bone in place are torn. Dislocations typically result from strong forces and are sometimes accompanied by bone fractures or other serious injuries. The patient is unable to use the joint because of pain and structural damage in the joint. Serious bleeding may result if nearby major blood vessels are injured. Nearby nerves may also be injured, causing altered sensation in the extremity, such as tingling or numbness. If the dislocation is severe, the joint or limb will look deformed **(Figure 14-6)**.

☑ **Sprains.** A sprain is a joint injury involving the stretching or tearing of ligaments. Sprains typically occur when the joint is overextended or forced beyond the range of normal movement. Sprains can range from mild to severe. The ankles, knees, wrists, and fingers are most often sprained. Swelling may be considerable and often occurs rapidly.

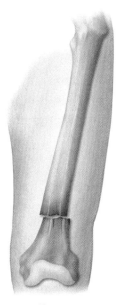 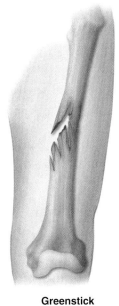 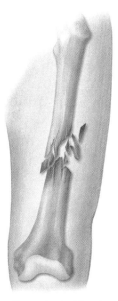 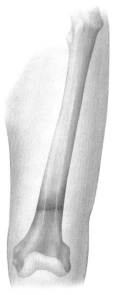 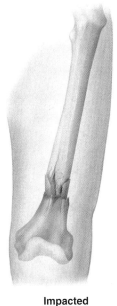

Transverse	**Greenstick**	**Comminuted fracture**	**Hairline fracture**	**Impacted**
The fracture line crosses the bone at a right angle.	An incomplete fracture and bending of bone that is more likely in children whose bones are soft.	The bone is broken into more than two fragments.	The bone fragments do not separate.	One fragment is driven into the bone of the other fragment.

Figure 14-4 Common types of fractures.

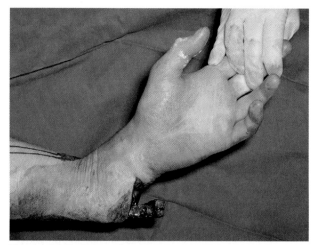

Figure 14-5 Open fracture.

☑ **Muscle Injuries.** Common muscle injuries include **strains, contusions,** and **cramps.** These injuries are usually less serious than fractures and joint injuries. Muscle injuries are typically caused by overexertion, careless or sudden uncoordinated movements, or poor body mechanics, such as lifting a weight with the back bent or twisted.

In some cases, the type of injury may be obvious, while in many cases you will recognize only that a musculoskeletal injury is present but will not know what kind. The emergency care for most patients with musculoskeletal injuries is the same regardless of the type.

Do You Understand?

1. Large forces are more likely to result in _____ or _____ (types of musculoskeletal injuries).

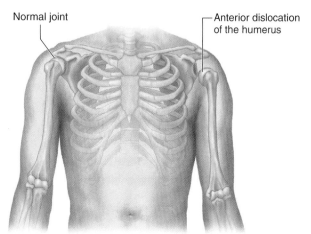

Normal joint   Anterior dislocation of the humerus

Figure 14-6 A deformity may occur with a dislocation.

2. An elderly patient suffering trauma is more likely than a younger patient to suffer a fracture because of _____.

3. What may result from a dislocation that can cause a serious or even life-threatening condition?

Assessment of Musculoskeletal Injuries

✔ Need to Know

Remember to perform the initial assessment of any patient and care for any life-threatening conditions before performing a physical examination. Musculoskeletal injuries are usually not life threatening, except in cases of severe bleeding, but may nonetheless be serious and result in pain and disability.

☑ Ask a responsive patient what happened and what he or she felt when the injury occurred.

☑ If large forces were involved in the injury, consider the potential also for a spinal injury. Particularly if the patient is unresponsive, do not move him or her unnecessarily to assess a musculoskeletal injury.

■ Need to Recognize

Perform the standard assessment:

1. Size up the scene before beginning emergency medical care.
2. Complete the initial assessment.
3. Perform a physical examination as appropriate.
4. Complete ongoing assessments.

In addition:

♦ Expose the injury site (control bleeding as needed).

♦ Recognize that the amount of pain or swelling is not a good indicator of the seriousness of the injury.

♦ Assess for circulation, sensation, and movement (CSM) below the injury site:
   ○ Check for a pulse below the injury (radial pulse in the wrist or pedal pulse in the foot) and for skin color and temperature.
   ○ Check for sensation by touching the patient's fingers or toes to determine whether the patient can feel your touch or feels a tingling sensation or numbness.

○ Check movement by asking the patient to wiggle the fingers or toes, unless doing so causes pain.

◗ A lack of circulation or possible nerve damage indicated by abnormal sensation or movement indicates a need for immediate medical treatment.

Signs and symptoms of musculoskeletal injuries **(Figure 14-7):**

◗ Deformity of the area or angulation of the extremity (compare to the other extremity)

◗ Pain and tenderness

◗ A feeling or sound of bone ends grating together (**crepitus**)

◗ Swelling

◗ Skin discoloration: Bruising or a pale or light blue skin color (an ashen color in dark-skinned individuals), along with cool skin, may indicate a lack of blood flow below the injured area.

◗ Bone ends exposed in an open wound

◗ Joint locked into position

◗ Abnormal sensation (numbness, tingling)

◗ Inability to move the area

◗ Difference in temperature from the opposite extremity

Emergency Care of Musculoskeletal Injuries

✔ Need to Know

Any movement of a musculoskeletal injury can cause further injury, pain, and swelling. With a fracture or dislocation, movement of the extremity could cause the bone to move, further injuring soft tissues such as blood vessels and nerves. Movement also generally increases blood flow, which may increase internal bleeding and swelling.

Manually stabilizing or splinting the injured area is therefore a key part of emergency care.

▶ Need to Do

Perform standard patient care:

1. Ensure EMS has been activated.

2. Take body substance isolation precautions.

3. Maintain the patient's airway and provide artificial ventilation if needed.

4. Comfort, calm, and reassure the patient while awaiting additional EMS resources.

In addition:

◗ After any life threats have been controlled, allow the patient to remain in a position of comfort.

◗ Cover open wounds with a sterile dressing.

◗ Put a cold pack on an area of painful, swollen, deformed extremity to reduce swelling and pain, except on an open fracture.

◗ Do not try to replace bones protruding from a wound.

◗ Stabilize an injured extremity manually, or have the patient manually support the area.
  ○ Support above and below an injury.
  ○ Pad the area to prevent pressure and discomfort.
  ○ When in doubt, manually stabilize the injury.

◗ Follow local protocol to administer oxygen if it is available and you are so trained.

◗ If appropriate, splint the extremity.

✎ Do You Understand?

1. What three things should you assess distal to a musculoskeletal injury?

_____ _____ _____

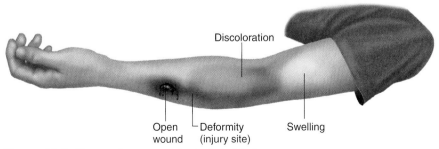

Discoloration

Open wound └Deformity (injury site) Swelling

Figure 14-7 Signs of a musculoskeletal injury.

2. In addition to a weak or absent pulse, what are other signs of impaired circulation below a musculoskeletal injury?

_____ _____

3. True or false: The greater the patient's level of pain, the more serious is the injury.

4. Why is a cold pack used on most musculoskeletal injuries?

_____

Splinting

✔ Need to Know

All musculoskeletal injuries should be stabilized to prevent movement. An injured extremity may be stabilized with a splint if there is a risk for movement of the injured area unless help is expected within a few minutes. An extremity is always splinted before the patient is transported. Splinting helps prevent further injury, reduces pain, and minimizes bleeding and swelling.

Types of Splints

A **splint** is any object used to help keep an injured body area from moving. Commonly used splints include rigid, soft, and improvised splints. **Figure 14-8** shows some examples of commercial splints.

☑ Rigid splints are made of many different materials and often resemble a padded board. Some can be contoured to fit the extremity more closely. Rigid splints are applied along an extremity in line with the bone.

☑ Soft splints may be made from a pillow, a folded blanket or towel, or a triangular bandage folded into a **sling.** Soft splints provide support for an injured joint such as the ankle or hand. Slings help immobilize the arm.

☑ Air splints, or inflatable splints, are like plastic sleeves that surround the lower leg or arm and become rigid when inflated by blowing into a tube. Air splints are a type of pneumatic splints, which also include vacuum splints.

☑ Vacuum splints are flexible bladder-like splints that are positioned around an extremity. When the air is suctioned out of the splint, it becomes rigid.

☑ Improvised rigid splints may be made from a board, a cane or walking stick, a broom

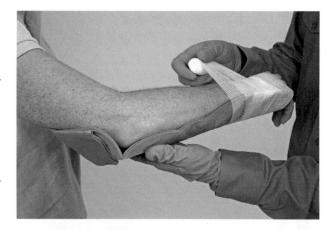
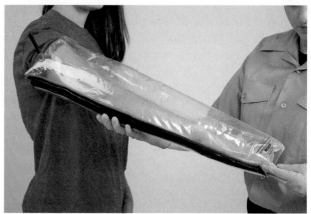
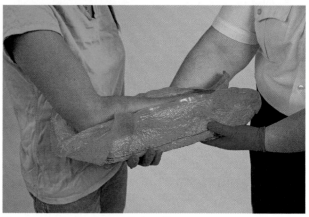

Figure 14-8 Commercial splints.

handle, a piece of plastic or metal, a rolled newspaper or magazine, or thick cardboard. Improvised splints can be tied in place with bandages, belts, neckties, or strips of cloth torn from clothing.

☑ Improvised anatomic splints involve splinting one part of the body with another part, such as an injured leg to the uninjured leg or splinting fingers together, or splinting the arm to the chest to immobilize the shoulder.

Splints are usually secured by wrapping bandages, strips of cloth (often called **cravats**), Velcro® straps, or other materials around the splint and extremity.

☑ Use knots that can be untied because you may have to loosen or remove the splint if it interferes with circulation to the limb.

☑ Do not secure a splint with tape, which can be difficult to remove, unless no other material is available; if used, do not tape the skin directly but put a dressing or other material over the skin first.

Guidelines for Splinting

▶ Need to Do

Regardless of the specific type of injury and its location, always follow these general guidelines for splinting. Later sections in this chapter show how to use these guidelines when splinting specific extremity injuries.

◆ Put a dressing on open wounds before splinting the area.

◆ Assess circulation, sensation, and movement before applying the splint.

◆ Splint an injury only if it does not cause more pain for the patient. Splinting usually involves touching and perhaps manipulating the injured area, which may cause pain and may worsen the injury. If the patient complains, stop the splinting and manually immobilize the area until additional EMS personnel arrive.

◆ Splint the injury in the position you find it **(Figure 14-9)**. Trying to straighten out an extremity or joint could worsen the injury. Blood vessels or nerves near a fracture or dislocation could be damaged by moving the bone ends. The extremity should be straightened only if the patient is in a remote location and will not receive medical attention for a long time and if circulation has been cut off in the extremity by the injury. Follow your local protocols.

◆ Splint to immobilize the entire injured area. The splint should extend to the joints above and below the injured area. With a bone fracture near a joint, assume that the joint too is injured, and extend the splint well beyond the joint to keep it immobilized as well as the fracture site.

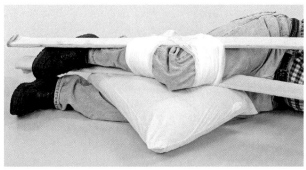

Figure 14-9 Splint an injury in the position found, such as this knee injury. Do not try to straighten an injured extremity to splint it.

◆ Put padding, such as cloth, between the splint and the skin, especially with rigid splints, which otherwise might press into soft tissues and cause pain and further injury. Use materials that will conform to the space between the splint and the body part. Pad body hollows and ensure the area of the splint close to the injury is well padded **(Figure 14-10)**.

◆ Put splints on both sides of a fractured bone if possible. If the injury makes this difficult or splinting materials are limited, splint one side.

◆ Do not secure the splint on an open wound because the securing bandage or strap could cut into or irritate the wound. Tie the bandages or other materials used to hold the splint in place on both sides of the wound.

◆ Elevate the splinted extremity if possible, but do not move the injured area to elevate it if it causes the patient pain or may worsen the injury.

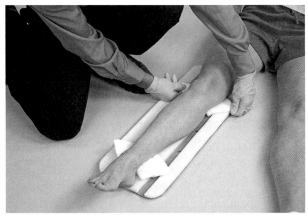

Figure 14-10 Pad areas between the splint and the skin.

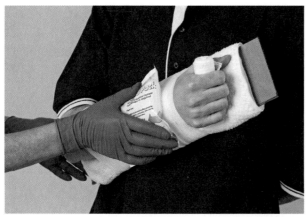

Figure 14-11 Apply a cold pack to the injured area around the splint.

- Apply a cold pack to the injury around the splint. The ice or cold pack must be removed after 20 minutes, so it should not be positioned inside the splint. Splint the injury first and then position the cold pack as near the injury as possible around the splint **(Figure 14-11)**.

- With a splinted extremity, do not completely bandage over the fingers or toes, and assess them frequently after splinting for CSM. Swelling, a pale or bluish discoloration, tingling or numbness, and cold skin are signs and symptoms of reduced circulation. If any of these occurs, loosen the bandages, holding the limb to the splint.

Guidelines for Slings

▶ Need to Do

A sling is used to prevent movement of the arm and shoulder with most upper extremity injuries, including shoulder, upper and lower arm, elbow, and wrist injuries.

- A sling is best made from a large triangular bandage but can be improvised with many other materials, such as strips of cloth torn from clothing, neckties, and so on. Cloth or a soft, flexible material is usually best.

- A swathe, also called a binder, is used along with the sling to provide additional support **(Skill 14-1)**.

Follow these guidelines when using a sling:

- Splint the injury first, when appropriate. A fracture of the upper or lower arm or a dislocation of the elbow or wrist should be splinted to prevent movement of the extremity. Then apply a sling.

- If you splint the injury in the position found and this position makes the use of a sling impossible or difficult, do not try to use a sling.

- Do not move the arm into position for a sling if this causes the patient more pain. If moving the arm causes pain, splint the arm in the position found, not using a sling, and keep the arm immobilized.

- A cold pack can be used inside the sling.

- Do not cover the fingers inside the sling. Periodically assess CSM.

✎ Do You Understand?

1. List at least three common materials you may use to improvise a rigid splint if needed.

_____   _____

_____

2. True or false: Always elevate a splinted extremity.

3. When should you splint an injury in the position in which you find it?

_____

4. You plan to splint a patient's forearm and then put the arm in a sling. Will you use a cold pack on the injury? If so, where should the pack be placed?

_____

Splinting Upper Extremity Injuries

Shoulder Injuries

✓ Need to Know

Shoulder injuries can fracture the **clavicle** (collarbone), the **scapula** (shoulder blade), or joint structures.

- ☑ The clavicle is the most frequently fractured bone in the body.

- ☑ Fractures of the scapula are rare.

- ☑ Dislocations of the shoulder are common.

▶ Need to Do

The goal of splinting the shoulder is to stabilize the area from the trunk to the upper arm.

1. Use a soft, not rigid, splint for shoulder injuries. Do not move the extremity.

2. Assess for circulation, sensation, and movement in the hand and fingers.

Skill 14-1 **Applying an Arm Sling and Swathe**

1 Secure the point of the bandage at the elbow.

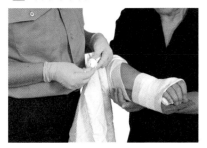

2 Position the triangular bandage.

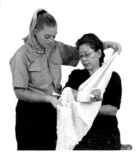

3 Bring up the lower end of the bandage to the opposite side of the neck.

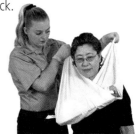

4 Tie the ends.

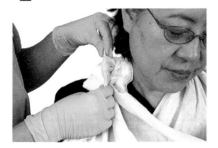

5 Tie a swathe bandage over the sling and around the chest.

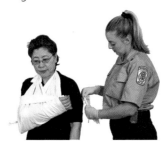

3. Pad the hollow between the body and the arm with a small pillow or towels, and apply a sling and swathe to support the arm and immobilize it against the chest **(Figure 14-12)**. If moving the arm closer to the chest causes pain, use a larger pillow between the arm and the trunk.

4. Follow the general guidelines for safe splinting. Check the fingers periodically for CSM.

Upper Arm Injuries

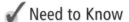 **Need to Know**

Fractures of the **humerus,** the bone of the upper arm, are immobilized with a rigid splint except for fractures near the shoulder, which should be treated identically to shoulder injuries with soft splinting. The goal of splinting is to stabilize the bone between the shoulder and the elbow.

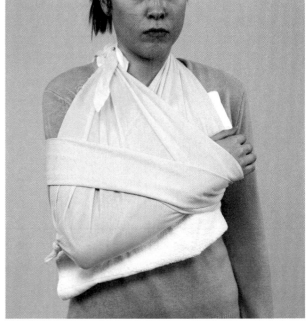

Figure 14-12 Immobilize a shoulder injury with a sling and swathe.

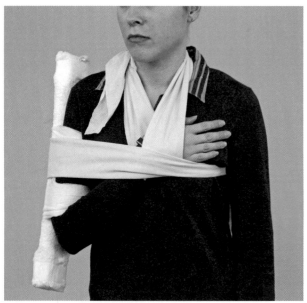

Figure 14-13 Immobilize an upper arm injury with a splint, sling, and swathe.

Need to Do

1. Assess for circulation, sensation, and movement in the hand and fingers.
2. Apply a rigid splint along the outside of the upper arm, tied above the injury and at the elbow.
3. Support the wrist with a sling, and then apply a wide swathe to support the arm and immobilize it against the chest **(Figure 14-13)**. (Be careful not to apply the swathe directly over the fracture site.) If it causes the patient pain to raise the wrist for a sling, a long rigid splint may be used that supports the arm in a straighter position.

4. Follow the general guidelines for safe splinting. Check the fingers periodically for CSM.

Elbow Injuries

Need to Know

Sprains and dislocations are the most common injuries to the elbow joint, along with fractures of the bones above or below the elbow. The patient is unable to move the joint and may say the joint is "locked." The goal of splinting the elbow is to stabilize the joint from the arm to the forearm in the position found.

- ☑ If the elbow is bent, a soft splint with sling and swathe may be sufficient, but a rigid splint provides greater stability.
- ☑ If the elbow is straight, a rigid splint should be applied.

Need to Do

1. Assess for circulation, sensation, and movement in the hand and fingers.
2. If the elbow is bent, apply a rigid splint from the upper arm to the wrist as shown in **Figure 14-14a**. If more support is needed, use a sling at the wrist and a swathe around the chest at the upper arm.
3. If the elbow is straight, apply a rigid splint from the upper arm to the hand as shown in **Figure 14-14b**. If more support is needed, swathes may be used around the chest and upper arm and around the lower arm and waist.
4. Follow the general guidelines for safe splinting. Check the fingers periodically for CSM.

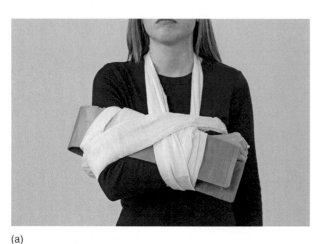

(a)

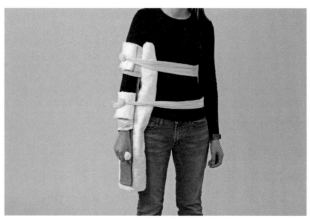

(b)

Figure 14-14 Immobilize an elbow injury with a rigid splint in the position found. (a) Splinting a bent elbow. (b) Splinting a straight elbow.

Skill 14-2 **Splinting the Forearm**

1 Support the arm. Check circulation, sensation, and movement.

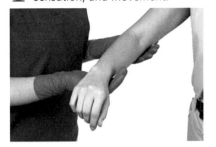

2 Position the arm on a rigid splint.

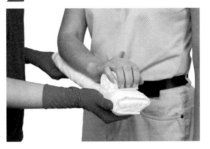

3 Secure the splint.

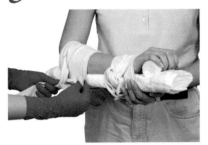

4 Put the arm in a sling, and tie a swathe over the sling and around the chest.

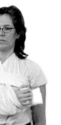

5 Assess for circulation, sensation, and movement.

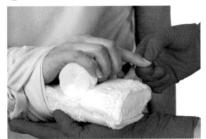

Forearm Injuries

✓ Need to Know

The forearm is frequently injured by direct blows that may fracture either or both the bones (the **radius** and **ulna**). The goal of forearm splinting is to stabilize and support the area from the elbow to the hand with a rigid splint on the palm side of the forearm or on both sides **(Skill 14-2)**.

Wrist Injuries

✓ Need to Know

Common wrist injuries include sprains and fractures. The goal of splinting is to stabilize the area from the forearm to the hand.

☑ In some cases, a soft splint is sufficient, with the area supported with a sling.

☑ A rigid splint provides more support, and the joint is stabilized in a manner similar to a forearm injury.

▶▶ Need to Do

1. Assess for circulation, sensation, and movement in the hand and fingers.

2. Apply a rigid splint on the palm side of the arm from the forearm past the fingertips, tied above and below the wrist. Leave the fingers uncovered.

3. Support the forearm and wrist with a sling, and then apply a swathe around the upper arm and chest **(Figure 14-15)**.

4. Follow the general guidelines for safe splinting. Check the fingers periodically for CSM.

Hand and Finger Injuries

✓ Need to Know

The hand may be injured by a direct blow. Fractures often occur when the patient punches something with a closed fist. The goal is to immobilize the hand with a soft or rigid splint.

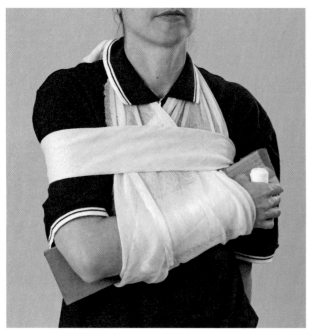

Figure 14-15 Immobilize an injured wrist with a splint, a sling, and a swathe.

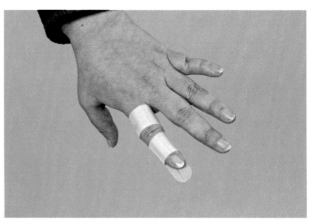

(a)

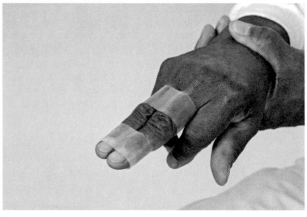

(b)

Figure 14-16 Splint a finger injury. (a) Rigid splint. (b) Anatomic splint.

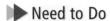 **Need to Do**

1. Place a roll of gauze or similar padding in the palm, allowing the fingers to take a naturally curled position. Then bandage the entire hand.

2. Place a rigid splint on the palm side of the hand extending from above the wrist to the fingers, the same as with a wrist injury. Pad the area well between the hand and the splint.

3. Support the injury further with a sling and swathe.

Finger injuries include fractures and dislocations, common in sports and industrial injuries. Often a splint is not required, but a patient with a painful injury will benefit from splinting.

- Use a soft splint if the finger cannot be straightened without pain. Do not try to manipulate the finger to move a bone into its normal position.

- Use a rigid splint, such as a tongue depressor or ice cream stick secured in place with tape, or an anatomic splint by taping the finger to an adjoining finger with gauze in between (**Figure 14-16**).

Splinting Lower Extremity Injuries

✓ **Need to Know**

Because the bones of the thigh and lower leg are larger than those of the arm, typically larger forces are involved in injuries, which may result in a spinal injury as well.

☑ Assess the patient, being careful not to move the extremity.

☑ A fracture of the femur can damage the large femoral artery and cause life-threatening bleeding.

Hip and Pelvis Injuries

✓ **Need to Know**

The hip is the joint where the top of the **femur** meets the pelvis. Pelvis and hip injuries include fractures and, less commonly, hip dislocations.

☑ A hip fracture is a fracture of the top part of the femur.

☑ Fractures are more common in the elderly, whose bones are often more brittle because of osteoporosis. Bleeding and pain may be severe.

☑ Hip dislocations can occur at any age, resulting from falls, vehicular crashes, and blows to the body.

▶ Need to Do

1. Do not move the patient, and immobilize the leg and hip in the position you find it.

2. If the patient's legs are together, you can immobilize the area by padding between the legs with a soft pillow or blanket and gently bandaging them together, unless this causes more pain **(Figure 14-17)**.

3. Treat the patient for shock but do not elevate the legs.

Upper Leg Injuries

✔ Need to Know

Fractures of the femur are serious because, even with a closed injury, bleeding can be profuse. The patient experiences severe pain and may be in shock.

☑ Keep the patient from moving. If the patient is lying down with the leg supported by the ground, a rigid splint may be unnecessary.

☑ Provide additional support with folded blankets or coats to immobilize the leg in the position found.

☑ If help may be delayed, splinting helps stabilize the injury. To use an anatomic splint, pad between the legs, move the uninjured leg beside the injured one, and carefully tie the legs together.

☑ A rigid splint provides better support if needed.

▶ Need to Do

1. Assess for circulation, sensation, and movement in the foot and toes.

2. If possible, put a rigid splint on each side of the leg. Pad bony areas and voids between the leg and the splints. The inside splint should extend from the groin past the foot, and the outside splint from the armpit past the foot.

3. Tie the splints with cravats or bandages **(Figure 14-18)**.

4. Follow the general guidelines for safe splinting. Check the toes periodically for CSM.

Traction Splint for Leg Injuries

✔ Need to Know

With fractures of the femur, the muscles of the thigh often spasm and contract, shortening the leg and causing pain and potential circulation or nerve problems. A traction splint works by maintaining a continual pull on the femur to keep the bone ends in approximately normal position. Although First Responders usually do not apply traction splints on their own, they may assist other EMS personnel in applying a traction splint to a patient with a closed fracture of the femur **(Figure 14-19)**.

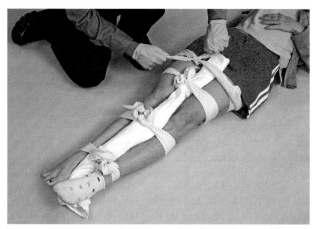

Figure 14-17 Immobilizing the legs for a hip or pelvis injury.

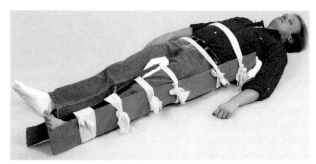

Figure 14-18 Splinting a fractured femur.

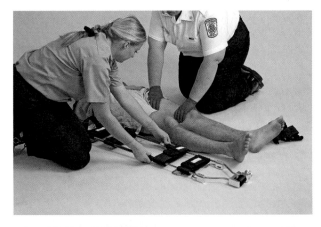

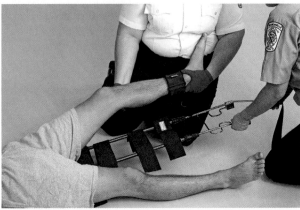

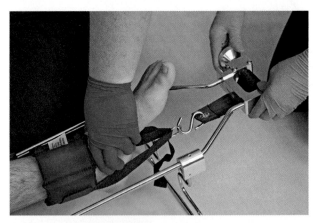

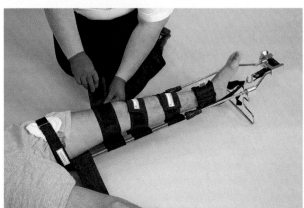

Figure 14-19 Assisting with applying a traction splint.

Knee Injuries

✓ Need to Know

The most common knee injuries are sprains, but dislocations also occur. These injuries commonly result from sports injuries, motor vehicle crashes, and falls. Fractures of the end of the femur or the **tibia** or **fibula** can be indistinguishable from other knee injuries. Dislocations of the **patella** (kneecap) may also occur.

☑ Any knee injury should be splinted in the position found.

☑ A soft splint can be applied by rolling a blanket or placing a pillow around the knee.

☑ If the knee is straight, you can make an anatomical splint by tying the upper and lower leg to the unaffected leg.

☑ Rigid splints provide additional support. If the knee is straight, ideally two splints are applied along both sides of the knee. If the knee is bent, splint the joint in the position found.

▶ Need to Do

1. Assess for circulation, sensation, and movement in the foot and toes. Knee dislocations resulting from vehicular crashes often cause vascular injury behind the knee, so it is important to assess the lower leg pulses.

2. If possible, put a rigid splint on each side of the leg in the position found. Pad bony areas and voids between the leg and the splints.

3. Tie the splints with cravats or bandages **(Figure 14-20)**.

4. Follow the general guidelines for safe splinting. Check the toes periodically for CSM.

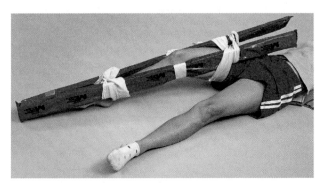

Figure 14-20 Splinting a knee injury.

Skill 14-3 | Anatomic Splinting of Leg

1 Check circulation. Gently slide 4 or 5 bandages or strips of cloth under both legs.

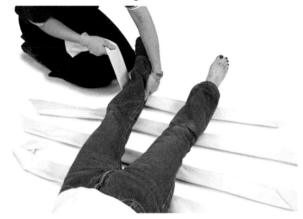

2 Put padding between the legs.

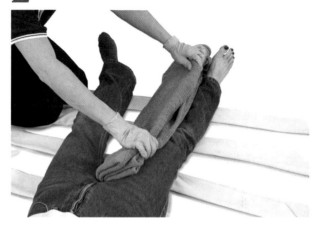

3 Gently slide the uninjured leg next to the injured leg.

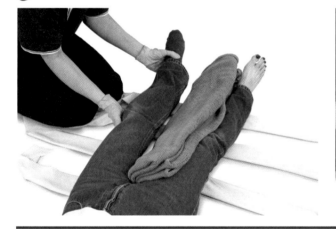

4 Tie the bandages. Check circulation, sensation, and movement.

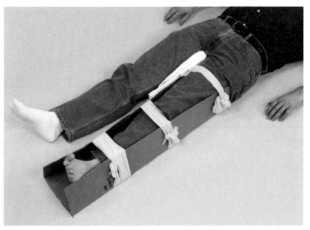

Lower Leg Injuries

✔ Need to Know

Injuries to the leg commonly result from sports, motor vehicle crashes, and falls. Either or both of the bones of the lower leg can be fractured. The goal of splinting is to stabilize the area from the knee to the ankle.

- ☑ A rigid splint is applied the same as for a knee injury; a three-sided cardboard splint can also be used **(Figure 14-21)**.

- ☑ A leg fracture can also be splinted using an anatomic splint if necessary **(Skill 14-3)**. A similar anatomic splint can be used for an

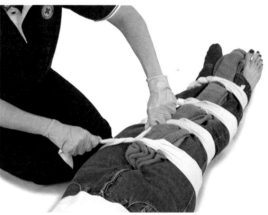

Figure 14-21 Rigid splinting of a lower leg fracture using cardboard.

upper leg fracture, with the bandages tied higher (including the hips).

Ankle Injuries

✓ Need to Know

The most common ankle injury is a sprain, which typically occurs when the foot is forcefully twisted to one side. Fracture or dislocation may also occur, often involving torn ligaments and possibly also nerve and blood vessel damage. Usually a soft splint is best for ankle injuries.

▶ Need to Do

1. Assess for circulation, sensation, and movement in the toes.
2. Position the foot in the middle of a soft pillow and fold the pillow around the ankle.
3. Using cravats or bandages, tie the pillow around the foot and lower leg **(Figure 14-22)**.
4. Follow the general guidelines for safe splinting. Check the toes periodically for CSM.

Foot Injuries

✓ Need to Know

Foot injuries most commonly result from direct blows to the foot or from falls. Foot injuries may involve almost any bone or ligament of the foot.

☑ Treat foot injuries the same as ankle injuries.

▶ Need to Do

Fractures of the toes can be very painful.

◆ Usually no splinting is required.

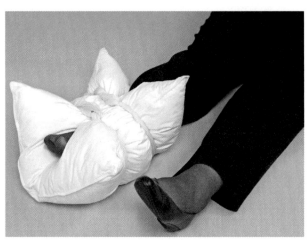

Figure 14-22 Soft splint for an ankle injury.

◆ If the toe is significantly bent, more than one toe is involved, or the foot is very painful, a pillow splint can be used as for an ankle injury.

Splinting Rib Injuries

✓ Need to Know

Rib fractures typically result from blunt trauma to the chest. Rib fractures are more common in the lower ribs and along the side.

☑ Rib fractures usually cause severe pain, discoloration, and swelling at the site of the fracture.

☑ The pain is often sharper upon breathing in, and the patient may be breathing shallowly and often is holding or supporting the area.

▶ Need to Do

The goal of splinting is primarily supportive:

1. Have the patient sit or stand in position of easiest breathing.
2. Support the ribs with a pillow or soft padding loosely bandaged over the area and under the arm.
3. If helpful, immobilize the arm with a sling and swathe to prevent movement and ease pain **(Figure 14-23)**.
4. Monitor the patient's breathing.

✎ Do You Understand?

1. An injured elbow, when the arm is straight, should be splinted from the _____ to the _____.
2. The one injury of the upper extremity in which you do not need to leave the fingers exposed to check CSM is an injury of the _____.
3. True or false: A rigid splint should be used with an injury of the pelvis.
4. What kind of splint is used for rib fractures?

Conclusion

You do not have to determine the type of musculoskeletal injury to provide effective emergency care. Care for open wounds and stabilize the injured area either manually or with a splint. When the nature of the injury indicates significant forces were involved, consider the possibility also of a spinal injury, the care for which is described in the next chapter.

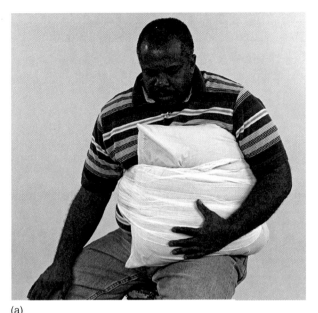
(a)

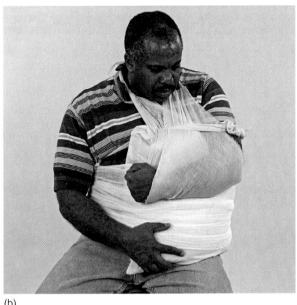
(b)

Figure 14-23 (a) For a rib injury do not wrap a bandage tightly. (b) Immobilizing the arm helps prevent movement of rib area.

Key Terms

clavicle (p. 228)

closed injury (p. 223)

contusion (p. 224)

cramp (p. 224)

cravat (p. 227)

crepitus (p. 225)

dislocation (p. 223)

femur (p. 232)

fibula (p. 234)

fracture (p. 223)

humerus (p. 229)

ligament (p. 221)

open injury (p. 223)

osteoporosis (p. 222)

patella (p. 234)

radius (p. 231)

scapula (p. 228)

sling (p. 226)

splint (p. 226)

sprain (p. 223)

strain (p. 224)

tendon (p. 221)

tibia (p. 234)

ulna (p. 231)

Review Questions

1. Usually the most important need for First Responder emergency care for a musculo-skeletal injury involves

   a. nerve damage.

   b. severe bleeding.

   c. pain.

   d. swelling.

2. With an extremity musculoskeletal injury, assess below the injury for circulation,

   a. skin temperature, and skin color.

   b. tingling, and numbness.

   c. skin temperature, and numbness.

   d. sensation, and movement.

3. Which of the following is *not* done with most musculoskeletal injuries?

    a. Stabilizing the area in the position found

    b. Applying a cold pack after dressing an open wound

    c. Moving bone ends back into normal position

    d. Taking body substance isolation precautions

4. If you discover signs of reduced circulation below an injury after applying a splint, you should

    a. loosen the bandages or cravats holding the splint to the extremity.

    b. remove the splint entirely and use manual stabilization.

    c. leave the splint in place and report this to arriving EMTs.

    d. massage the extremity on both sides of the splint to promote circulation.

5. When is it appropriate to apply two splints to an extremity with an obvious fracture?

    a. With closed injuries only

    b. Whenever possible

    c. When help will be delayed 20 minutes or more

    d. Never

6. Which statement is true about how splints should be applied?

    a. Tape the splint tightly in place.

    b. For greatest support, tie a cravat directly over the wound.

    c. Straighten the limb as much as possible before splinting.

    d. Dress an open wound before splinting the area.

7. Which is a sign of reduced circulation below an injury?

    a. Cold skin

    b. Hot skin

    c. Red skin

    d. Itching skin

8. How is an injured elbow splinted when you find it in a bent position?

    a. Gently straighten the arm and use a long, rigid splint from shoulder to hand.

    b. Gently bend the elbow to 90 degrees and put it in a sling.

    c. Keep the elbow in its original bent position and use a rigid splint from the upper arm to the hand.

    d. Do not splint the arm, but bind it directly to the chest with bandages.

9. How is an injured hand positioned for splinting?

    a. Let the fingers curl naturally around a soft padding in the palm.

    b. Ask the patient to make a fist before bandaging the hand.

    c. Straighten out the fingers on the surface of a rigid splint.

    d. Keep the fingers spread with bandaging and padding between them.

10. When treating a patient with a possible hip fracture for shock,

    a. cover the patient with as many blankets as are available.

    b. do not raise the patient's legs.

    c. apply direct pressure, even with a closed injury, because bleeding may be profuse.

    d. position the patient in the recovery position.

Chapter 15

Injuries to the Head and Spine

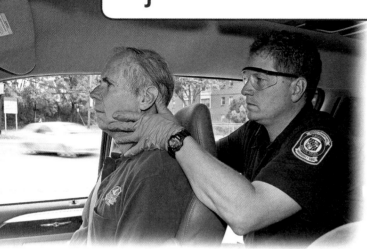

Chapter Preview

- Mechanisms of Injury to the Head and Spine
- Injuries to the Head
- Assessing Head and Spinal Injuries
- Emergency Care for Head Injuries
- Injuries to the Spine
- Emergency Care for Spinal Injuries

You Respond To ...

a scene in a warehouse where a man has fallen from a high ladder. He is lying unresponsive on his side on the concrete floor. Without moving his head, you can see a small amount of blood on the floor under his head. According to the dispatcher, EMTs will arrive in approximately three minutes.

Introduction

Head and spinal injuries may be life threatening or cause permanent damage to the brain or spinal cord, producing nervous system deficits such as paralysis. Any trauma to the head, neck, or torso may result in a serious injury. Injuries that cause unresponsiveness or a loss of sensation in a body part are particularly likely to be serious, but even injuries without immediate obvious signs and symptoms may involve a potentially life-threatening problem. Any injury to the head may also injure the spine because of the forces involved.

Mechanisms of Injury to the Head and Spine

Need to Recognize

Assessing a patient with a potential head and spinal injury begins with considering the mechanism of injury and the forces involved. In the scene size-up and general impression, you should recognize the possibility of a head or spinal injury because this possibility affects the immediate patient care.

- Any trauma to the head may cause a head or spinal injury.
- Spinal injuries may also be caused by forces to the back, chest, or even the pelvis or legs by indirect force.

Common mechanisms of head and spinal injuries include:

- Motor vehicle crashes (including whiplash injuries without direct impact to the head) and pedestrian-vehicle collisions
- Falls from a height of more than a few feet
- Diving emergencies involving impact to the head (even blows that do not cause bruises or wounds)

- Skiing incidents and other sports injuries
- Any forceful blunt or penetrating trauma to the head, neck, or torso
- Hanging incidents

Suspect a head or spinal injury with any unresponsive trauma patient or when wounds or other injuries to the body suggest large forces were involved. Observe the patient carefully and thoroughly for the signs and symptoms of a head or spinal injury even as you are carrying out the initial assessment.

Injuries to the Head

✓ Need to Know

- ☑ Head injuries may be open or closed.
- ☑ Bleeding from open scalp wounds may be profuse because of the large number of blood vessels in the scalp. Control bleeding with direct pressure unless there are signs of a skull fracture.
- ☑ Closed injuries may involve swelling or a depression at the site of a skull fracture.
- ☑ A brain injury involving bleeding inside the skull may occur with any head injury.

Assessing Head and Spinal Injuries

Although a head injury may occur in a patient without a spinal injury, and a spinal injury may occur in a patient without a head injury, the assessment of a patient with such injuries should look for both head and spinal injuries.

◼ Need to Recognize

Perform the standard assessment:

1. Size up the scene before beginning emergency medical care.
2. Complete the initial assessment.
3. Perform a physical examination as appropriate.
4. Complete ongoing assessments.

The general signs and symptoms of head and spinal injuries may overlap in patients with an injury of the head, neck, or back. Suspect a head or spinal injury in a patient if any of these signs and symptoms is present:

- Lump or deformity in the head, neck, or back
- Changing levels of responsiveness, drowsiness, confusion, dizziness

- Unequal pupils
- Headache
- Clear fluid from the nose or ears
- Stiff neck
- Inability to move any body part
- Tingling, numbness, or lack of feeling in the feet or hands
- Pain or tenderness in area of injury or associated with movement (but do not move or ask the patient to move)
- Continuous or intermittent pain along the spinal column or extremities independent of movement and palpation

Noting any of these signs and symptoms in the initial assessment or physical examination of a patient should lead to a more specific assessment, looking for a head or spinal injury.

- **During the initial assessment,** if you have to position the patient to open the airway, check breathing, give CPR or control bleeding, or allow fluid to drain from the mouth, take great care when moving or repositioning the patient. Unless necessary, do not move the patient.

- **If the patient is unresponsive** and the initial assessment does not reveal a life-threatening condition for which you must provide care, continue on to perform a limited physical examination for other injuries. Do not move the patient unless necessary. Check for serious injuries such as bleeding that must be controlled. Stabilize the patient's head and neck to prevent movement while waiting for additional EMS resources. Ask others at the scene what happened and what the patient's mental status was before becoming unresponsive.

- **If the patient is responsive** and the nature of injuries suggests the possibility of a spinal injury, carefully assess for the signs and symptoms of spinal injury during the physical examination. Ask the patient not to move more than you ask during the examination. Ask the patient:

  ◦ Does your neck or back hurt?

  ◦ What happened?

  ◦ Where does it hurt?

Skill 15-1 Assessing Head and Spinal Injuries

1 Gently feel the skull for bumps, depressions, and bleeding. Check the ears and nose for blood or a clear fluid. Check the pupils of both eyes, which should be of equal size and should respond to light.

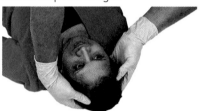

2 Check the neck for deformity, swelling, bleeding, and pain.

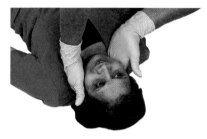

3 Touch the toes of both feet and ask the patient if the sensation feels normal.

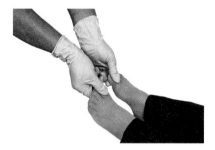

4 Ask the patient to point his or her toes.

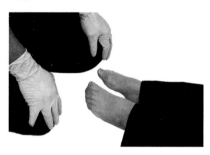

5 Ask the patient to push against your hands with both feet.

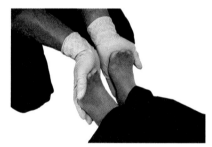

6 Touch the fingers of both hands and ask the patient if the sensation feels normal.

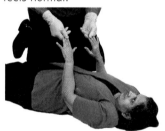

7 Ask the patient to make a fist and curl (flex) it in.

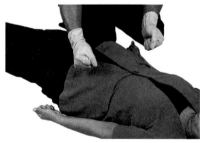

8 Ask the patient to squeeze both your hands.

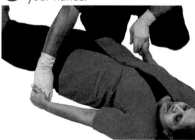

- ♦ **Perform the physical examination** as described in Chapter 6, checking for the signs and symptoms of a head or spinal injury **(Skill 15-1)**.
  - ◦ When checking the torso, observe the patient for impaired breathing or a loss of bladder or bowel control, which can be signs of nerve damage.
  - ◦ When assessing the extremities, compare strength from one side of the body to the other. Assess both feet, and both hands, at the same time.
  - ◦ Do not assume a patient without specific symptoms does not have a possible spinal injury. Consider the forces involved in the injury and, when in doubt, keep the patient's head immobile while waiting for additional EMS resources to arrive.

Brain Injuries

◼◼ Need to Recognize

Brain injuries may occur with a blow to the head with or without an open wound. A brain injury is likely with a skull fracture. Even if the signs and symptoms seem mild at first, swelling and/or bleeding in the brain may continue and the patient's condition may rapidly deteriorate and become life threatening. Swelling and bleeding in the brain can become very serious because the closed skull does not allow the brain to expand much with swelling. Any swelling or bleeding therefore puts pressure on nerve tissue, thereby threatening brain functions.

Signs and symptoms of a brain injury **(Figure 15-1)**:

- Severe or persistent headache
- Altered mental status (confusion, unresponsiveness)
- Lack of coordination, movement problems
- Weakness, numbness, loss of sensation, or paralysis of body areas
- Nausea and vomiting
- Seizures
- Unequal pupils

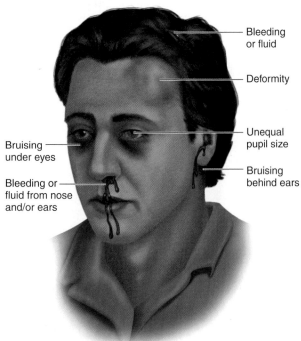

Figure 15-1 The signs of a brain injury.

- Problems with vision or speech
- Breathing problems or irregularities

The signs and symptoms of a brain injury may occur only hours or even days after the trauma. Do not assume a patient with a head injury does not have a brain injury if signs and symptoms are not immediately apparent.

Concussion

◼◼ Need to Recognize

A **concussion** is a brain injury that results in a temporary impairment of brain function but usually not permanent damage. Often there is no head wound, and the patient may not have many of the signs and symptoms of a more serious brain injury. The patient may have been "knocked out" by a blow to the head but regained consciousness quickly.

Signs and symptoms of a concussion:

- Temporary confusion
- Memory loss about the traumatic event
- A brief loss of responsiveness
- Mild or moderate altered mental status, including drowsiness
- Unusual behavior
- Headache

Although a patient with a concussion may seem to recover quickly, it is difficult to determine the seriousness of the injury. More serious signs and symptoms may occur over time. Patients with any suspected brain injuries require medical evaluation.

✎ Do You Understand?

1. Which of the following are common signs and symptoms of a head or spinal injury? (Check all that apply.)

☐ Changing levels of responsiveness

☐ Unequal pupils

☐ Cold fingers or toes

☐ Headache

☐ Clear fluid from the nose or ears

☐ Irregular pulse

☐ Paradoxical breathing patterns

☐ Tingling, numbness, or a lack of feeling in the feet or hands

2. List at least four common mechanisms of injury for head and spinal injuries.

_____ _____

_____ _____

3. True or false: With an unresponsive trauma patient, roll the patient facedown to carefully check the full length of the spine for bumps and depressions.

4. True or false: A patient briefly "knocked out" by a blow to the head but who has no signs or symptoms of a head or spinal injury does not require further medical evaluation.

Emergency Care for Head Injuries

▶ Need to Do

Perform standard patient care:

1. Ensure EMS has been activated.
2. Take body substance isolation precautions.
3. Maintain the patient's airway and provide artificial ventilation if needed.
4. Comfort, calm, and reassure the patient while awaiting additional EMS resources.

In addition:

- Use the jaw-thrust technique if necessary to open the airway.
- Follow local protocol to administer oxygen if it is available and you are so trained.
- Manually stabilize the head and neck, and do not let the patient move.
- Closely monitor the patient's mental status for deterioration.
- Control bleeding without putting pressure directly on a skull fracture.
- Monitor the patient's vital signs, and be prepared for changes in the patient's condition.
- Be prepared for vomiting.
- Provide additional care for a skull fracture.

Skull Fractures

■ Need to Recognize

With bleeding from the scalp, check carefully for a possible skull fracture before applying direct pressure to the wound. If the skull is fractured, direct pressure on the wound could push bone fragments into the brain, causing serious injury.

Signs of a skull fracture:

- A deformed area of the skull
- A depressed or spongy area in the skull
- Blood or fluid from the ears or nose
- Eyelids swollen shut or becoming discolored (bruising)
- Bruising under eyes (raccoon eyes)
- Bruising behind the ears (Battle's sign)
- Unequal pupils
- An object impaled in the skull

▶ Need to Do

1. Provide general care as for any head and spinal injury.
2. Do not clean the wound, press on it, or remove an impaled object.
3. Cover the wound with a sterile dressing.
4. If there is significant bleeding, apply pressure only around the edges of the wound, not on the wound. Use a ring dressing (Chapter 13) to apply pressure around the wound **(Figure 15-2)**.
5. Do not move the patient unnecessarily, because there may also be a spinal injury.
6. Do not raise the patient's legs.

Injuries to the Spine

✔ Need to Know

A fracture of the neck or back is always serious because of possible damage to the spinal cord.

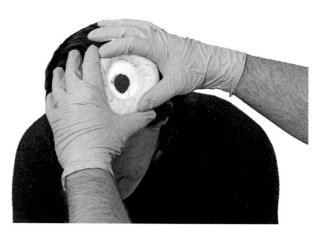

Figure 15-2 With a skull fracture, apply pressure to control bleeding only around the edge of the wound.

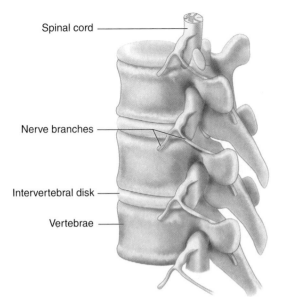

Figure 15-3 The spinal cord passes through openings in the vertebrae. Nerve branches exit the spinal cord to reach all body areas.

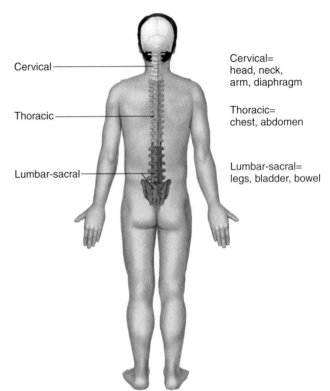

Figure 15-4 The signs and symptoms of a spinal cord injury depend on the level of the injury.

☑ Nerves from the spinal cord pass through openings in the **vertebrae,** the bones of the neck and back **(Figure 15-3)**. Even a small displacement or fracture of these bones can damage the soft tissue of the spinal cord or nerves leading from the cord to other parts of the body.

☑ Nerve damage may result in paralysis in all or part of the body and in breathing problems. The signs and symptoms of a spinal cord injury depend on the level of the injury **(Figure 15-4)**.

▇ Need to Recognize

Assess patients with potential spinal injuries as described earlier: "Assessing Head and Spinal Injuries."

Emergency Care for Spinal Injuries

▶ Need to Do

Perform standard patient care:

1. Ensure EMS has been activated.

2. Take body substance isolation precautions.

3. Maintain the patient's airway and provide artificial ventilation if needed.

4. Comfort, calm, and reassure the patient while awaiting additional EMS resources.

In addition:

▶ Provide general care as for any head and spinal injury.

▶ Establish and maintain constant manual stabilization until additional EMS resources have secured the patient to a backboard with the head stabilized; if possible, support the head in the position found **(Figure 15-5)**.

▶ Without moving the patient's head, whenever possible, maintain an airway and provide ventilations when needed.

▶ If the patient must be positioned to give ventilations or CPR, keep the head in line with the body while you move the patient with assistance from others.

Positioning a Spinal Patient

▶ Need to Do

Move the patient only if absolutely necessary:

▶ You may have to roll a patient who vomits to one side to drain the mouth.

▶ You may have to roll a facedown patient onto his or her back to provide ventilations or CPR.

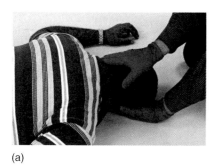
(a)

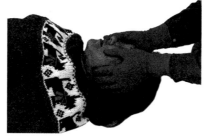
(b)

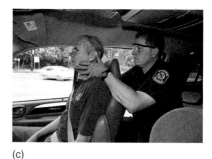
(c)

Figure 15-5 Support the head in the position in which you find the patient.

◆ Along with other rescuers, use the log roll to turn the patient while keeping the head in line with the body (Chapter 5).

◆ If you are alone and the patient vomits, move him or her into the HAINES recovery position, supporting the head and neck at all times.

Removing a Helmet

If an injured victim is wearing a helmet, *it should be removed only if absolutely necessary to care for a life-threatening condition,* because removal involves the risk of moving the victim's head or neck and possibly worsening a spinal or head injury. Leave the helmet in place for arriving EMS professionals. The one circumstance in which a First Responder may have to remove a helmet, following local protocol, occurs when the faceguard of a full-face helmet prevents giving a nonbreathing patient ventilations.

With many sports helmets and some newer motorcycle helmets, the faceguard can be removed or pivoted out of the way so that the helmet can be left on while ventilations are given. Motorcycle helmets with nonpivoting faceguards, however, must be removed to provide ventilations.

Two rescuers are needed to safely remove a victim's helmet. In an athletic helmet (such as a football helmet), first unsnap and remove the jaw pads by placing a flat object between the helmet and the

pad and gently separating them. This reduces the amount of head and neck movement during helmet removal. For all helmets:

1. The first rescuer slides one hand under the victim's neck to provide support at the base of the skull and holds the lower jaw with the other **(Figure 15-6a)**.

2. The second rescuer tilts the helmet back slightly as the first rescuer prevents movement of the head. The second rescuer pulls the helmet back until the chin is clear of the mouth guard section **(Figure 15-6b)**.

3. The second rescuer tilts the helmet forward slightly and moves the helmet back past the base of the skull, then slides it straight off **(Figure 15-6c)**.

Cervical Collars

Cervical collars are used to help stabilize the head and neck in patients with suspected spinal injuries. Most First Responders do not apply cervical collars by themselves but may assist EMTs or other emergency personnel in applying cervical collars, and therefore should be familiar with their use and application.

Several different types of cervical collars are available **(Figure 15-7)**. If you will apply cervical collars, you will learn how to apply the type used in your EMS system.

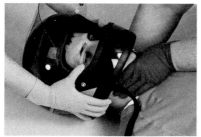
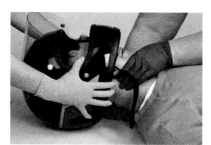
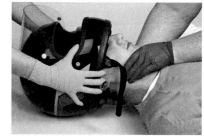

Figure 15-6 Removing a motorcycle helmet.

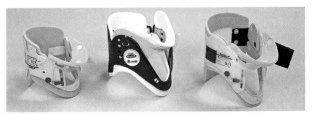
Figure 15-7 Different types of cervical collars.

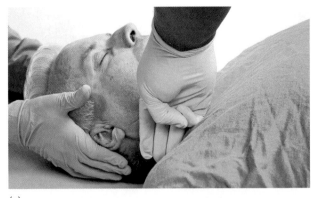
(a)

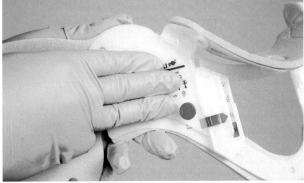
(b)

The following is the general process for applying a cervical collar to a supine patient:

1. Choose the correct size cervical collar by measuring with your fingers from the top of the shoulder to the bottom of the chin **(Figures 15-8a and b)**.

2. The first rescuer maintains the head in line while the second rescuer slips the back section of the open cervical collar under the patient's neck **(Figure 15-8c)**.

3. Correctly position the cervical collar to fit the chin and neck **(Figure 15-8d)**. Then close the collar with the Velcro attachment. Ensure the collar fits correctly, following the manufacturer's instructions.

4. Continue to manually support the head and neck in line.

Backboarding

Patients with potential spinal injuries are usually immobilized on a backboard before being moved to a stretcher for transport. Most First Responders do not use backboards by themselves but may assist EMTs or other emergency personnel in positioning a patient on a backboard, and therefore should be familiar with this process.

Many different types of backboards are available **(Figure 15-9)**. Short backboards are usually used for patients found in a seated position (such as in a vehicle) or a confined space; long backboards are used in most other situations. If you will assist with backboarding patients, you will learn about the type used in your EMS system.

The following is the general process for positioning a patient on a long backboard:

1. Three or more rescuers are needed. Position the long backboard beside the patient **(Figure 15-10a)**.

2. While one rescuer maintains the patient's head in line, the other rescuers take position to log roll the patient toward them and away from the backboard **(Figure 15-10b)**.

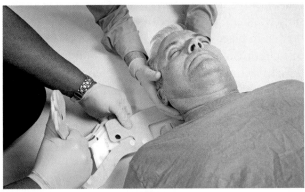
(c)

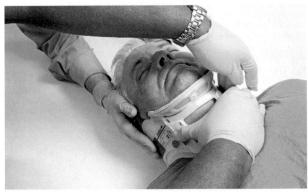
(d)

Figure 15-8 Applying a cervical collar. (a) Measure the patient for the collar. (b) Select the correct size collar. (c) Slip the open collar under the patient's neck. (d) Position and close the collar.

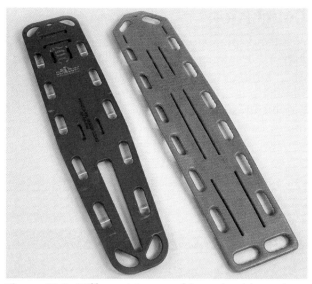

Figure 15-9 Different types of long backboards.

3. Following the instructions of the rescuer at the patient's head, the other rescuers roll the patient toward them as one unit **(Figure 15-10c)**.

4. The backboard is slid next to the patient. Following the instructions of the rescuer at the patient's head, the other rescuers roll the patient as one unit back into a supine position on the backboard **(Figure 15-10d)**.

5. The patient is secured to the backboard using the straps **(Figure 15-10e)**.

Do You Understand?

1. Describe how to open the airway of a patient with a suspected spinal injury.

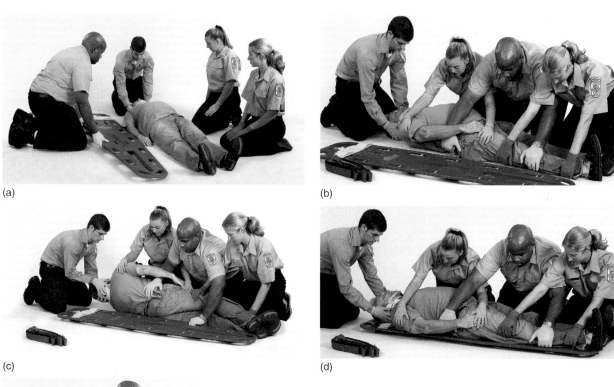

(a)

(b)

(c)

(d)

(e)

Figure 15-10 Positioning a patient on a long backboard. (a) Position the backboard. (b) Rescuers take position. (c) Logroll the patient away from the backboard. (d) Roll the patient onto the backboard. (e) Secure the patient to the backboard.

2. What is the best kind of dressing to use when controlling bleeding from a skull fracture?

_____

3. How long should you manually stabilize the head and neck of an unresponsive patient with a suspected spinal injury?

_____

Conclusion

Head and spinal injuries are common in trauma patients. Emergency care should always focus on maintaining the patient's airway and providing ventilations if needed, while manually stabilizing the head and neck and preventing patient movement.

Key Terms

concussion (p. 242)

vertebrae (p. 244)

Review Questions

1. Assessing a patient with a potential head or spinal injury includes
   a. considering the mechanism of the injury.
   b. asking the patient to turn his or her head to the side.
   c. assessing how the patient holds his or her head when sitting.
   d. comparing skin color in different parts of the body.

2. Which of the following is *not* a sign or symptom of a possible head or spinal injury?
   a. Unequal pupils
   b. A sudden, red rash around the neck
   c. Tingling in the hands
   d. Headache

3. What is the best way to stop bleeding from the scalp at the site of a skull fracture?
   a. Apply direct pressure on the wound.
   b. Apply indirect pressure on the pulse point in the neck.
   c. Apply pressure only around the edges of the wound.
   d. Tightly bandage the wound but do not apply pressure at all.

4. What is the one sure way to know whether a head injury patient has a serious brain injury?
   a. The patient feels temporarily confused.
   b. The patient is acting unusually.
   c. The patient was briefly unconscious.
   d. There is no certain way to know.

5. In what circumstance can you move a patient suspected to have a spinal injury?
   a. To check the back for bleeding if the patient is responsive and has no pain
   b. To position an unresponsive patient on the side in case vomiting occurs
   c. To provide CPR
   d. To roll the patient to put a blanket beneath the body if shock occurs

6. What action is *not* performed when assessing a patient with a suspected head or spinal injury?
   a. Comparing strength in the extremities from one side to the other
   b. Checking the patient's fingers and toes for feeling
   c. Asking the patient to turn the head to each side
   d. Checking the pupils of both eyes

7. Which of the following statements is true about the signs and symptoms of a brain injury?

   a. Seldom appear until about four hours after the injury.

   b. May begin mild and then intensify.

   c. Usually begin with intensity but may quickly diminish.

   d. Frequently come and go in repeated short cycles.

8. Signs of a skull fracture include

   a. bruising behind the ears.

   b. a sudden high body temperature.

   c. clear fluid from the mouth.

   d. bleeding from the eyes.

9. What action is *not* performed for a patient with suspected head and neck injuries?

   a. Covering the patient with a blanket

   b. Raising the patient's legs

   c. Providing ventilations if needed

   d. Manually stabilizing the head and neck

10. Nerve damage from a spinal injury may cause

   a. muscle spasms.

   b. anaphylactic shock.

   c. extensive internal bleeding.

   d. breathing problems.

Unit 6
Childbirth and Children

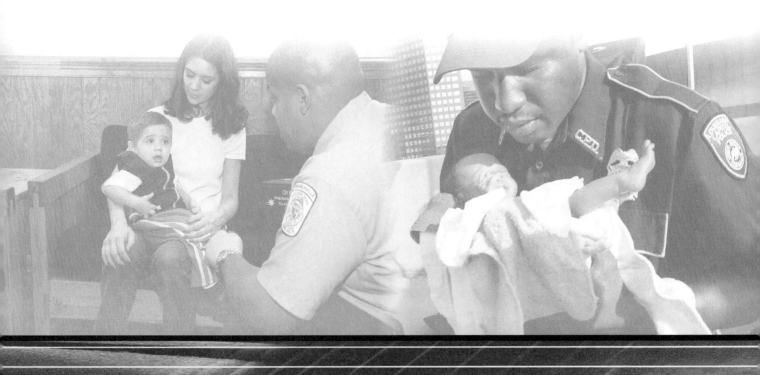

Chapter 16

Childbirth

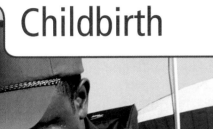

Chapter Preview

- Pregnancy and Labor
- Emergency Care During Pregnancy
- Childbirth
- Assisting With Delivery

- Care of the Mother After Delivery
- Care of the Newborn
- Childbirth Problems

You Respond To ...

a rural home in which a pregnant woman, attended only by a friend, has gone into labor and is having frequent, intense contractions. You assess her contractions and recognize childbirth is imminent and will likely occur soon. EMTs are on the way but will not arrive for about 10 minutes.

Introduction

Childbirth sometimes occurs outside a planned setting, so a First Responder may be called upon to assist. Delivery rarely becomes a medical emergency because childbirth usually takes place without problems or complications, with only minimal assistance required. In some cases, however, complications become emergencies. In addition, medical problems may occur earlier during pregnancy that require emergency care.

Pregnancy and Labor

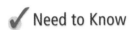 Need to Know

Pregnancy begins with fertilization of the ovum, or egg cell, by a sperm cell. Growth and development proceed in an orderly manner for about 40 weeks and culminate in childbirth. The pregnancy is usually considered in three stages, followed by labor and delivery.

Stages of Pregnancy

Pregnancy is often divided into three trimesters of roughly three months each.

- ☑ Within the first few days, the single cell resulting from fertilization divides into a mass of many cells.

- ☑ After it implants in the **uterus** at five to seven days, and thereafter for the first eight weeks, the developing human is called an **embryo;** thereafter it is called a **fetus.**

- ☑ The fetus develops inside the **amniotic sac,** which contains **amniotic fluid** (often called "water").

- ☑ The embryo is attached to the woman's **placenta,** an organ that develops in pregnancy to supply the embryo and fetus with oxygen and nutrients and to remove wastes through the **umbilical cord (Figure 16-1).**

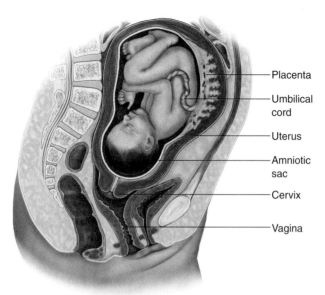

Figure 16-1 The fetus at 8 months.

☑ By eight weeks, the embryo has developed all major organ systems. Through the rest of the pregnancy, the fetus continues to grow and develop.

☑ By week 36, the fetus is fully formed, weighs about 6 1/2 pounds, and often can live outside the mother without advanced medical intervention.

☑ Near the end of pregnancy, the head of the fetus is positioned downward in the woman's pelvis. The woman's uterus has expanded high in the abdomen and presses on the lungs, possibly causing a slight shortness of breath. The pregnant woman may also experience backache, heartburn, constipation, and frequent urination.

☑ During childbirth, the fetus passes through the dilated **cervix** and **vagina.** The structures from the lower uterus to the vaginal opening are often called the **birth canal. Crowning** refers to the visibility of the infant's presenting part, usually the head, as it presses against the expanding vaginal opening before emerging.

Stages of Labor and Delivery

✓ Need to Know

Labor and delivery occur in three stages beginning with the first uterine contractions.

☑ **Stage 1: Labor to Cervical Dilation.** During pregnancy, a mucus plug forms in the cervix

to protect the uterus from possible infection from the vagina. During labor, or up to 10 days before the beginning of contractions, the mucus plug is released; this is sometimes called "the show" or "**bloody show**" but is often unnoticed. Uterine contractions, which mark the beginning of labor, eventually push the infant's head into the dilating cervix, the lower part of the uterine opening to the vagina. Contractions gradually become stronger and more frequent. The amniotic sac ruptures either shortly before or during the first stage of labor, causing the fluid to either rush or trickle out the vaginal opening; this is often referred to as "water breaking." The first stage may last from a few hours up to a day in a woman who has not given birth before, but sometimes occurs in only a few minutes in a woman who has previously given birth. Contractions initially are usually 10 to 15 minutes apart and shortly before childbirth may be only 2 to 3 minutes apart.

☑ **Stage 2: Delivery.** In the second stage, the infant is delivered. This stage typically lasts 1 to 2 hours but may happen more quickly in women who have given birth previously. The cervix has fully dilated, and contractions are powerful and often painful. The infant's head presses on the floor of the pelvis, and the woman feels a strong urge to push down. The vagina stretches open as the infant's head moves out of the uterus, and the top of the infant's head can now be seen (crowning) **(Figure 16-2)**. The vagina stretches more as the head emerges, often quickly, and the rest of the infant's body is typically pushed out rapidly.

☑ **Stage 3: Childbirth to Placenta Delivery.** In the third stage, the placenta separates from the uterus and is delivered, usually within 30 minutes after childbirth. The uterus then contracts and seals off bleeding vessels.

✎ Do You Understand?

1. The first stage of labor begins with _____.

2. The placenta is usually delivered within _____ minutes after childbirth.

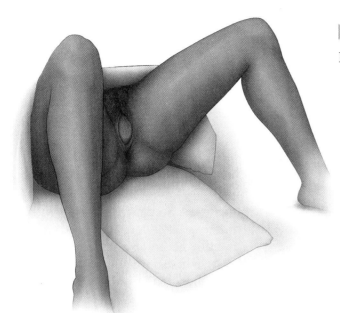

Figure 16-2 Crowning.

Emergency Care During Pregnancy

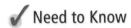 Need to Know

Most pregnant women receive regular care and are advised by their healthcare provider about what potential problems to watch for. Although rare, problems may occur that require emergency care before the woman receives medical attention.

Vaginal Bleeding

▉▉ Need to Recognize

Vaginal bleeding during pregnancy is abnormal:

- Bleeding may be caused by cervical growths or erosion, by a problem with the placenta, or by miscarriage.
- In the third trimester, vaginal bleeding may be a sign of potential preterm birth.
- The woman should see her healthcare provider immediately.

Perform the standard assessment:

1. Size up the scene before beginning emergency medical care.
2. Complete the initial assessment.
3. Perform a physical examination as appropriate.
4. Complete ongoing assessments.

In addition:

- Take repeated vital signs.

▶ Need to Do

Perform standard patient care:

1. Ensure EMS has been activated.
2. Take body substance isolation precautions.
3. Maintain the patient's airway and provide artificial ventilation if needed.
4. Comfort, calm, and reassure the patient while awaiting additional EMS resources.

In addition:

- Have a female assistant present if possible.
- Position the patient lying on her left side.
- Do not attempt to control bleeding by keeping the patient's legs together.
- Give the patient a towel or sanitary napkins to absorb the blood, but do not try to pack the vagina. Save any expelled material to give to arriving medical personnel.
- Follow local protocol to administer oxygen if it is available and you are so trained.
- Treat for shock.

Miscarriage

✓ Need to Know

Miscarriage, also called **spontaneous abortion,** is loss of the embryo or fetus, usually occurring in the first 14 weeks of pregnancy.

- ☑ An estimated 20-25% of all pregnancies end in miscarriage, a natural way that the body manages a potential problem in the pregnancy.
- ☑ Miscarriage may result from a genetic disorder or fetal abnormality, from some factor related to the woman's health, or from no known cause.
- ☑ Most women who have a miscarriage do not have problems with later pregnancies.

▉▉ Need to Recognize

Perform the standard assessment:

1. Size up the scene before beginning emergency medical care.
2. Complete the initial assessment.
3. Perform a physical examination as appropriate.
4. Complete ongoing assessments.

In addition:

◆ Take repeated vital signs.

Signs and symptoms of miscarriage:

◆ Vaginal bleeding

◆ Abdominal pain or cramping

▶ Need to Do

◆ Provide the same emergency care as for vaginal bleeding in pregnancy.

◆ Retain any expelled materials for EMS personnel.

◆ Because the possibility of miscarriage is often very distressing, be calm and reassuring.

Trauma in Pregnancy

▪ Need to Recognize

A woman's blood volume increases significantly in pregnancy, so blood loss due to internal or external bleeding caused by trauma may not immediately cause signs of shock.

◆ Blood flow is reduced to the fetus, potentially causing unseen fetal problems.

◆ Signs of internal blood loss may not be as apparent as in a nonpregnant patient.

▶ Need to Do

Perform standard patient care:

1. Ensure EMS has been activated.

2. Take body substance isolation precautions.

3. Maintain the patient's airway and provide artificial ventilation if needed.

4. Comfort, calm, and reassure the patient while awaiting additional EMS resources.

In addition:

◆ Assume any pregnant woman with trauma may have internal bleeding, and treat accordingly.

◆ Treat for shock.

◆ Follow local protocol to administer oxygen if available and you are so trained.

◆ If possible, do not let a patient late in pregnancy lie flat on her back but raise her right side higher (left lateral recumbent position) to reduce the pressure of the fetus on the vena cava (a large vein from which blood flows into the heart).

Other Possible Problems

▪ Need to Recognize

In addition to emergency situations, a pregnant woman should see her healthcare provider for any of the following:

◆ Abdominal pain, which may result from miscarriage or a problem with the placenta. The woman should rest until she receives medical advice.

◆ Persistent or severe headache, especially in the last trimester, which may be a sign of a serious condition called *toxemia*. Toxemia may also cause unusual weight gain, blurred vision, and swollen fingers or face.

◆ Sudden leaking of water from the vagina, unless the woman is close to the time of labor, which may indicate premature rupture of the amniotic sac.

◆ Other serious signs and symptoms, which include persistent vomiting, chills and fever, convulsions, and difficulty breathing. All should be reported immediately to the healthcare provider.

◆ Persistently elevated blood pressure may be a sign of a condition requiring medical attention.

◆ Signs or symptoms related to diabetes. Some women who did not previously have diabetes may develop it during pregnancy.

✎ Do You Understand?

1. The early signs of a possible miscarriage include

   a. vaginal bleeding.

   b. high fever.

   c. altered mental status.

   d. All of the above.

2. Check off the signs and symptoms that may indicate a possible problem during pregnancy:

   ___ abdominal pain   ___ persistent headache

   ___ chills and fever   ___ convulsions

   ___ difficulty   ___ water leaking from
   breathing   vagina in 20th week

3. What is different about the potential risks of bleeding due to trauma for a pregnant woman?

   _____

   _____

Childbirth

✓ Need to Know

In the United States, childbirth has occurred predominantly in hospitals for so long that many assume it is a difficult or dangerous process that always requires full medical care. If a woman is unable to reach medical care when childbirth may be imminent, she and significant others are likely to panic and be fearful and distressed. Coping with these stresses may be more difficult than assisting with the childbirth.

However, childbirth is not an emergency. Childbirth is a natural process that seldom involves complications or requires elaborate medical care except when rare complications occur. In the great majority of cases, care is relatively simple during the short time before additional EMS resources arrive.

Is Delivery Imminent?

■ Need to Recognize

Labor usually lasts for several hours, allowing the woman to be transported to the hospital or other planned childbirth location or for other assistance to arrive.

- In rare cases, labor may proceed unexpectedly fast or transportation may be delayed.
- If your assessment indicates delivery may be imminent, you will need to prepare to assist in the childbirth.
- Labor may begin potentially many weeks before the woman is due, resulting in a premature birth. A premature infant is more likely to need medical care after birth, so it is important to recognize the first signs of labor at any point in the pregnancy.

The following assessments can help determine whether delivery may be imminent:

- Gather information from the woman:
  - Her name, age, and due date.
  - Her physician's name and telephone number.
  - Ask if she has given birth before. If she has given birth in the past, labor is likely to proceed more quickly this time.
  - Ask if she knows whether she may be having twins or triplets—most women have learned this during their prenatal care.
  - Ask if her water has broken, and if so, to describe it. Normal amniotic fluid is clear. Rupture of the amniotic sac often occurs hours before delivery, so this is not a reliable sign that childbirth is imminent.
  - Ask if she has experienced any bleeding.
  - Ask about any past or present medical problems.
  - Give this information to arriving EMS personnel.

- Assess the contractions. When did they begin? How close together are they, and how long does each last? As labor progresses, contractions generally become stronger, last longer, and come more frequently. If contractions are less than five minutes apart and each lasts 45 to 60 seconds, delivery may occur soon, and preparations should begin.

- Ask whether the woman feels a strong urge to push or feels like she is having a bowel movement. This may mean delivery is approaching.

- If other signs are suggestive, check whether the infant's head is crowning. If possible, ask a woman present at the scene to check this. Once the top of the head is visible through the vaginal opening, be prepared for delivery very soon.

Assisting During Labor

▶ Need to Do

If labor has begun but delivery is not imminent, give supportive care to the expectant mother:

- Ensure that a plan is in place for the woman's transport to the planned childbirth location or for arrival of the planned attendant.

- Help the woman rest in whatever position is most comfortable for her.

- Provide any desired comfort measures, such as massaging the lower back (which may help reduce pain). Although the woman should not eat or drink, she may suck on small ice chips or have her lips moistened if her mouth is dry.

- Do not let the woman have a bath if the amniotic sac has ruptured, because of the risk of infection.

- Time the length of contractions and the interval between them, and write down this information.

- Help remind the woman to control her breathing: short, quick breaths (panting) during contractions, and deep, slow breaths between.

- Continue to help the woman stay calm and provide reassurance. Anxiety and fear will only add to her pain. Regular deep breathing in through the nose and out through the mouth may help her relax. (Using the same technique yourself, in synch along with the woman, may help.)

Assisting with Delivery

▶ Need to Do

If signs are present that delivery may be imminent, prepare to assist with the delivery. Ensure that someone stays with the woman while preparations are being made. If possible, another woman should be present—preferably a friend or family member.

Gather the items needed or helpful for the delivery. Many First Responders carry a commercial OB kit that includes most items needed **(Figure 16-3)**. If not available, improvise with the following items:

- A clean blanket or coverlet
- Several pillows
- A plastic sheet (or shower curtain) or stack of newspapers (to cover the bed surface)
- Clean towels and washcloths

- Sanitary napkins or pads made of clean folded cloth
- Medical exam gloves (use plastic bags on your hands if gloves are unavailable)
- Plastic bags (for afterbirth and clean-up)
- A bowl of hot water (for washing—but not the infant)
- An empty bowl or bucket (in case of vomiting)
- A clean handkerchief (to wear as face mask)
- A clean, soft towel, sheet, or blanket (to wrap the newborn)
- A bulb syringe (to suction the infant's mouth and nose), or sterile gauze
- If help may be delayed: clean, strong string, shoelaces, or cloth strips to tie the cord
- If help may be delayed: sharp scissors or a knife sterilized in boiling water for 5 minutes or held over a flame for 30 seconds (to cut the cord)

Follow these steps to prepare for childbirth:

1. Prepare the birthing bed with clean sheets over a rubber or plastic sheet (or shower curtain or thicknesses of newspaper) to protect the mattress.

2. If a bed is not present, prepare a clean place on the floor or ground, making a padded area of newspapers, clothes, or blankets.

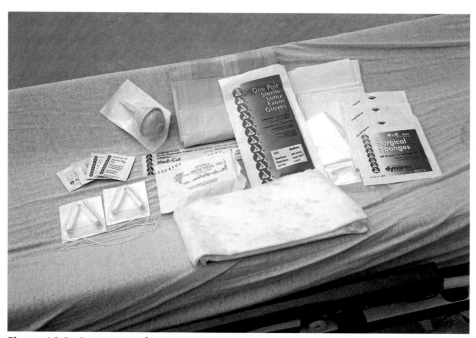

Figure 16-3 Contents of a commercial OB kit.

3. Roll up your sleeves, wash your hands thoroughly for about 1 minute, and put on medical exam gloves.

4. If possible, protect your eyes, mouth, and nose from likely splashes of blood and other fluids; a handkerchief can be tied over your mouth and nose.

5. Do not let the woman go to the bathroom.

6. Do not touch vaginal areas except during delivery and when a partner is present.

7. Call dispatch or the woman's healthcare provider so that additional instructions can be given over the phone during or after the childbirth if necessary.

8. When crowning occurs, move the woman into the birthing position and assist with delivery (see **Box 16.1** Childbirth Care: Assisting with Delivery).

Care of the Mother After Delivery

▶ Need to Do

- After the delivery, continue to support and comfort the mother.
- Ensure that she is warm and comfortable.
- Monitor her pulse and breathing.
- Replace any blood-soaked sheets and blankets, and dispose of used supplies, while awaiting transport.
- The mother may drink water now and may find it comforting to have her face wiped with cool water.

Bleeding After Delivery

✓ Need to Know

It is normal for bleeding to occur with childbirth and with delivery of the placenta.

- ☑ Up to 300-500 mL of blood loss is generally well tolerated.
- ☑ Place sanitary napkins or folded clean cloths against the vaginal opening to absorb the blood but do not apply pressure.
- ☑ Usually bleeding stops soon after the placenta is delivered.
- ☑ Reassure the mother that this blood loss is normal.

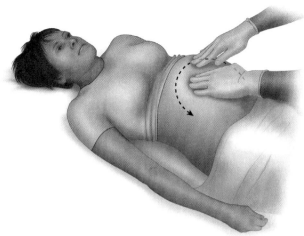

Figure 16-4 Massage the uterus to stimulate contraction to control bleeding.

▶ Need to Do

- To stimulate the uterus to contract and reduce bleeding, massage the mother's abdomen below the level of the navel, where you should feel the uterus as a mass about the size of a softball. Explain to the mother that this will help stop the bleeding.
- Massage with your palms using a kneading motion **(Figure 16-4)**.

If bleeding persists:

- Be sure you are kneading, not rubbing, with your palms.
- Keep the mother still and try to calm her while waiting for additional EMS resources. Treat her for shock.
- Follow local protocol to administer oxygen if available and you are so trained.
- Encourage breastfeeding, which stimulates contraction of the uterus.

Care of the Newborn

▶ Need to Do

- Dry but do not try to wash the newborn, whose skin may be covered with a protective, white, cheesy-looking coating called **vernix.**
- Ensure that the infant stays wrapped, including the head, to stay warm.
- Support the newborn's head if it must be moved for any reason.

BOX 16-1

CHILDBIRTH CARE: ASSISTING WITH DELIVERY

1 Help the woman to lie on her back with knees bent and apart and feet flat on the bed. (If she feels faint or dizzy, use pillows or blankets under her right side to position her slightly on her left side.) She may have been trained already in other acceptable birthing positions. Ensure that she is not wearing undergarments or other clothing that may get in the way. If she prefers, cover her above the knees with a blanket or sheet. Place folded towels or a blanket under her buttocks. Do not try to delay the birth by having the woman hold her legs together or any other maneuver. Talk to the woman and tell her what is happening throughout the process.

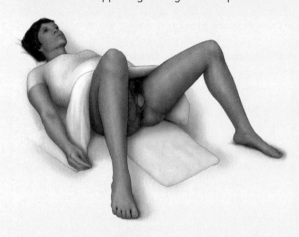

2 As the infant's head appears, have your gloved hands ready to receive and support the head, which may emerge very quickly. Do not interfere with the childbirth or touch the infant until the head is completely out. Check that the head is not covered by the amniotic sac; if so, pull it away as the mouth and nose emerge.

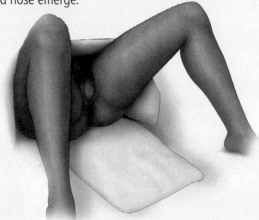

4 After the head is out, have the woman stop pushing and breathe in a panting manner. Often there is a delay before the shoulders emerge, during which you can suction the newborn's mouth and nose (as described later). Support the infant as its body emerges, often quickly after the head. Do not pull on the head or shoulders. Usually the infant turns to the side as the shoulder emerges. Newborns are usually very slippery and should be handled carefully. Note the time of birth. If the mother is having multiple births, prepare for the delivery of the second infant. Note the time of delivery to tell medical personnel later.

3 As the head emerges (usually face down), support the head. If the umbilical cord is wrapped around the infant's neck, carefully slip it over the head or shoulder to prevent strangulation.

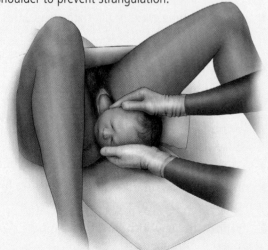

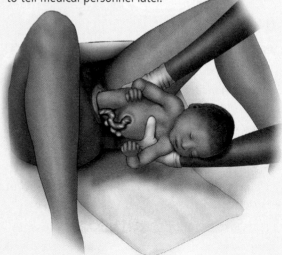

5 Position the newborn on its side, at the level of the vagina, with head lower than the feet for secretions to drain from the nose and mouth. Use the bulb syringe to gently suck secretions from the mouth first and then the nose, or wipe both with sterile gauze. The newborn normally begins to cry. If the infant is not crying, gently flick the bottom of its feet with a finger or gently rub its back. If the newborn is still not crying, check for breathing and give ventilations if needed (as described later).

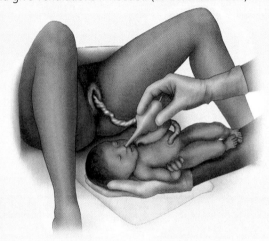

6 Gently dry and wrap the infant in a towel or blanket to prevent heat loss, keeping the cord loose. Do not try to wash the infant's skin, eyes, or ears. Keep the infant at the level of the vagina or place it on the mother's abdomen, lying on its side with its head low for the nose and mouth to drain. Ensure the infant stays warm and continues to breathe. Skin-to-skin contact of mother and infant also helps the infant stay warm. The mother can begin nursing the infant immediately, which will help the uterus contract and stop bleeding.

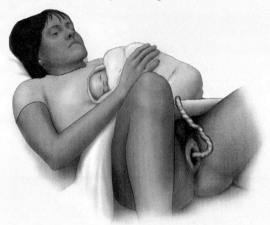

7 Follow your local protocol to clamp or tie the umbilical cord or leave it intact for arriving EMS personnel. In many situations, it is not necessary to tie or cut the umbilical cord, even after the placenta has been delivered, because more advanced medical help will arrive soon. If help may be delayed, clamp or tie and cut the cord before delivery of the placenta. Wait until the cord stops pulsating. Clamp or tie a tight knot around the cord about 4 inches from the infant, using strips of gauze, string, or thin strips of cloth. Clamp or tie a second knot 2 to 4 inches farther away from the infant, and cut the cord between the two ties with sterilized scissors or a sterile scalpel.

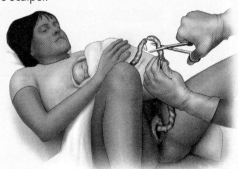

8 Wait for the delivery of the afterbirth, the placenta, and umbilical cord, which usually occurs with milder contractions in 10 to 30 minutes. Do not pull on the umbilical cord in an attempt to pull out the placenta. Typically there is a gush of blood as the placenta detaches from the uterus. Save the placenta in a plastic bag or towel for healthcare providers to examine it later. Place a sanitary pad over the vaginal opening to help control bleeding, and lower the woman's legs together.

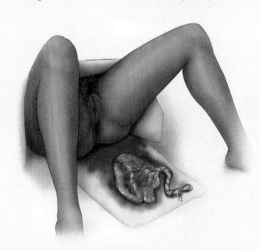

◆ Continue to check that the newborn is breathing well and that the airway is clear.

◆ Assess the newborn:
  ◦ Note skin color, movement, and whether crying is strong or weak.
  ◦ The normal respiratory rate for a newborn is more than 40 breaths/minute.
  ◦ The normal pulse for a newborn is more than 100 beats/minute (taken at the umbilical cord or the brachial artery).
  ◦ Note any changes over time. Provide this information to arriving EMS personnel.

Note: A very small or premature infant born significantly before the mother's due date is at greater risk for complications after birth. It is crucial to keep a small newborn warm. There is also a greater likelihood that resuscitation may be needed.

Nonbreathing Newborn

▶ Need to Do

If the newborn is not crying, gently flick the bottom of its feet with a finger or gently rub its back. If it is still not crying, check for breathing. If the infant is not breathing:

◆ Provide two gentle ventilations mouth to mask or using a BVM of the correct size **(Figure 16-5)**.

◆ Assess breathing and pulse.

◆ If breathing is absent, slow, or very shallow, provide ventilations at a rate of 40-60 breaths/minute. Follow local protocol to administer 100% oxygen if it is available and you are so trained.

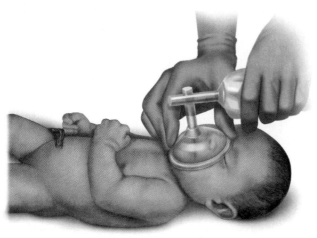

Figure 16-5 Use the correct size BVM to provide ventilations to an infant when needed.

◆ If the pulse is between 60 and 100 beats/minute, continue to give ventilations.

◆ If the newborn's pulse is less than 60 beats/minute, start chest compressions at a rate of 120/minute using the thumb-encircling method if a second responder is present. Use a ratio of 3 compressions and 1 breath.

◆ Reassess breathing and pulse after 30 seconds. If the pulse is more than 100 and respiration has improved, gradually discontinue ventilations.

✎ Do You Understand?

1. List at least five questions you should ask the woman when assessing whether delivery is imminent.

_____

_____

_____

_____

_____

2. The clearest sign that childbirth is imminent is _____.

3. If there is a delay between the emergence of the infant's head and the shoulders, what should you do?

_____

4. Describe what to do if the mother continues to bleed after childbirth.

_____

5. If the newborn has a pulse of 80 and the breathing rate is slow, what action do you take?

_____

6. List at least three things you should *not* do when assisting with childbirth.

_____

_____

_____

Childbirth Problems

Most deliveries occur without problems or complications, but you should be prepared to manage a problem if one does occur. The most common problems involve the presentation of the infant (its position at emergence) or maternal bleeding after delivery.

Meconium Staining

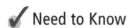 Need to Know

In some cases, the infant may defecate before or during childbirth. The feces, called **meconium,** may mix with amniotic fluid, staining it brown or green. The newborn may inhale this fluid with its first breath, causing a lung infection. If the mother describes the amniotic fluid as having color or if you observe this, report it to arriving EMS personnel. Meconium staining often results from fetal or maternal distress, so this may be a sign of another problem.

Breech or Limb Presentation

✔ Need to Know

A **breech presentation** occurs when the infant's buttocks or feet appear in the birth canal rather than the head **(Figure 16-6)**. This can become an emergency because

- ☑ as the head enters the birth canal, the umbilical cord is squeezed and blood flow may stop
- ☑ if the infant's head becomes lodged in the birth canal and the infant tries to breathe, it may suffocate because the face is pressed against the vaginal wall

▶ Need to Do

- Tell the woman not to push. Calm and reassure her.
- Update responding EMTs.
- Support the infant's body as it emerges, but do not try to pull the head out, which may cause injury and will not speed up the birth.

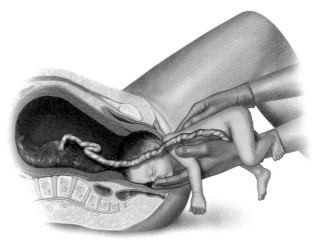

Figure 16-7 Make a breathing space around the infant's nose during a breech birth.

- If the head does not emerge soon after the body, you may need to open a breathing space:
  - Carefully insert one hand alongside the infant's head, palm against the face, and make a "V" with two fingers positioned on each side of the infant's nose **(Figure 16-7)**.
  - Press against the birth canal to allow air to reach the infant's nose while waiting for the head to be delivered.
- Check the infant immediately, and be prepared to give CPR if needed.

Very rarely, one arm or leg may emerge first from the birth canal, which is an emergency that requires immediate medical assistance.

- Move the woman to the knee-chest position with her head and chest down **(Figure 16-8)**. This position minimizes pressure on the cord.
- Do not try to pull the infant out or push the arm or leg back inside the woman.

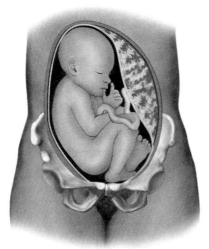

Figure 16-6 Breech presentation.

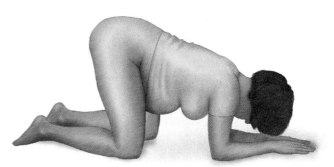

Figure 16-8 The knee-chest position for limb presentation or prolapsed cord.

◗ Tell the woman not to push. Calm and reassure her.

◗ Update responding EMTs.

Prolapsed Cord

✓ Need to Know

The umbilical cord is said to be **prolapsed** when a segment of it protrudes through the birth canal before childbirth **(Figure 16-9)**. This is an emergency because the cord will be compressed as the infant begins to move through the birth canal, cutting off blood flow.

▶ Need to Do

◗ Follow local protocol to position the woman either in the knee-chest position, to reduce pressure on the cord, or lying on the left side.

◗ Place dressings soaked in sterile or clean water on the cord.

◗ Follow local protocol to administer oxygen to the woman if available and you are so trained.

◗ Do not try to push the cord back inside the mother.

◗ If medical personnel have not arrived when the infant presents and begins to emerge, follow your local protocol. Carefully insert your sterile gloved hand into the birth canal and attempt to gently push the presenting part away from the cord while allowing the birth to continue. This is the only time you put your hand in the mother's vagina. If this cannot be done, open a breathing space

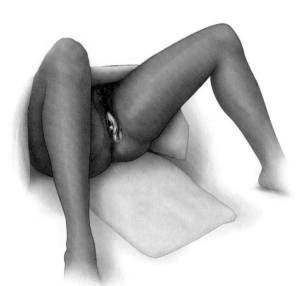

Figure 16-9 Prolapsed cord.

with your fingers the same as for a breech presentation.

◗ Check the infant immediately, and be prepared to give CPR if needed.

Cord Around the Neck

▶ Need to Do

◗ If the umbilical cord is wrapped around the infant's neck when the head emerges, try to slip it over the head or shoulder to allow the infant to emerge without strangling on the cord.

◗ Rarely, it may be wrapped so tight that you cannot release the infant's head and the cord is strangling the infant and preventing emergence of the body. If medical personnel are not present, you must tie or clamp the cord and cut it and then unwrap it from around the infant's neck.

Premature Infant

An infant born more than two weeks before the due date should be considered premature.

▶ Need to Do

◗ It is critical to keep a premature newborn warm.

◗ Be prepared to provide ventilations or CPR if needed.

◗ Follow local protocol to provide blow-by oxygen.

Stillborn Infant

Rarely, infants are born dead or die shortly after birth.

▶ Need to Do

◗ Use all resuscitation measures available, and continue efforts until relieved by arriving EMS personnel.

◗ Provide comfort for the mother and significant others present.

✎ Do You Understand?

1. Describe what to do in a breech birth if the head does not deliver soon after the body has emerged.

_____

2. Into what position should you place the woman if the cord is prolapsed?

_____

3. What should you do if the umbilical cord is tightly wrapped around the infant's neck when the head emerges and you are unable to free it?

Conclusion

Remember that although complications can occur with childbirth, they are rare. In most cases, childbirth is a natural process that requires only your assistance rather than emergency medical care. Childbirth outside a planned facility can be a stressful, emotional situation, and providing comfort and reassurance to the mother is often as important as emergency care. Though problems are rare, it is important to know what actions to take in emergency situations, such as when maternal bleeding does not stop or the newborn is not breathing.

Key Terms

amniotic fluid (p. 251)
amniotic sac (p. 251)
birth canal (p. 252)
bloody show (p. 252)
breech presentation (p. 261)
cervix (p. 252)
crowning (p. 252)
embryo (p. 251)
fetus (p. 251)
meconium (p. 261)
miscarriage (p. 253)
placenta (p. 251)
prolapsed cord (p. 262)
spontaneous abortion (p. 253)
umbilical cord (p. 251)
uterus (p. 251)
vagina (p. 252)
vernix (p. 257)

Review Questions

1. The first stage of labor begins with
   a. crowning.
   b. uterine contractions.
   c. cervical dilation.
   d. rupture of the amniotic sac.

2. When the amniotic sac ruptures after contractions begin, which of these statements is true?
   a. Childbirth may occur soon.
   b. The infant must be delivered immediately before suffocation occurs.
   c. The infant's lungs are likely to become infected if childbirth does not occur soon.
   d. The mother needs care to prevent dehydration.

3. Shortly before childbirth occurs, contractions usually occur
   a. every 30 seconds.
   b. every 2 to 3 minutes.
   c. every 5 to 10 minutes.
   d. irregularly, varying from 1 to 10 minutes.

4. Emergency care for a pregnant woman with vaginal bleeding includes
   a. massaging the abdomen with a kneading motion.
   b. packing the vagina with a pad made from sterile dressings.
   c. absorbing the blood with a towel or sanitary napkin.
   d. controlling the bleeding with direct pressure on the abdomen.

5. During labor, you can support the woman by

 a. urging her to push with each contraction.

 b. massaging her uterus.

 c. helping her control her breathing.

 d. holding an ice pack against her abdomen.

6. How should you position the newborn immediately after birth?

 a. On its side at the level of the vagina

 b. On its back at the level of the vagina

 c. Facedown above the height of the uterus

 d. Facedown at the level of the vagina

7. If the newborn is not crying or breathing immediately after birth, first

 a. start care for an airway obstruction.

 b. blow air into his or her mouth using the bulb syringe.

 c. give back slaps.

 d. flick the bottom of his or her feet with your finger.

8. How much maternal blood loss after childbirth is normal and generally well tolerated?

 a. Up to 100 mL   c. 100-300 mL

 b. 100-200 mL   d. 300-500 mL

9. In a situation when the umbilical cord can be seen protruding from the birth canal before childbirth occurs, what should you do?

 a. Cut the cord and wait for childbirth.

 b. Push the cord back inside the mother.

 c. Position the mother to reduce pressure on the cord.

 d. Pull on the cord to speed up the birth.

10. Give CPR to a newborn with a

 a. pulse below 100 beats/minute.

 b. pulse below 60 beats/minute.

 c. pulse below 100 beats/minute and a slow breathing rate.

 d. lack of respirations.

Chapter 17

Infants and Children

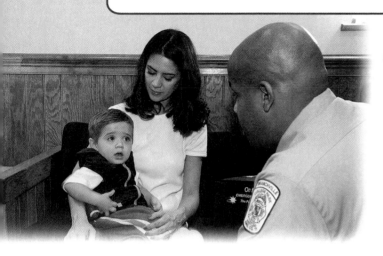

You Respond To ...

a scene where a father is holding a toddler on his lap. From 20 feet away, you can tell the toddler is seriously ill. As you approach, you see she is listless, barely responsive, pale, and breathing slowly. Her eyes are fixed and glassy.

Introduction

Because 5-10% of emergency responses involve children, you will often be called upon to care for an ill or injured child. Children are not small adults but have unique needs and require special care. Children, especially young children, may not be able to tell you what is bothering them or what happened. In addition to the ill or injured child, you must also deal with the child's often emotional caretakers. As well, the child's physical size and anatomical difference from adults often make emergency care somewhat different. This chapter focuses on common childhood emergencies and appropriate emergency care.

Chapter Preview

- Interacting with Infants, Children, and Caretakers
- Developmental Stages
- Differences in Anatomy and Physiology
- Assessing Infants and Children
- Common Emergencies in Infants and Children
- First Responder Stress

Interacting with Infants, Children, and Caretakers

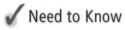 **Need to Know**

How you interact with pediatric patients and their caretakers is important. You must try to prevent anxiety and panic in the child, caretakers, or both. Follow these guidelines during assessment and treatment:

- ☑ **Tell the child your name and say you are there to help him or her.**

- ☑ **When a child is away from caretakers, be especially sensitive to the child's feelings.** Ensure a parent or caretaker has been called and that the child knows they are on the way. Try to stay at the child's level, and be friendly and calm. Ensure the child understands what you are saying by asking questions and giving the child an opportunity to speak.

- ☑ **A young child is often comforted by being allowed to hold a favorite toy or other object.** In addition, some children may be comforted by touch, whereas others are fearful of strangers—observe the child for clues about how best to be reassuring.

- ☑ **Always be honest with the child and caretakers.** If they detect a lie, you will lose the child's trust.

265

☑ **Keep the patient and caretakers informed, using appropriate language.** Explain what you are going to do before you do it. Be sure to use words appropriate for the age of the child.

☑ **Do not separate the child from a caretaker unless absolutely necessary.** This is especially true for younger children. Often, it is advantageous to have the caretaker hold the child while you assess and treat the child **(Figure 17-1)**. Approach slowly from a safe distance.

☑ **Talk with both the caretaker and the child.** When you can calm caretakers, the child will calm down as well. Explain to them what you think is wrong and what you are planning to do.

☑ **Observe the child and caretaker before touching the child.** You can gain much information while forming a general impression, including the respiratory rate and effort, the level of responsiveness, and apparent injuries. These may change once you touch the child, who may then become anxious or upset.

☑ **Remain calm.** Caring for children, especially those who are seriously ill or injured, can be very stressful. Your calmness will show confidence and be reassuring to the caretaker.

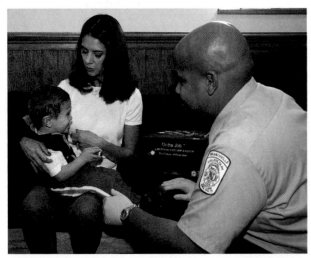

Figure 17-1 Help calm a pediatric patient by allowing the caretaker to hold the child. When possible, stay at the child's level, and speak to both the child and the caretaker.

Developmental Stages

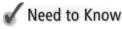 Need to Know

Children at different developmental stages perceive and behave differently. **Table 17-1** describes key differences along with suggestions of how to interact successfully with children at different ages.

Differences in Anatomy and Physiology

Remember that infants and children are not small adults. The following are some key issues related to differences from adult anatomy and physiology:

■ Need to Recognize

Head and Neck

◆ The smaller airway is easily blocked by secretions and swelling. The tongue is relatively larger and can easily block the airway in an unresponsive infant or child.

◆ When opening the airway of an infant or younger child, take care not to hyperextend the neck. Because of the relatively larger head size, a young child lying flat on the back may have the neck flexed forward (chin to chest) obstructing the airway. Placing padding under the shoulders makes it easier to keep the airway open **(Figure 17-2)**.

◆ Infants are nose breathers, so suctioning secretions from the nose can improve breathing problems.

◆ The head of an infant or young child is relatively larger and heavier, so it is more likely to be injured by trauma.

◆ The "soft spots" (fontanels) of an infant put the head at greater risk for serious injury from trauma.

Chest and Abdomen

◆ Children can compensate well for respiratory problems and shock for short periods by increasing breathing rate and the effort of breathing. Compensation is followed by rapid **decompensation** with respiratory muscle fatigue.

◆ In respiratory distress, the use of accessory muscles to aid the respiratory effort—causing

Table 17-1

Children's Characteristics in Different Developmental Stages

	Young Infant	Older Infant	Toddler	Preschooler	School-Age Child	Adolescent
Developmental Stage	Birth to 3-6 months	3-6 months to 1 year	1 to 3 years	3 to 5-6 years	5-6 to 12 years/ puberty	12 years/ puberty to 18-21 years
Common Characteristics	Usually not bothered by strangers Alert to environment Crying from discomfort, hunger, or pain	Alert, watchful Often uncomfortable around strangers and may cry and cling to caretaker	Curious, active Frequently uncooperative or distrustful May become concerned that they will be separated from caretaker	Alert, active, engaged in environment Understands language at a simple level Relatively easy to examine if approached properly	Varying levels of language comprehension Usually cooperative and a good source of information about what happened More familiar with strangers and doctors	Typically acts more like an adult than a child Concerned with privacy May need a sense of independence
Interacting with Child	Relatively easy to examine Prefers warmth and being held Unlikely to provide clues about location of injury or symptoms	Assess and treat in the arms of a caretaker May be distracted by a toy	Distracted by fun activity (assessment, equipment) Assess and treat in the arms of a caretaker Reassurance by caretaker may be needed	Explain things in appropriate language Allow to inspect and play with your equipment to allay fears and provide distraction Involve caretakers in assessment and treatment	Converse with both the child and caretakers Ask child's permission before touching When possible, give child some control and a role in decisions	Talk with patient rather than caretaker (but allow caretaker's input) Accurate history may not be possible if caretakers are present Respect the child's modesty at all times Treat with respect

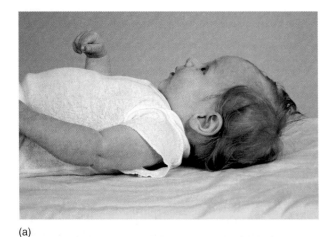

(a)

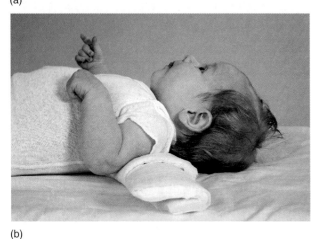

(b)

Figure 17-2 (a) Because of relatively larger head size, in a young child lying flat the neck flexes forward (chin to chest), obstructing the airway. (b) A pad under the shoulders makes it easier to keep the airway open.

retractions around the neck and shoulders and between the ribs—is more apparent in children and a clear sign of a breathing problem (Figure 17-3).

⬥ Infants and children are more susceptible to hypothermia because they have a higher ratio of body surface area to volume, and their temperature-regulating mechanisms are not fully developed.

⬥ The same blood loss that would be tolerated by an adult may be fatal for a child because of the small volume of blood in infants and children.

⬥ Infants and children are more easily dehydrated by losing fluid by diarrhea or vomiting.

⬥ With a thinner abdominal wall and a more pliable chest wall, internal injuries are more

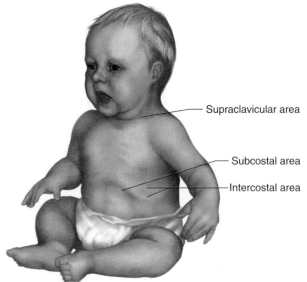

Figure 17-3 Obvious retractions of the accessory muscles of breathing in a child is a sign of respiratory distress.

likely with trauma in an infant or a child, often with minimal external signs.

Extremities

⬥ Bones of the extremities are easily fractured by trauma in an infant or a child.

Assessing Infants and Children

✓ Need to Know

The assessment of pediatric patients follows the same steps as for adults. Any problems that threaten the child's airway, breathing, or circulation are corrected as soon as found. Your approach to pediatric patients varies somewhat based on the child's age and the nature of the problem.

Scene Size-Up

▓ Need to Recognize

As always, begin the assessment by observing the scene as you approach.

⬥ Note how the child and caretakers interact.

⬥ Gather information from caretakers about what happened and how the child has been acting.

⬥ Observe the environment for clues about the mechanism of injury, such as substances present that may have caused a poisoning or signs of neglect or possible child abuse.

General Impression

▣ Need to Recognize

Even from some distance away you can often form an impression of how ill or how severely injured a child is.

- ◆ Consider the child's appearance.
  - ◦ Skin color (normal pink or pale, blue, flushed, or mottled)
  - ◦ Body position (normal movement or limp, unresponsive)
  - ◦ Eyes (normal moving about or fixed, glassy)
- ◆ Mental status may be revealed by how the child is interacting with others and the environment.
  - ◦ Quality of crying or speaking (energetic or weak)
  - ◦ Emotional state (crying, upset, frightened)
  - ◦ Behavior (appropriate for age, playing, and moving, or listless, motionless)
  - ◦ How the child responds to caretakers (comforted, responsive, or combative, irritable, inattentive)
  - ◦ How attentive the child is to you (makes eye contact, or is disinterested)
- ◆ The child's effort of breathing may be obvious.

Initial Assessment

▣ Need to Recognize

The initial assessment follows the same ABC steps as in an adult:

Airway

- ◆ Be careful not to hyperextend the neck when using the head tilt–chin lift to open the airway of an infant, which can obstruct the airway.
- ◆ Put a folded towel under the shoulders of an infant or young child for better positioning of the airway.
- ◆ Look inside the mouth of an unresponsive infant for an obstructing object.
- ◆ Use the jaw-thrust technique for a trauma patient.
- ◆ Suction the airway if needed.

Breathing

- ◆ With the airway opened, check for breathing by looking, listening, and feeling for breathing.
- ◆ If the infant or child is not breathing when the airway is opened, immediately provide ventilations and check the pulse.
- ◆ If the child is breathing, assess the adequacy of breathing:
  - ◦ Respiratory rate
  - ◦ Chest expansion and symmetry of movement
  - ◦ Effort of breathing: nasal flaring, retractions, grunting
  - ◦ Abnormal sounds due to mild obstruction: stridor (high-pitched sound on inspiration), crowing

Circulation

- ◆ Check the pulse as described in Chapter 6. Begin CPR if the pulse is less than 60 beats/minute in an infant or child if there are signs of poor circulation.
- ◆ Compare central and peripheral pulses to assess a potential circulatory problem (e.g., brachial and radial pulses).
- ◆ Assess skin color, temperature, and condition. Reduced circulation may be indicated by:
  - ◦ Pale, ashen, or cyanotic skin color
  - ◦ Cool, clammy skin
  - ◦ Capillary refill time of more than 2 seconds
- ◆ Control external bleeding immediately with direct pressure, remembering that decompensation can occur quickly in an infant or child with blood loss.

History and Physical Examination

▣ Need to Recognize

- ◆ In the physical examination, maintain spinal immobilization in trauma and unresponsive patients. Always support an infant's head when moving the infant.
- ◆ Gather the same assessment information as with an adult.
- ◆ When taking the history, try to communicate at an appropriate level with the child when possible, but also gather information from caretakers or others at the scene.

♦ Examine a child toe to head to gain acceptance, at first staying away from areas of pain and tenderness.

♦ Remember that vital signs of infants and children are normally different from adults **(Table 17-2)**. Changes may occur quickly in infants and children, especially with decompensation. Falling blood pressure is a late sign of shock.

♦ Assess the anterior **fontanel** on top of the infant's skull. Bulging may indicate a brain injury and swelling; a depression may indicate dehydration.

✎ Do You Understand?

1. List at least three things you can do to help calm a young child who is fearful about care.

_____

_____

_____

2. True or false: Children can compensate well for shock for a time.

3. List at least three things you can evaluate to assess mental status in a child too young to talk.

_____

_____

_____

4. In your initial assessment, you find that an unresponsive toddler is breathing slowly and has a pulse of 40 along with signs of poor perfusion. What should you do?

_____

Common Emergencies in Infants and Children

Airway Management

Airway management issues in infants and children include opening the airway, suctioning, and the use of airway adjuncts. Opening the airway was described earlier in the initial assessment.

Suctioning

▶ Need to Do

♦ Clear liquids you see in the mouth using a gauze pad to sweep the mouth or suctioning with the appropriate device.
  ○ Chapter 8 describes the basic technique for suctioning and safety guidelines.

♦ Do not insert the tip of a rigid catheter deeper than the base of the child's tongue.

♦ With a newborn, do not suction for longer than three to five seconds at a time.

♦ With an older infant or child, do not suction for longer than 10 seconds at a time.

Airway Adjuncts

▶ Need to Do

Use an oral airway to maintain the airway open in an unresponsive child without a gag reflex. Remove the airway if the child gags, coughs, or otherwise responds to an attempt to insert it.

♦ Use the oral airway to maintain an open airway but not for initial ventilations.

Table 17-2

Normal Vital Signs

Patient	Infant	Child	Adult
Normal Respiratory Rate at Rest	20-30	18-30	12-20
Normal Pulse Rate at Rest	80-150	70-130	60-100
Normal Blood Pressure (systolic/diastolic)	84-106/56-70	98-124/50-80	118-140/60-90

- Remember that the patient's airway must be opened before the airway device is inserted; the device does not open the airway but will help to keep it open.
- Select the proper size: Measure from the corner of the patient's lips to the bottom of the earlobe.
- Nasal airways are not usually inserted in children by First Responders.

Insert an oral airway in the upright position in which it will remain—do not rotate it 180 degrees as with an adult:

1. Open the child's mouth.
2. Use a tongue blade to press the base of the tongue down, and insert the airway in the upright (anatomic) position **(Figure 17-4)**.
3. If a tongue blade is not available, use your index finger to press the base of the tongue down to allow proper positioning of the oral airway.

Respiratory Emergencies

✔ Need to Know

Respiratory emergencies are common in infants and children, including:

- ☑ **Airway obstructions**
- ☑ **Respiratory distress and arrest**
- ☑ **Respiratory infections**
- ☑ **Asthma**

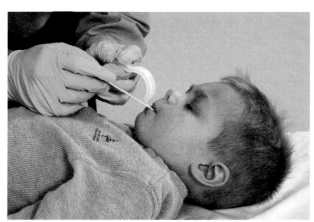

Figure 17-4 Insert an oral airway in a child in the upright position, *not rotated as for an adult.*

Airway Obstructions
Mild Airway Obstructions

■■ Need to Recognize

- Infant or child is alert and sitting
- May hear stridor, crowing, or noisy breathing
- May see retractions on inspiration
- Skin is pink with good peripheral perfusion
- Strong pulse

▶ Need to Do

- Allow the child to assume a position of comfort; assist a younger child to sit up, not lie down. The child may sit on a caretaker's lap.
- Do not agitate the child.
- Encourage continued coughing to attempt to dislodge the obstruction.
- Follow local protocol to administer oxygen if it is available and you are so trained.

Severe Airway Obstructions

■■ Need to Recognize

- No crying or speaking; a weak and ineffective cough
- Cyanosis
- A cough that becomes ineffective
- Increased respiratory difficulty and stridor
- Altered mental status; the child loses responsiveness

▶ Need to Do

For a severe obstruction, attempt to clear the airway as described in Chapter 7.

- Use alternating back slaps and chest compressions in a responsive infant.
- Use abdominal thrusts in a responsive child.
- Give CPR to an unresponsive infant or child. Check for an object in the mouth before you give a breath, and remove any object you see. Never perform a blind finger sweep of the mouth. Attempt artificial ventilations with mouth-to-mask technique.

Respiratory Distress and Arrest

Respiratory distress is difficulty breathing, which frequently leads to respiratory arrest (the stopping of breathing).

Assessing Respiratory Distress

■ Need to Recognize

Perform the standard assessment:

1. Size up the scene before beginning emergency medical care.
2. Complete the initial assessment.
3. Perform a physical examination as appropriate.
4. Complete ongoing assessments.

Signs and symptoms of respiratory distress:

- Respiratory rate of more than 60 breaths/minute in infants or 30-40 breaths/minute in children
- Nasal flaring
- Intercostal retractions (between the ribs), supraclavicular retractions (neck muscles), subcostal retractions (below the margin of the rib)
- Stridor, grunting, or noisy breathing
- Cyanosis
- Altered mental status (irritable, decreased mental status, unresponsive)

Emergency Care for Respiratory Distress

▶ Need to Do

Perform standard patient care:

1. Ensure EMS has been activated.
2. Take body substance isolation precautions.
3. Maintain the patient's airway and provide artificial ventilation if needed.
4. Comfort, calm, and reassure the patient while awaiting additional EMS resources.

In addition:

- Allow the child to assume a position of comfort; assist a younger child to sit up, not lie down. The child may sit on a caretaker's lap.

- Ensure the appropriate position of the child's head and neck to keep the airway open.
- Follow local protocol to administer oxygen if it is available and you are so trained.

An infant or child in respiratory distress needs oxygen, but a responsive patient may resist having a mask placed on his or her face. Use the **blow-by oxygen** delivery technique if necessary:

1. Connect high-flow oxygen to a mask and start the flow.
2. Have a caretaker hold the mask about 2 inches from the infant's or child's face.
3. If the child is still agitated by the mask, try connecting the oxygen tubing to a hole punched in the bottom of a paper cup, and hold it near the child's mouth **(Figure 17-5)**. Do not use a Styrofoam cup because the child may inhale small, loose pieces of Styrofoam when the hole is made.

Assessing Respiratory Arrest

■ Need to Recognize

Perform the standard assessment:

1. Size up the scene before beginning emergency medical care.
2. Complete the initial assessment.

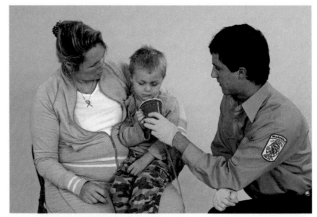

Figure 17-5 Administering blow-by oxygen through a paper cup may distract a young child who otherwise would not accept an oxygen mask near the face.

3. Perform a physical examination as appropriate.

4. Complete ongoing assessments.

Signs and symptoms of respiratory arrest:

- A breathing rate of less than 20 breaths/minute in an infant or less than 10 breaths/minute in a child
- Limp muscle tone
- Unresponsiveness
- A slow or absent pulse
- Weak or absent distal pulses
- Cyanosis

Emergency Care for Respiratory Arrest

▶ Need to Do

Perform standard patient care:

1. Ensure EMS has been activated.

2. Take body substance isolation precautions.

3. Maintain the patient's airway and provide artificial ventilation if needed.

4. Comfort, calm, and reassure the patient while awaiting additional EMS resources.

In addition:

- Provide ventilations by mouth or mask or by using the appropriate size BVM, as described in Chapter 8.
- Follow local protocol to administer oxygen if it is available and you are so trained.
- Monitor the patient's pulse and provide CPR if needed.

Respiratory Infections

✓ Need to Know

Respiratory tract infections are common in childhood, ranging from minor upper respiratory infections (the common cold) to serious, life-threatening infections. Respiratory problems can affect the upper or lower airways. They can result from infection, foreign bodies, or allergic conditions.

■ Need to Recognize

Signs and symptoms of respiratory problems include:

- Rapid breathing
- Noisy breathing
- Retractions
- Mental status changes

Croup

✓ Need to Know

Croup is a viral infection of the upper and lower airway that causes a swelling of the tissues below the voice box. It frequently occurs in the winter months and in the evening. Croup is more common in younger children and is often preceded by a day or two of being ill with or without fever. Croup generally is not life-threatening.

■ Need to Recognize

Perform the standard assessment:

1. Size up the scene before beginning emergency medical care.

2. Complete the initial assessment.

3. Perform a physical examination as appropriate.

4. Complete ongoing assessments.

Signs and symptoms of croup:

- Hoarseness
- Stridor
- A "barking" cough
- Difficulty breathing

▶ Need to Do

Perform standard patient care:

1. Ensure EMS has been activated.

2. Take body substance isolation precautions.

3. Maintain the patient's airway and provide artificial ventilation if needed.

4. Comfort, calm, and reassure the patient while awaiting additional EMS resources.

In addition:

- It is difficult to distinguish croup from the life-threatening emergency epiglottitis, so the child should be evaluated by a physician if the croup is severe or persistent.
- Give care for respiratory distress.
- Follow local protocol to administer humidified oxygen if it is available and you are so trained.

Epiglottitis

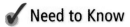 **Need to Know**

Epiglottitis is a rare, life-threatening infection of the epiglottis. The epiglottis is the flap of tissue that protects the airway during swallowing. When it becomes infected, it can swell to the point where the airway is completely obstructed. Epiglottitis occurs more frequently in children 4 years of age or older but can occur in younger children.

◼◼ Need to Recognize

Perform the standard assessment:

1. Size up the scene before beginning emergency medical care.

2. Complete the initial assessment.

3. Perform a physical examination as appropriate.

4. Complete ongoing assessments.

Signs and symptoms of epiglottitis:

◗ The child appears ill and frightened.

◗ High fever.

◗ The child is sitting up to breathe.

◗ Saliva may drool from the child's mouth because swelling of the epiglottis prevents swallowing.

▶▶ Need to Do

Perform standard patient care:

1. Ensure EMS has been activated.

2. Take body substance isolation precautions.

3. Maintain the patient's airway and provide artificial ventilation if needed.

4. Comfort, calm, and reassure the patient while awaiting additional EMS resources.

In addition:

◗ Do not attempt to examine the mouth or place an oropharyngeal airway.

◗ Allow the child to remain in a comfortable position.

◗ Give care for respiratory distress.

◗ Follow local protocol to administer oxygen if it is available and you are so trained.

◗ Ensure immediate transport.

Bronchiolitis

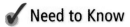 **Need to Know**

Bronchiolitis is a common cause of respiratory distress in young children. Also called RSV, for respiratory syncytial virus (a common cause of this illness in the winter months), bronchiolitis is a viral infection of the smaller airways in the lungs that causes respiratory distress and occasional hypoxia.

◼◼ Need to Recognize

Perform the standard assessment:

1. Size up the scene before beginning emergency medical care.

2. Complete the initial assessment.

3. Perform a physical examination as appropriate.

4. Complete ongoing assessments.

Signs and symptoms of bronchiolitis:

◗ Fever

◗ Nasal congestion

◗ Increased work of breathing with retractions and use of accessory muscles

◗ Markedly abnormal lung sounds with crackles (bubbling or crackling sounds) and wheezes together

◗ May be cyanotic

▶▶ Need to Do

Perform standard patient care:

1. Ensure EMS has been activated.

2. Take body substance isolation precautions.

3. Maintain the patient's airway and provide artificial ventilation if needed.

4. Comfort, calm, and reassure the patient while awaiting additional EMS resources.

In addition:

◗ Give care for respiratory distress.

◗ Follow your local protocol to administer humidified oxygen if it is available and you are so trained.

◗ If the patient has an asthma medication inhaler, follow local protocol to assist with its use if needed, as described in Chapter 11.

Asthma

✓ Need to Know

Asthma, a common medical problem in children, causes periodic attacks of difficulty breathing. Asthma results from an abnormal spasm of the lower airways. Asthma attacks range from minor to life-threatening.

Need to Recognize

Perform the standard assessment:

1. Size up the scene before beginning emergency medical care.
2. Complete the initial assessment.
3. Perform a physical examination as appropriate.
4. Complete ongoing assessments.

Signs and symptoms of asthma attack:

- Difficulty breathing, rapid irregular breathing
- Coughing, wheezing
- Exhaustion
- In severe attack:
  - Altered mental status
  - Cyanosis

Need to Do

Perform standard patient care:

1. Ensure EMS has been activated.
2. Take body substance isolation precautions.
3. Maintain the patient's airway and provide artificial ventilation if needed.
4. Comfort, calm, and reassure the patient while awaiting additional EMS resources.

In addition:

- Give care for respiratory distress.
- Follow local protocol to administer humidified oxygen if it is available and you are so trained.
- If the patient has an asthma medication inhaler, follow local protocol to assist with its use if needed, as described in Chapter 11.

Do You Understand?

1. Do not suction a newborn for longer than _____ seconds at a time.

2. What are the signs and symptoms of a *mild* airway obstruction in a child? (Check off all that apply.)

☐ Unresponsiveness
☐ Stridor or crowing
☐ Cyanosis
☐ Retractions
☐ Normal skin color
☐ Inability to cough

3. In what circumstance should you perform a blind finger sweep of a child's mouth when you suspect an obstruction?

_____

4. True or false: When providing blow-by oxygen to a fussy child, the mask must be held within a half inch of the child's mouth and nose for the technique to be successful.

5. True or false: A child having a breathing problem due to a respiratory infection should be calmed and then taken by caretakers to his or her usual pediatrician.

Shock

✓ Need to Know

In infants and children, shock commonly occurs from bleeding, traumatic injury, and fluid loss from prolonged vomiting or diarrhea.

☑ Shock may occur rapidly in infants and become quickly life-threatening.

☑ Shock may be delayed in children, who compensate well at first but then suddenly decompensate.

☑ Shock is a common cause of cardiac arrest in infants and children.

Need to Recognize

Perform the standard assessment:

1. Size up the scene before beginning emergency medical care.
2. Complete the initial assessment.
3. Perform a physical examination as appropriate.
4. Complete ongoing assessments.

Signs and symptoms of shock:

- Rapid (early) or slow (late) weak pulse
- Unequal central and peripheral pulses

◗ Poor skin perfusion, delayed capillary refill (longer than 2 seconds)

◗ Cool, clammy skin that is pale (ashen in dark-skinned individuals)

◗ Altered mental status

▶▶ Need to Do

Perform standard patient care:

1. Ensure EMS has been activated.

2. Take body substance isolation precautions.

3. Maintain the patient's airway and provide artificial ventilation if needed.

4. Comfort, calm, and reassure the patient while awaiting additional EMS resources.

In addition:

◗ Follow local protocol to administer oxygen if it is available and you are so trained.

◗ Monitor the pulse carefully for cardiac arrest and provide CPR if needed.

◗ Raise the legs if a spinal or traumatic injury is not suspected.

◗ Keep the patient warm but not overheated.

◗ Monitor vital signs frequently while awaiting additional EMS resources.

Seizures

✓ Need to Know

Seizures in infants and young children may result from many causes, including high fever, epilepsy, infections, head injuries, poisoning, low oxygen levels, low blood sugar, and other cases. View seizures as potentially life threatening. You do not need to know the cause of a seizure to provide emergency care.

☑ **Febrile seizures** (caused by high fever) are most common in children less than 5 years of age.

☑ Most seizures will be over by the time you arrive at the scene. If you witness the seizure, protect the child from injury and observe carefully so that you can describe the seizure to arriving EMS personnel.

☑ After a seizure (except a febrile seizure), the child usually appears very sleepy or confused.

■■ Need to Recognize

Perform the standard assessment:

1. Size up the scene before beginning emergency medical care.

2. Complete the initial assessment.

3. Perform a physical examination as appropriate.

4. Complete ongoing assessments.

In addition:

◗ Assess for injuries that may occur during the seizure.

◗ Gather the history from caretakers:
   - Has the child had prior seizure(s)?
   - If yes, is this the child's usual seizure pattern? How long did it last?
   - Does the child take a seizure medication?
   - Could the child have ingested any other medication or other potential toxins?

Signs and symptoms of seizures:

◗ Altered mental status

◗ Muscle twitching, convulsions, rigid extremities

◗ May be brief or prolonged

◗ Loss of bowel and bladder control

▶▶ Need to Do

Perform standard patient care:

1. Ensure EMS has been activated.

2. Take body substance isolation precautions.

3. Maintain the patient's airway and provide artificial ventilation if needed.

4. Comfort, calm, and reassure the patient while awaiting additional EMS resources.

In addition:

◗ Protect the patient from the environment.

◗ Loosen any constricting clothing.

◗ Ask bystanders (except caretakers) to leave the area.

◗ Assure that the airway remains open.

◗ Never attempt to restrain the patient.

◗ Do not put anything in the patient's mouth.

◗ If the patient is bluish, ensure the airway is open and give ventilations.

◆ After the seizure, place an unresponsive patient in the recovery position.

◆ Seizure patients often have significant oral secretions, so be prepared to suction to maintain the airway.

◆ Follow local protocol to administer oxygen if it is available and you are so trained.

◆ Report your assessment findings to additional EMS personnel.

Altered Mental Status

✓ Need to Know

Altered mental status in infants and children may result from many causes, including:

- ☑ Low blood sugar
- ☑ Poisoning
- ☑ Seizures
- ☑ Infection
- ☑ Head trauma
- ☑ Any condition that causes decreased oxygen levels

▦ Need to Recognize

Perform the standard assessment:

1. Size up the scene before beginning emergency medical care.

2. Complete the initial assessment.

3. Perform a physical examination as appropriate.

4. Complete ongoing assessments.

In addition:

◆ Ask caretakers about any history of diabetes, seizures, or recent trauma.

◆ Monitor the patient's vital signs.

Signs and symptoms of altered mental status in an infant or child:

◆ Drowsiness

◆ Confusion, agitation

◆ Behavior described as unusual by caretakers

▶ Need to Do

Perform standard patient care:

1. Ensure EMS has been activated.

2. Take body substance isolation precautions.

3. Maintain the patient's airway and provide artificial ventilation if needed.

4. Comfort, calm, and reassure the patient while awaiting additional EMS resources.

In addition:

◆ Place an unresponsive patient, or one who cannot protect the airway, in the recovery position (unless trauma is suspected).

◆ Follow local protocol to administer oxygen if it is available and you are so trained.

Sudden Infant Death Syndrome (SIDS)

✓ Need to Know

Sudden infant death syndrome (SIDS) is the unexpected and sudden death of a seemingly normal and healthy infant that occurs during sleep. The causes of SIDS are not well understood.

- ☑ It is the leading cause of death between 1 week and 1 year of age in the United States.
- ☑ The peak incidence occurs between 2 and 4 months of age.
- ☑ It is more common during winter months and in males.
- ☑ It is not due to external suffocation from blankets or pillows.
- ☑ It is not related to child abuse or vomiting and aspiration of stomach contents.

▦ Need to Recognize

Perform the standard assessment:

1. Size up the scene before beginning emergency medical care.

2. Complete the initial assessment.

In addition, ask the caretakers about the circumstances with questions such as these:

◆ When was the infant put to bed? When was he or she last seen?

◆ What position was the infant in when found?

◆ How did the infant look when found?

◆ Was there anything unusual in the environment?

◆ What has been the infant's general health recently?

Signs and symptoms of SIDS:

- The infant is in cardiac and respiratory arrest.
- The skin is often cyanotic or mottled.
- The infant is most commonly discovered in the early morning.

▶ Need to Do

Perform standard patient care:

1. Ensure EMS has been activated.
2. Take body substance isolation precautions.

In addition:

- Try to resuscitate the infant unless the body is stiff (follow local protocol). Assure the caretakers that everything possible is being done.
- Parts of the infant in contact with the bed may look bruised, a condition called *lividity* caused by blood pooling after death. These are not a sign of abuse.
- While awaiting additional EMS resources, comfort, calm, and reassure the caretakers, who will likely be experiencing emotional distress, remorse, and guilt. If available, another responder should be assigned to assist the caretakers and to explain what is being done.
- Avoid any comments that might suggest blame to caretakers. Assure them that there is nothing they could have done to prevent the death.

✎ Do You Understand?

1. In a child, the pulse is usually _____ in early shock, becoming _____ in late shock.
2. How is a febrile seizure in a child treated?

   _____

   _____

   _____

3. List at least four causes of altered mental status in infants and children.

   _____   _____

   _____   _____

4. True or false: When an infant dies of sudden infant death syndrome, do not ask the parents questions about how they put the infant to bed because they will be made to feel guilty and to blame.

Trauma

✔ Need to Know

Trauma is a common emergency in childhood and the leading cause of death in children. Blunt trauma causes the most injuries, and the pattern of injury may be different from that in adults. Common causes include:

- ☑ Motor vehicle crashes
  - ◦ Unrestrained infants and children have head and neck injuries.
  - ◦ Restrained infants and children have abdominal and lower spine injuries.
  - ◦ Infant and booster seats are often improperly fastened, resulting in head and neck injuries.
- ☑ Being struck by a vehicle while riding a bicycle, causing head, spinal, abdominal injuries
- ☑ Being struck by a vehicle while walking, causing abdominal injuries with internal bleeding, extremity fractures, and head injuries
- ☑ Falls from a height or diving into shallow water, causing head and neck injuries
- ☑ Burns
- ☑ Sports injuries to the head and neck
- ☑ Child abuse and neglect

Anatomical differences in children make certain types of injury more likely **(Figure 17-6)**:

- ☑ In younger children, the head is heavy and proportionally larger than in older children and adults, making the chances of head injury more likely.
- ☑ Children have soft, pliable ribs, so there may be significant internal injuries without external signs.
- ☑ The abdomen is a more common site of injury in children than in adults and often the site of a hidden injury.
- ☑ Extremity injuries are managed in the same manner as for adults.
- ☑ Burns are more likely to be life-threatening to infants and children because the effects of the loss of body fluid are so serious.

▪ Need to Recognize

Perform the standard assessment:

1. Size up the scene before beginning emergency medical care.

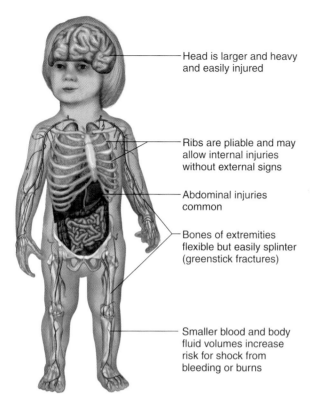

Head is larger and heavy and easily injured

Ribs are pliable and may allow internal injuries without external signs

Abdominal injuries common

Bones of extremities flexible but easily splinter (greenstick fractures)

Smaller blood and body fluid volumes increase risk for shock from bleeding or burns

Figure 17-6 The anatomy of children increases the risk for certain types of injury.

2. Complete the initial assessment.

3. Perform a physical examination as appropriate.

4. Complete ongoing assessments.

In addition:

◆ Examine a responsive child toe to head.

◆ Suspect certain types of injuries based on the mechanism of injury.

◆ Remember that smaller amounts of blood loss can result in shock in infants and children, and that the signs of shock may occur later in children.

▶ Need to Do

Perform standard patient care:

1. Ensure EMS has been activated.

2. Take body substance isolation precautions.

3. Maintain the patient's airway and provide artificial ventilation if needed.

4. Comfort, calm, and reassure the patient while awaiting additional EMS resources.

In addition:

◆ In all trauma patients, use the jaw thrust to open the airway. Use the head tilt–chin lift if you cannot successfully open the airway with the jaw thrust.

◆ Suction the airway as needed.

◆ Manually stabilize the head and neck.

◆ Manually stabilize extremity injuries.

◆ Treat shock by elevating the legs, if a spinal injury is not suspected, and maintaining body warmth.

◆ Follow local protocol to administer oxygen if it is available and you are so trained.

◆ Ensure transport as soon as possible.

Suspected Child Abuse and Neglect

✔ Need to Know

Abuse is an intentional improper or excessive action that injures or causes harm to someone under the abuser's power, such as a child, an elder, or a spouse. **Neglect** is a caretaker's failing to provide for the basic needs of someone who has a claim to care.

☑ First Responders should be aware of the characteristics of abuse and neglect to be able to recognize the problem.

☑ Abuse may include psychological abuse and sexual abuse, but physical abuse and neglect are the forms of child abuse that First Responders are most likely to encounter.

Any child may be abused, although some are more likely to experience abuse:

☑ A child seen as "special" or different from others

☑ Premature infants

☑ Twins

☑ Children with special needs

☑ Boys are more frequently abused than girls

The child abuser can come from any geographic, religious, ethnic, occupational, educational, or socioeconomic group.

☑ The abuser is usually a caretaker or someone in the role of a parent.

☑ Most abusers of children were themselves abused as children.

◼ Need to Recognize

Signs and Symptoms of Abuse

- Multiple bruises or burns in various stages of healing
- An injury inconsistent with the mechanism described by caretakers
- Bite marks
- Suspicious patterns of injury or marks on skin **(Figure 17-7)**:
  - Cigarette burns
  - Whip marks
  - Hand prints
  - Injuries to genitals, inner thighs, or buttocks
  - Rope burns
- Repeated calls to the same address
- Unusual burns:
  - Scalding
  - A glove or dip pattern (protected areas when a child was immersed in scalding water)

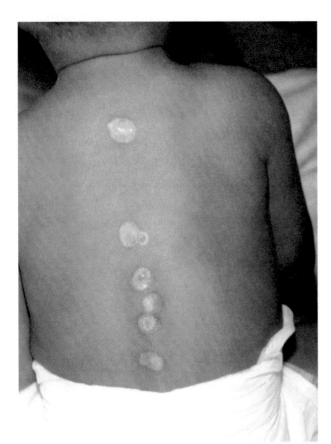

Figure 17-7 Suspicious skin marks may be a sign of child abuse.

- Burns inconsistent with the history presented
  - Untreated burns
- Caretakers inappropriately unconcerned
- Caretakers with uncontrollable anger
- Conflicting stories
- Fear of the child to discuss how the injury occurred
- Child's obvious fear of the caretaker
- Obvious or suspected fractures in a child younger than two years of age
- More injuries than are usually seen in children of the same age
- Injuries scattered on many areas of the body

Signs and symptoms of neglect:

- Lack of adult supervision
- A child who appears malnourished
- Clothing inappropriate for the environment
- An unsafe living environment
- Signs of drug or alcohol abuse
- Untreated chronic illness, for example, asthmatic with no medications
- Untreated soft-tissue injuries
- Delayed call for help

Perform the standard assessment:

1. Size up the scene before beginning emergency medical care.
2. Complete the initial assessment.
3. Perform a physical examination as appropriate.
4. Complete ongoing assessments.

In addition:

- Obtain as much information as possible, asking questions in a nonjudgmental manner.
- Document all information on the patient report.

Emergency Care When Abuse is Suspected

▶ Need to Do

Perform standard patient care:

1. Ensure EMS has been activated.
2. Take body substance isolation precautions.
3. Maintain the patient's airway and provide artificial ventilation if needed.

4. Comfort, calm, and reassure the patient while awaiting additional EMS resources.

In addition:

- Do not accuse caretakers in the field. It is not your role to accuse a caretaker, and accusation and confrontation delays transport of the patient.

- Treat the patient's injuries appropriately.

- Protect the child from further abuse, if necessary.

- Report objective information to the responding EMS unit.

- Save any evidence of physical or sexual abuse.

- File a report as required by state law and local protocol:
  - Remain objective.
  - Report what you see and what you hear.
  - Do not comment on what you think.

- Maintain confidentiality about the call.

Shaken Baby Syndrome

Need to Recognize

Shaken baby syndrome is a pattern of injury that typically results when a caretaker becomes frustrated with a crying infant and shakes the infant. This is a common, specific form of child abuse that may occur as well with young children.

- Although there may be no evidence of external injuries, the infant may have severe internal injuries, including brain or spinal injuries.

- The infant may be unresponsive or experiencing seizures.

Need to Do

Perform standard patient care:

1. Ensure EMS has been activated.

2. Take body substance isolation precautions.

3. Maintain the patient's airway and provide artificial ventilation if needed.

In addition:

- Manually stabilize the head and neck.

- Follow local protocol to administer oxygen if it is available and you are so trained.

- Ensure transport as soon as possible.

Do You Understand?

1. What kinds of injuries may result from a motor vehicle crash in an infant or child who was properly restrained?

    _____   _____

2. In what trauma situations should you use the jaw thrust technique to open a child's airway?

    _____

3. List several patterns of injury or marks on the skin of a child that may result from child abuse.

    _____   _____

    _____   _____

    _____   _____

4. True or false: If you suspect child abuse, it is better to confront caretakers right away to elicit a confession before they have time to make up a plausible story.

First Responder Stress

Need to Recognize

The death or serious injury of a child is a critical incident that can cause strong emotional reactions and stress that may persist long after the incident. This is especially true in instances of serious child abuse or neglect. It is stressful also to provide care while family members or caretakers also are very emotional because of the child's injury or death.

- Realize that a patient, family member, or bystander experiencing strong emotions is reacting to the stress caused by the emergency. Do not react personally to their emotions or behavior.

- Realize that many patients may die regardless of the care you provide. It is only human to feel guilt, anxiety, or anger, but these feelings are unjustified. If they persist, seek help.

- Chapter 2 describes some ways you can reduce stress resulting from incidents occurring while providing emergency care.

- In some instances, you may find that you cannot solve the problem alone or with the help of family members. There is no shame in seeking help from those professionally trained in reducing stress and handling other emotional problems.

◆ Remember that programs of critical incident stress management (CISM) are available in most public safety departments or EMS systems. A critical incident stress debriefing (CISD) can help emergency personnel cope with the severe stress associated with a child's severe injury or death.

Conclusion

Emergency care for infants and children is somewhat different from care for adults because of differences in physical size and anatomy. Follow the same steps for assessment, paying special attention to the airway and breathing, and consider the child's developmental stage when interacting with the child. Time is often especially critical for injured or ill infants or children, whose condition can deteriorate rapidly.

Key Terms

abuse (p. 279)

asthma (p. 275)

blow-by oxygen (p. 272)

croup (p. 273)

decompensation (p. 266)

epiglottitis (p. 274)

febrile seizure (p. 276)

fontanel (p. 270)

neglect (p. 279)

retractions (p. 268)

shaken baby syndrome (p. 281)

sudden infant death syndrome (SIDS) (p. 277)

Review Questions

1. In an injured child whose breathing rate initially increased, respiratory muscle fatigue may lead to
   a. decompensation.
   b. muscle paralysis.
   c. fluid in the lungs.
   d. increased retractions.

2. Which action will make it easier to keep the airway open in a responsive child who is lying down?
   a. Having the child lie facedown
   b. Hyperextending the neck
   c. Placing a folded towel under the head
   d. Placing a folded towel under the shoulders

3. Check whether a child is breathing by
   a. feeling with your hand on the abdomen just below the diaphragm.
   b. looking, listening, and feeling for breaths.
   c. holding the rib cage on each side and feeling for retractions.
   d. listening for lung sounds with a stethoscope.

4. If a child has signs of poor circulation, begin CPR if the pulse is less than _____ beats/minute.
   a. 20
   b. 40
   c. 60
   d. 80

5. With an older infant or child, what is the maximum period you can suction at one time?

  a. 3 seconds

  b. 5 seconds

  c. 7-8 seconds

  d. 10 seconds

6. To select the correct size oral airway for a 6-year-old, measure from the

  a. corner of the lips to the bottom of the earlobe.

  b. bottom outside edge of the nose to the bottom of the earlobe.

  c. corner of the lips to the outside corner of the eye.

  d. tip of the nose to the tip of the chin.

7. In a child in respiratory distress, intercostal retractions may be seen

  a. just below the bottom ribs.

  b. between the ribs.

  c. at the base of the neck.

  d. between the neck and shoulders.

8. An infant with a respiratory rate of 12 breaths/minute is said to be in

  a. respiratory distress.

  b. respiratory arrest.

  c. compensation.

  d. shock.

9. Which of the following actions should you *not* take for a child having a seizure?

  a. Loosen clothing around the neck.

  b. Give ventilations if the child looks cyanotic.

  c. Hold the child's body still to better assess breathing.

  d. Follow local protocol to administer oxygen.

10. Which of the following is *not* a sign of possible child abuse in a young child?

  a. The child is fearful of being touched by the First Responder.

  b. The child is reluctant to talk about what happened.

  c. The caretaker seems unconcerned about the injury.

  d. The caretaker's description of what happened does not match the injury.

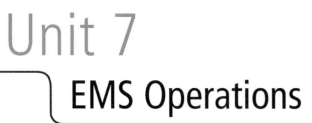

Unit 7

EMS Operations

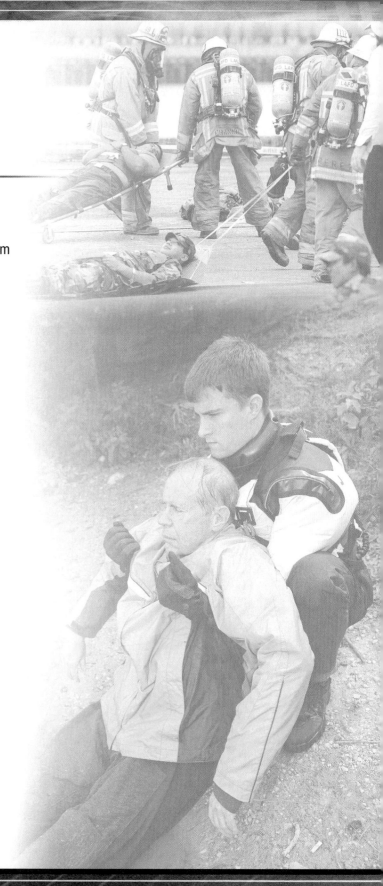

Chapter 18

EMS Operations

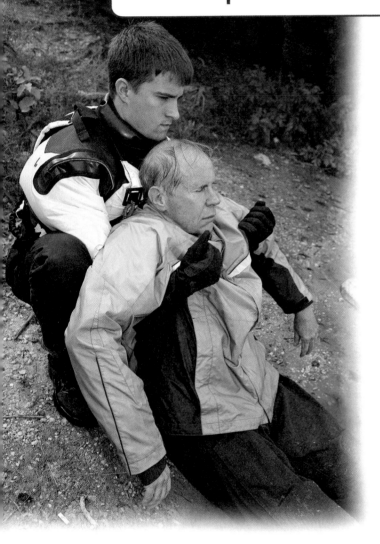

Chapter Preview

- Phases of a Response
- Helicopter Transport and Evacuation
- Patient Extrication
- Hazardous Materials Incidents
- Water and Ice Rescue
- Special Response Situations

You Respond To ...

a call involving an overturned truck on a local secondary road. The citizen who called 911 said it was a big truck and that it looked like the driver was still inside. Apparently no other vehicles are involved, but as you drive toward the scene, you are reviewing your local protocol for managing the scene if a hazardous material may be present.

Introduction

As a First Responder, it is important to understand your role within the EMS system, especially in complex operations. While you may be the first to respond to the emergency scene, many other personnel are usually involved. This chapter provides an overview of First Responders' responsibilities through the phases of a call and examines special operational factors involved in situations that include air transport, extrication of patients from wreckage, hazardous material incidents and the need for other special response teams, and rescue situations such as water and ice rescues. This chapter is *only* an introduction to special rescue situations, not a comprehensive discussion—advanced training is almost always required for these emergencies.

Always remember that your personal safety is the first priority. Many of the emergencies discussed in this chapter involve hazards. First Responders should consider these while en route, when arriving at the scene, and throughout the call with a continuous scene size-up.

Phases of a Response

✓ Need to Know

Chapter 1 described the complete process of the EMS response to a medical emergency from the initial occurrence and recognition of the emergency through to transfer to an in-hospital care system. This chapter discusses only those phases typically involving First Responders, from being prepared for the call to the transfer of the patient to the ambulance and post-run activities.

Preparation for the Call

Being prepared to respond to a call includes:

- ☑ Personal preparedness
- ☑ Keeping the response vehicle ready to respond and properly equipped
- ☑ Daily checks of your equipment and supplies

Oxygen cylinders must be kept full. Dressings, bandages, and other equipment must be replaced after being used. Follow your agency's guidelines and local protocol for equipment to carry and maintaining your response vehicle, based on the requirements of your EMS system as well as state regulations. Your instructor will inform you of

requirements affecting your daily preparations. The following equipment may be used by First Responders:

Medical equipment and supplies

- ☑ Personal protective equipment: medical exam gloves, pocket mask, eye protection, gown
- ☑ Basic supplies, including scissors, cold packs
- ☑ Basic wound care supplies: dressings, bandages, adhesive tape
- ☑ Oral and nasal airways
- ☑ Suction equipment
- ☑ Oxygen equipment
- ☑ AED
- ☑ Splints
- ☑ Backboard
- ☑ Cervical collars
- ☑ Bag mask
- ☑ Obstetrical kit
- ☑ Blanket

Miscellaneous equipment and supplies

- ☑ Planned routes or comprehensive street maps
- ☑ Flashlight
- ☑ DOT *Emergency Response Guidebook*
- ☑ Extrication equipment
- ☑ Flares, cones, reflective triangles
- ☑ Fire extinguisher

Being prepared includes, when appropriate, ensuring other personnel are available to assist when needed. Another important preparation involves **preplanning.** Preplanning is a response plan prepared in anticipation of an emergency.

- ☑ Many industrial plants have prearranged plans for emergency response in the event of different types of emergencies. These plans identify key personnel, the locations of supplies, the mechanism for **notifying** EMS, and evacuation routes for removing patients.
- ☑ Many fire departments and EMS systems also preplan responses to areas at high risk for an emergency, such as sports stadiums, theatres, public buildings, and industrial plants. The preplan involves inspection of the site, noting any potential hazards present, and planning an incident response.

Dispatch

✔ Need to Know

The EMS dispatch center, reached by citizens and others by dialing 911 or the local emergency number, is staffed 24 hours a day by personnel trained to obtain key information from the caller and to dispatch the appropriate emergency personnel. In some cases, you may contact the dispatch center to request assistance.

Depending on your position and facility, the dispatch center may dispatch you to the emergency scene via a variety of communication devices, including telephone, pager, radio, computer, and other devices. Generally, the dispatcher will provide you with at least the following information:

- ☑ Nature of the call
- ☑ Name, location, and callback number of caller
- ☑ Location of patient(s)
- ☑ Number of patients
- ☑ Severity of the problem
- ☑ Other pertinent information, such as help being given to the patient

Write down this information so that it is accessible to you en route.

En Route to the Scene

▶ Need to Do

When dispatched, gather any necessary medical equipment and depart for the scene. Many First Responders use a vehicle equipped with warning equipment, such as emergency lights and sirens, while others use their private vehicle. Follow these guidelines en route to the scene:

- Follow local laws and guidelines for use of the emergency warning equipment.
- In a private vehicle, obey all traffic laws and signs and drive safely.
- Wear seat belts and shoulder harnesses.
- Notify dispatch that you are en route.
- Confirm you have the essential information about the emergency, including its nature and the exact location. Check with dispatch if anything is not clear.

Arrival at the Scene

▶ Need to Do

- Park safely where your vehicle will not be in the way of ambulances and other EMS vehicles. If there is a possible hazardous material spill, park upwind of the scene.
- Keep emergency lights or flashers on.
- Notify dispatch when you arrive at the scene.
- Update the dispatcher with any information that differs from the original dispatched information, such as apparent additional patients, the presence of hazards, or a different location from that reported.

Size up the scene before approaching the patient. Check for hazards such as hazardous substances, downed wires, unstable vehicles, risk for fire or explosion, and so on. Notify dispatch of any special conditions not previously reported.

As you approach, consider these factors:

- The need for body substance isolation precautions (medical exam gloves, gowns, and eyewear when appropriate)
- Any need to move the patient because of hazards at the scene
- The mechanism of injury or medical emergency
- The need for additional help
- The number of patients in a mass-casualty incident (begin triage; see Chapter 19)

Update dispatch if you discover that unanticipated additional help or special equipment is needed. Then care for the patient until other EMS personnel arrive and take over patient care.

Transferring the Patient

▶ Need to Do

1. When additional EMS personnel arrive, provide all pertinent patient assessment and treatment information.
2. Remain with the patient for the time being, and assist other EMS personnel as required.
3. If CPR or other labor-intensive procedures are necessary, you may be asked to stay with the patient while he or she is being transported.

Following stabilization, the patient is prepared for transport in a process termed **patient packaging.** You may assist with this process or moving the "packaged" patient to the ambulance for transportation to the appropriate hospital emergency department.

After the Run

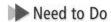 Need to Do

After the call, first complete any required documentation. Then prepare for the next call:

◆ Clean and disinfect equipment.

◆ Restock disposable supplies that were used.

◆ Refuel your vehicle if needed.

◆ Notify dispatch that you are ready for the next call.

 Do You Understand?

1. List five or six types of information the dispatcher will typically give you when you are dispatched to an emergency.

_____ _____

_____ _____

_____ _____

2. List four or five considerations as you approach the emergency scene.

_____ _____

_____ _____

_____

Helicopter Transport and Evacuation

 Need to Do

Air medical transport by helicopter is used to transport patients when time is critical and to evacuate patients from locations inaccessible to an ambulance. The First Responder's responsibilities may include

◆ Determining that air medical transport is required for the patient and making the request

◆ Preparing the patient for transport

◆ Setting up the helicopter landing zone

Requesting Air Transport

 Need to Do

Follow your local protocols and guidelines for requesting a helicopter. Consider the following general factors when deciding if air transport is needed:

◆ Will ground transport of a critical patient take too long to reach the appropriate specialty center or medical facility?

◆ Will patient extrication be prolonged for an unstable patient?

◆ Is ground access to the patient impossible or may be delayed?

Preparing the Patient

 Need to Do

Helicopter transport involves conditions different from transport by ambulance. While the responding helicopter crew is responsible for patient packaging, you should be aware of special considerations:

◆ If the patient is near the landing zone, secure anything that may be disturbed by high winds, such as blankets and equipment.

◆ Protect the patient, and yourself, against debris and dirt blown by the helicopter rotor wash. Use eye protection and protect exposed skin.

◆ Assist the helicopter crew to secure the patient to the stretcher along with any accompanying equipment.

◆ If an ambulance is present and the patient is some distance from the landing zone, the patient may be placed in the ambulance in preparation for transport to the helicopter after it arrives.

Setting Up the Landing Zone

Need to Do

The helicopter landing zone should be set up by trained personnel following local protocols, state requirements, and other recommendations. The following are general guidelines:

◆ The landing zone should be a flat area free of obstructions such as trees, power lines, and buildings.

- It should be a safe distance from the emergency scene.

- Ideally, the zone is at least 100 feet by 100 feet.

- Try to select an area free of loose objects, including stones and dirt, that will be blown by the rotor wash. Remove any objects that pose a risk if blown.

- Mark the corners of the landing zone with clearly visible objects such as traffic cones or flags. At night, mark the corners with strobe lights, chemical light sticks, or flares if there is no fire risk (but not railroad flares). Do not point vehicle headlights toward the center of the zone. If police vehicles are present, they may be used to mark the corners with their emergency red lights.

- Communicate with the pilot and describe the landing zone and the corner markings, as well as any nearby obstructions or hazards that may not be obvious. The pilot makes the final approval or rejection of the landing zone.

Helicopter Safety Guidelines

▶ Need to Do

- Keep other rescuers and bystanders far away from the landing zone.

- Close doors and windows of nearby vehicles before the helicopter approaches.

- At night, the headlights of parked vehicles away from the landing zone should face into the wind.

- Do not let any bright lights, including flashlights, shine upward or toward the helicopter as it lands, which could affect the pilot's vision. Ensure that bystanders do not photograph the landing helicopter, because a flash can blind the pilot.

- Never approach a helicopter until the pilot signals that it is safe to do so.

- Approach only from the front, avoiding the tail area where the rotor may be invisible.

- Stay low when approaching the helicopter, and do not raise your arms over your head. On a slope, approach from downhill.

 Do You Understand?

1. True or false: The length of time it may take to extricate a critical patient may be a factor when determining whether to ask for air transport.

2. A night landing zone should be at least _____ feet square.

3. Which side of a helicopter should you approach after landing?

Patient Extrication

✓ Need to Know

Injured patients are frequently trapped inside wrecked vehicles, building structures, and other settings. **Extrication** is the general term for accessing and removing a patient from wreckage or another entanglement. Your responsibility in such emergencies may include assisting with the extrication as well as providing patient care before and after extrication. Special training is required for all but simple forms of patient extrication.

This section focuses on patient extrication from a wrecked vehicle. A patient may be trapped within a vehicle because of damage to the vehicle's doors. If the patient is pinned by the wreckage, the rescue becomes more complicated.

- ☑ Your personal safety is the highest priority, followed by the safety of the patient.

- ☑ As a general rule, always administer necessary care to the patient before extrication, unless delayed movement would endanger the life of the patient or rescuer.

- ☑ Ensure that the patient is removed in a way to minimize further injury.

In many cases, you will be working with other emergency personnel to stabilize the vehicle and extricate the patient. A chain of command should be established to ensure patient care priorities.

Assess the Extrication Scene

◼ Need to Recognize

Your first concern when you arrive at the emergency scene should always be your safety and that of bystanders.

- Approach carefully. If at anytime the scene appears unsafe for you to manage, retreat to a safe distance, notify additional personnel, and wait for their arrival.

 ♦ Assess the scene to determine
   ◦ What happened
   ◦ How many patients may be present
   ◦ Whether any hazards are present
   ◦ What specialized rescue personnel, equipment, and tools will be required

▶ Need to Do

After this assessment, you call dispatch for additional personnel that are needed and decide whether to access the patient yourself or await the arrival of specially trained rescuers. *Never attempt a rescue for which you are not trained. Never attempt a rescue with improper or inadequate safety and rescue equipment.* Follow these guidelines:

 ♦ Evaluate the scene to ensure your safety and the safety of bystanders. Recognize dangers and potential dangers. Unless you have had special training and have the necessary equipment, stay away from a hazardous materials spill, a downed power line, or a vehicle on fire.

 ♦ Wear appropriate protective devices.

 ♦ Do not attempt to do anything you are not trained to do. Know what resources are available to help.

 ♦ Get the help you need. If you have not already done so, call for additional personnel. Be able to describe the scene and the types of help you need.

 ♦ Check the scene for other patients, such as someone who may have been hit by or thrown from the vehicle.

 ♦ Control the scene, and manage traffic control if appropriate, while waiting for other rescuers.

Stabilizing the Vehicle

▶ Need to Do

Before attempting to access the patient, ensure the vehicle is stable:

 ♦ If the vehicle is upright, check to see if it is stable. If you can do so safely, put the vehicle's automatic transmission in park or set the emergency brake; remove the key from the ignition.

 ♦ If it may move in any way, try to stabilize the wheels with blocks, rocks, boards, or similar items you find at the scene.

Head and neck injuries are common in crashes in which the vehicle has rolled onto its side.

 ♦ Do not attempt to return the car to an upright position before removing patients.

 ♦ If possible, stabilize the vehicle using ropes, tires, blocks, or materials available at the scene.

 ♦ Do not climb on top of the vehicle to try to open a door or window; instead, break the rear window as described in the following section.

A vehicle that has flipped upside-down is often difficult to access.

 ♦ Do not attempt to right the vehicle, and prevent bystanders from doing so.

 ♦ If fuel is leaking, clear the scene.

 ♦ Do not allow smoking anywhere near a rescue operation.

 ♦ After stabilizing the vehicle, you can try to access the patient.

Gaining Access to the Patient

✔ Need to Know

The second step is to gain **access** to the patient so that basic emergency care can be rendered. Gaining access may require the use of simple equipment and hand tools such as these (**Figure 18-1**):

 ☑ Protective clothing, leather gloves, and protective goggles
 ☑ Pliers
 ☑ Pocket knife
 ☑ Jack
 ☑ Jack handle
 ☑ Rope
 ☑ Screwdriver
 ☑ Hammers
 ☑ Hacksaw
 ☑ Pry bar
 ☑ Spring-loaded center punch
 ☑ Slim Jim

You may have access to other rescue tools and may use them if you are so trained. As a rule, use the simplest and safest tool that will accomplish the task at hand.

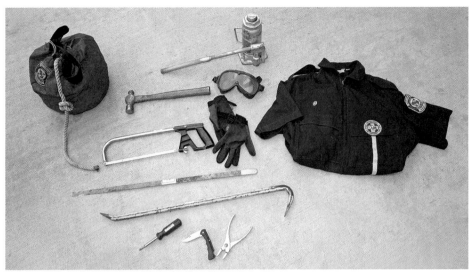

Figure 18-1 Hand tools and equipment used in patient extrication.

Need to Do

After stabilizing the vehicle, try the safest and easiest route of entry:

- Try the vehicle doors first. If one is locked, check the others.

- If all doors are locked, ask the patient to unlock one if he or she is able. If not, you may use a special tool (e.g., Slim Jim) designed for unlocking vehicle doors, if available. Many law enforcement officers and firefighters carry these special tools. You should become familiar with its use if you carry one.

If you cannot access the patient through a door, try to enter through a window.

- Ask the patient to open the window if possible. If not, the window must be removed.

- Breaking glass is dangerous for both the patient and the rescuer.

- Windshields have a layer of plastic within the glass that remains when the glass is shattered.

- Side windows are often made of tempered safety glass that does not include a plastic sheet. However, when the window is shattered, pieces of glass fly all over the inside of the automobile. Although the broken glass has relatively dull edges, pieces may get into open wounds, causing patient care problems.

If you must break safety glass to access the patient, do so only with proper protective equipment. If protective equipment is unavailable and you must break a window to rapidly access

a patient to deliver life-saving care, follow these guidelines:

1. Cover the window with a blanket, coat, or tarp.

2. Use a pointed object such as the pointed tip of the jack handle or a commercial punch to puncture the glass. A blunt object would propel glass throughout the car, endangering the patient.

3. Make the entry in a corner of the window farthest from the patient. If possible, tape the window first to minimize glass pieces striking the patient.

4. Once you have made entry, remove the glass until the opening is large enough to reach the door lock or enter.

5. Once inside, you may be able to unlock or force open a door to provide additional access.

It is also possible to remove the windshield or rear window to access a patient:

- Use a screwdriver or pry bar to remove the liner around the windshield. You will see the glass resting on a rubber gasket or glue.

- Pry the window free and remove it.

If you cannot access a patient safely by breaking or removing a window, wait for additional rescuers and rescue equipment to arrive. It may be necessary to cut doors open, remove parts of the roof, or perform other complex maneuvers. Such skills require special training.

If a patient is pinned under a motor vehicle, wait for a rescue squad with special equipment. If the patient's life is in imminent danger, however, with the help of several other responders, you may attempt to lift the car slightly and slide the patient out. If a patient in imminent danger is trapped by a wheel or the vehicle's frame, try jacking the car up, blocking it, and sliding the patient out. *Never* crawl under the vehicle yourself.

Once you have accessed inside the vehicle, turn off the ignition to reduce the risk of fire.

Providing Emergency Care

 Need to Do

After gaining access to the patient:

- Provide basic emergency care while the patient is still in the vehicle.

- Perform any Basic Life Support skills required, including controlling severe bleeding.

- Unless an explosion is possible, you may administer supplemental oxygen if it is available and you are so trained.

- If the scene is dangerous or if you must move the patient to access another more seriously injured patient, consider an emergency move (Chapter 5). Use an emergency move only if the benefits outweigh the potential risks. Ideally, wait until additional personnel are available to assist.

- Continue to provide life support care until additional EMS personnel arrive.

Disentanglement and Removal of the Patient

 Need to Know

Disentanglement involves freeing patients from the entrapment site. This may require sophisticated and specialized rescue equipment and is generally not a First Responder responsibility. During a prolonged disentanglement process, Paramedics may initiate Advanced Life Support procedures, such as administering intravenous fluids, while the patient is still trapped. Remain at the scene during the disentanglement process to assist as required.

The patient is then removed from the wreckage, ideally after being stabilized and packaged.

The spine is immobilized and critical interventions given. If the patient has life-threatening head, chest, or abdominal trauma, however, EMS personnel may remove the patient immediately for transport. **Removal** is not a First Responder responsibility, but you may be asked to assist.

 Do You Understand?

1. True or false: The highest priority when considering patient extrication is the patient's safety.

2. Which window in a vehicle should be broken when necessary to access a critical patient?

_____

3. At what point in the extrication process is the patient removed?

_____

Hazardous Materials Incidents

 Need to Know

Hazardous materials are common in our society and pose a special hazard for emergency personnel. **Hazardous materials** include:

- ☑ Poisonous substances
- ☑ Explosives
- ☑ Flammable gases, liquids, and solids
- ☑ Chemicals and substances that react with other substances
- ☑ Radioactive materials

Need to Recognize

When you approach the emergency scene and survey the scene, always check for clues that indicate the presence of a hazardous material. You may see a spilled chemical or liquid, or notice smoke or vapors. You may smell fumes—but remember that some hazardous gases and fumes may be odorless and invisible.

Hazardous materials are not limited to industrial sites or vehicles transporting substances. Homes also contain many potentially hazardous materials, including natural gas, gasoline, kerosene, pesticides, and many others. Never assume that a scene is safe because you do not smell an odor. Remember that some hazardous materials are explosion hazards.

Persons who transport or store hazardous materials are required to post placards that identify the hazardous material. If you do not see a placard but suspect a hazardous material may be present:

- Try to obtain additional information before approaching the scene.

- Do not enter the scene. Instead, retreat to a safe distance and call for help.

- Most fire departments have specially trained hazmat teams for managing hazardous materials incidents.

- Hazardous materials spills are now under the jurisdiction of the National Incident Management System (NIMS), which may require specific actions to be taken (see Chapter 19).

When a hazardous material is present at the emergency scene, First Responders' primary responsibility, as always, is personal safety, along with maintaining safety for bystanders and the patient when possible. Manage the emergency scene and prevent bystanders and other First Responders from entering the scene while awaiting the arrival of the hazmat team. If you can do so safely, try to identify the hazardous substance involved, as described later, and give this information to dispatch and arriving emergency personnel. Remain upwind of the scene.

Need to Do

Do not attempt to manage the hazardous substance unless you have advanced specialized training. Following are typical levels of training:

- Hazardous materials awareness training, frequently provided to First Responders, prepares responders to recognize a hazardous materials incident and help manage the scene from a safe distance.

- Hazardous materials operations training, at a higher level, includes how to establish a safety zone around a hazardous materials emergency scene and control the perimeter.

- A hazardous materials technician, a member of the hazmat team, is trained to stop the release of the hazardous material and control the exposure.

- A hazardous materials specialist has the highest level of training and takes command of the emergency and provides support activities.

The safety regulations and guidelines followed by hazardous materials technicians and specialists are mandated by the Occupational Safety and Health Administration (OSHA).

Managing the Scene

Need to Do

- Never enter a scene where hazardous materials may be present unless you are trained as a hazardous materials technician and are fully protected.

- Park upwind or uphill from the incident, at a safe distance.

- Your goal is to isolate the area and keep unnecessary people away.

- Avoid any contact with the hazardous material.

- If there is any chance of a hazardous material being present, be careful not to provide an ignition source. Even turning on a light switch or using a telephone or radio may generate a spark and start a fire or explosion. When you call for help, make certain that the telephone or radio you use is well clear of the scene.

- If patients are at risk for exposure to the hazardous material, you may move patients to a safe area but only if you can do so without risking exposure yourself. Otherwise, wait for the scene to be declared safe, or for patients to be brought from the scene by hazardous materials technicians.

- A patient who has been exposed to the hazardous material should first be decontaminated by hazardous materials technicians.

- Responsive patients and others potentially exposed to the hazardous material should not be allowed to leave the scene until they have been decontaminated.

Once a patient is removed from the hazard, perform basic care. Pay particular attention to the patient's airway and breathing. Provide Basic Life Support and treat any chemical burns.

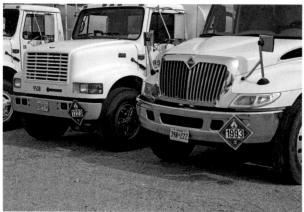

Figure 18-2 Hazard warning placards must be posted on hazardous materials storage sites and transportation vehicles.

Identifying the Hazardous Material

▪▪ Need to Recognize

When you are the First Responder at an emergency scene, try to identify the specific hazardous material present if you can do so safely.

- Federal regulations require that hazardous materials in storage areas and being transported be clearly labeled **(Figure 18-2)**.

- Drivers of vehicles carrying hazardous materials must also have shipping papers that identify the specific substance.

- All vehicles transporting hazardous materials must be marked with placards that identify the material and the hazards **(Figure 18-3)**.

The placard's color and design indicate the particular hazard, such as an explosive, flammable gas, or poison. A four-digit number on the placard identifies the specific material. Try to read the placard from a safe distance using binoculars, and report this information to the hazmat team and other personnel on site.

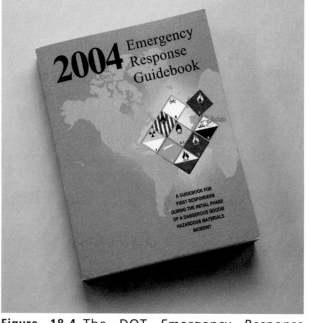

Figure 18-4 The DOT *Emergency Response Guidebook*.

The *Emergency Response Guidebook*, published by the United States Department of Transportation (DOT), identifies hazardous materials according to the codes used on warning placards and gives instructions for emergency procedures **(Figure 18-4)**. Keep a copy in your vehicle.

The National Fire Protection Association (NFPA) system for hazard warnings is often used on storage and industrial buildings where hazardous materials are present **(Figure 18-5)**. These placards identify the specific hazard by color:

Red   - flammable

Blue   - health hazard

Yellow   - instability hazard such as explosive or unstable material

White   - other information

Figure 18-3
Hazardous materials warning placards.

Explosives

Gases

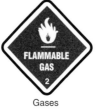
Flammable liquids

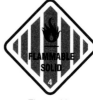
Flammable solids

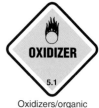
Oxidizers/organic peroxides

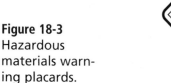
Toxic materials

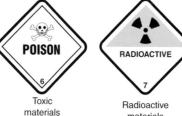
Radioactive materials

Corrosive materials

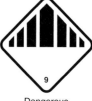
Dangerous goods

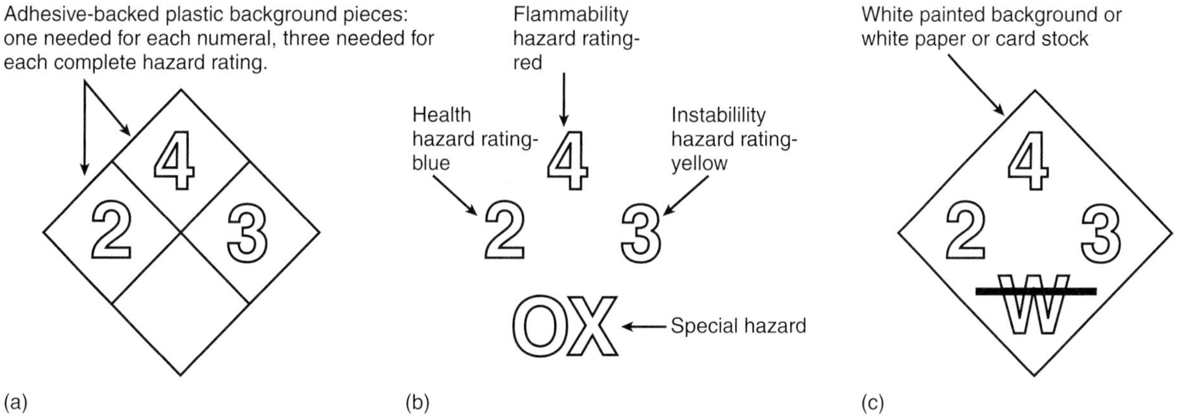

Adhesive-backed plastic background pieces: one needed for each numeral, three needed for each complete hazard rating.

Flammability hazard rating-red

Health hazard rating-blue

Instabilility hazard rating-yellow

← Special hazard

White painted background or white paper or card stock

(a)   (b)   (c)

Figure 18-5 The NFPA system for hazard placards. (a) For use when specified color background is used with numerals of contrasting colors. (b) For use where white background is necessary. (c) For use where white background is used with painted numerals or for use when hazard rating is in the form of sign or placard. Reprinted with permission from NFPA 704 *System for the Identification of the Hazards of Materials for Emergency Response,* Copyright © 2001, National Fire Protection Association, Quincy, MA 02269. This warning system is intended to be interpreted and applied only by properly trained individuals to identify fire, health and reactivity hazards of chemicals. The user is referred to certain limited number of chemicals with recommended classifications in the *Fire Protection Guide to Hazardous Materials* which would be used as a guideline only. Whether the chemicals are classified by NFPA or not, anyone using the 704 system does so at their own risk.

The placards also include a single digit from 0 to 4 that rates the level of the hazard, ranging from a very low hazard (0) to a very high hazard (4).

✏ Do You Understand?

1. At a hazardous materials incident, where is it safest to park and manage the scene?

   _____

2. How should you attempt to identify a substance spilled in a hazardous materials incident?

   a. Get close enough to smell the fumes.

   b. With a transport vehicle, look for the shipping papers in the cab.

   c. Telephone the owner of the company involved.

   d. Read warning placards using binoculars.

3. If a patient was exposed to a hazardous material, to what should you pay special attention in your assessment?

   _____

Water and Ice Rescue

✓ Need to Know

Like hazardous materials incidents, an emergency involving a person in water or ice is dangerous for rescuers. If you cannot safely approach the person, stay away and call for specialized help. A crew with the appropriate training and equipment will be dispatched to rescue the victim safely.

Water Rescues

Water rescues are often needed to prevent drowning:

☑ A nonswimmer may have gotten into deep water.

☑ A swimmer may have sustained an injury or sudden illness, such as a heart attack or seizure, that prevents the person from reaching safety.

☑ Any victim of hypothermia, whether intentionally or unintentionally in the water, is at risk for drowning because mental and physical abilities quickly diminish.

Regardless of the reason, if someone in deep water cannot reach safety, immediate rescue is required. An unresponsive person in the water as a result of drowning, injury, or illness usually needs immediate Basic Life Support after rescue.

The choice of rescue technique depends on the

☑ Type of situation

☑ Equipment or objects at hand

☑ Circumstances

Resist the temptation to jump immediately into the water to save the person. An actively drowning person is in a state of panic that frequently leads to the person grabbing a would-be rescuer so forcefully and desperately that the First Responder may also become a drowning victim. The person may grab your head or arms in a way that you can neither swim back to safety nor tread water to keep both of you afloat. Lifeguards receive special training in how to manage such victims: They are trained to keep a rescue tube between themselves and the victim to prevent being grabbed and also how to break a victim's hold underwater when necessary. It may be appropriate to swim to an unresponsive victim, if you have no other means to reach the person quickly to provide rescue breathing or CPR if needed.

1. The safest and often most effective rescue technique is to reach to the person with some object that the person can grasp while you pull him or her to safety.

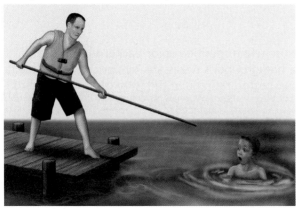

Reach

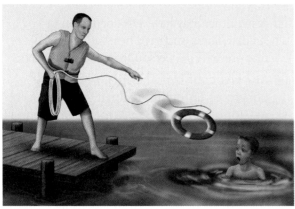

Throw

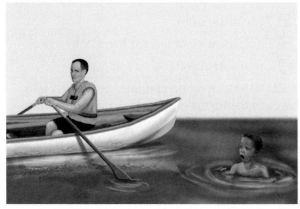

Go

Figure 18-6 The reach-throw-go priorities for water rescue.

2. The second most safe and effective technique is to throw something that floats to the person, preferably with a rope attached for pulling the person to safety.

3. The third and least safe and effective method is to go to the person.

This is called the reach-throw-go priority, which emphasizes which techniques to try first **(Figure 18-6)**.

"Reach" Rescue

▶ Need to Do

- Many pools have a rescue pole, which often has a hook at the end (called a shepherd's crook). This pole is usually long enough to reach a victim from the edge of the pool. Let a responsive person hold on to it while you slowly pull him or her to the edge. If the victim is unresponsive, hook the victim's body to pull him or her to the edge or shallow water.

- Use anything available to reach to the victim, such as a broom or rake handle, a fishing pole, a boat's oar, or a long branch.

- If the victim is close enough to the pool's edge, a dock, or the shore, you may also reach with your body; for example, you could hold on to something secure with your arms and extend your legs on the surface to the victim.

"Throw" Rescue

▶ Need to Do

If you cannot reach to the person, look for anything that floats that you can throw to a responsive person:

- Swimming pool or boating equipment may include a life ring, rescue tube, life jacket, or other devices.

- Some boats carry a throw bag, which has a coiled rope inside that uncoils when the bag is thrown to the person while you hold the other end.

- If no throwable rescue device is available, look around for anything that will float—such as a buoyant seat cushion, a water jug that can be mostly emptied (keep some water inside to give it weight for throwing), or even an empty soft drink cooler.

- If possible, tie a rope to the throwable device, hold it in one hand, coil the rope loosely, and throw with your stronger arm. Try to throw it over the person so that the line comes down beside him or her and can be easily grasped.

"Go" Rescue

▶▶ Need to Do

As noted earlier, entering the water to rescue a responsive victim is dangerous—so much so that unless you have training, you should not attempt this except with a small child or unresponsive victim.

- ◆ Look for other ways to go to the victim, such as on a surfboard, kayak, or other watercraft. Even if it is too small to support both of you, it likely has enough buoyancy to keep you both afloat until help arrives, or the person may be able to hold on to it for buoyancy while you tow him or her to shore.

- ◆ If possible, wear a personal flotation device when entering the water and take something with you that the person can hold on to instead of you.

Unresponsive Patients in Water

▶▶ Need to Do

An unresponsive patient found in the water, unless you are certain otherwise, should be assumed to have a potential spinal injury because of the likelihood of striking the head on the bottom or some other object. The patient's head and neck must be stabilized before the patient is removed from the water, if possible.

1. An unresponsive person not wearing a personal flotation device usually floats facedown. Your first action, therefore, is usually to turn the patient face up in the water to allow breathing or rescue breathing. If you are alone with the patient, support the patient's head in line with the body as you turn the patient on his or her back, using a technique such as the head splint **(Skill 18-1)**.

2. If the patient in the water is breathing, do not attempt to remove him or her from the water alone. Wait for other EMS personnel to bring a backboard into the water for immobilizing the patient prior to removal.

3. If alone, stabilize the patient's head and back as shown at the end of Skill 18-1.

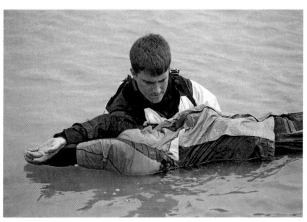

Figure 18-7 Inline stabilization of a patient in water.

4. If a second responder is present, one can hold the patient at shoulder and hips while the other supports the head and neck in line with the body **(Figure 18-7)**.

5. If the patient is not breathing and you are the only responder present, quickly float the patient into shallow water where you can provide rescue breathing once you can stand on the bottom **(Figure 18-8)**.

6. Check the patient's pulse, and do not remove a patient with a pulse but continue rescue breathing until additional EMS personnel arrive with a backboard.

7. If the patient does not have a pulse, you must remove him or her from the water to give CPR. Enlist the help of bystanders if possible and try to support the head while floating the patient from shallow water onto the shore. Alternately, you can remove the patient from a pool or deep water by the safest method possible given the circumstances.

8. Try to support the patient's head and spine during removal but do not delay potentially life-saving CPR.

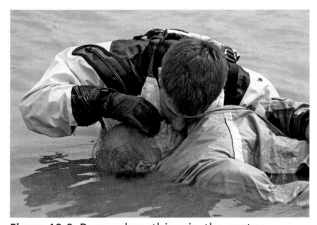

Figure 18-8 Rescue breathing in the water.

Skill 18-1 Turning A Patient in Water Using a Head Splint

1 From a position in the water beside the patient, bring the patient's arms along both sides of his or her head.

2 Holding both of the patient's arms against the sides of the head, rotate the patient toward you by pulling the farther arm up and toward you as you push the nearer arm down and away from you.

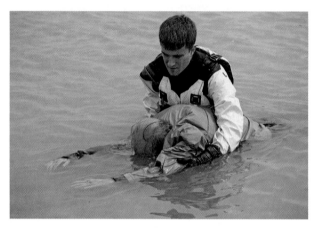

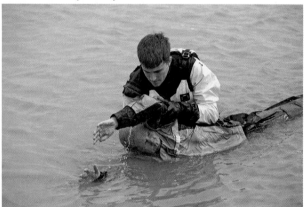

3 Maintain the head stabilization while assessing whether the patient is breathing. Use one hand and arm to hold the patient's arms along the head and the other under the patient's waist or hips for support.

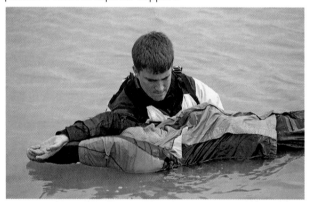

Walking Assist

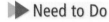 Need to Do

Many natural bodies of water gradually get deeper away from the shore. If a responsive person in the water is at a depth where he or she can stand, or if you can assist the person to that depth, you can help the patient exit the water with a walking assist:

1. Put the patient's arm around your shoulder and hold it at the wrist with your hand.

2. Put your other arm around the patient's waist.

3. Support the patient as you walk the patient out of the water.

Beach Drag

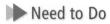 Need to Do

An unresponsive patient who is in or can be brought to shallow water with a gradual shoreline

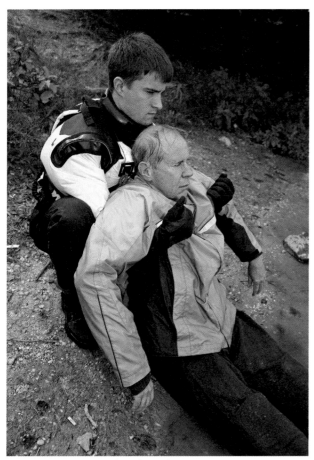

Figure 18-9 Use the beach drag to remove an unresponsive patient from shallow water when alone.

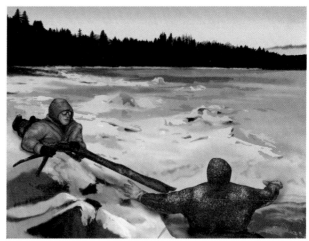

Figure 18-10 While remaining in a safe position, reach to a person who has fallen through ice.

can be taken from the water using a beach drag **(Figure 18-9)**. This rescue technique is similar to the shoulder drag used to move an unresponsive patient on land from a hazardous scene.

1. Reach under the patient's shoulders and hold the patient at the armpits.
2. Support the patient's head against your chest to prevent head or neck movement in case of a possible spinal injury.
3. Then slowly back out of the water, dragging the patient out.

Ice Rescue

▶ Need to Do

Ice rescues are dangerous and ideally should be performed only by those with special training and equipment. Cold-water immersion is very serious and can quickly doom even the best swimmers. Call immediately to summon appropriate emergency personnel.

If it is safe to do so and additional emergency personnel will not arrive in time, you may attempt an ice rescue using the same priorities as a water rescue: reach-throw-go.

1. Using a pole or tree limb, try first to reach to a person who has broken through ice **(Figure 18-10)**.
2. If you cannot reach to the victim, throw a rope or any buoyant object tied to a rope. As a last resort, throw any object that will float to help the person stay afloat, but be aware that in icy water hypothermia sets in very quickly and the victim will not be able to hold on to an object for long.
3. Only as an extreme last resort should you try to go to the person. Realize the ice may not hold your weight and that you too may become a victim. If you must go on the ice, lie down to distribute your weight over a larger surface area. Another person should hold your feet and be prepared to pull you out if the ice under you breaks. If possible, push a branch or other object ahead of you to the victim to minimize the distance you must go onto the ice.

Following ice rescue, the patient is likely to need treatment for hypothermia (Chapter 11).

Do You Understand?

1. Number these ways to rescue a person in water in order of safety.

   _____ Throw a rope to the person.

   _____ Swim to the person.

   _____ Reach to the person with an oar.

2. True or false: When attempting to rescue a person in the water, it does no good to throw a floating object unless you have a rope to tie to it.

3. How can you support the patient's head for a potential spinal injury when you are alone with the patient in deep water?

   _____

4. If you must go onto ice to reach to a victim who has broken through the ice, how should you position yourself?

   _____

Special Response Situations

 Need to Know

Many other types of emergencies and rescues require response from teams with special training and equipment. The following sections serve only to introduce such emergencies and the teams trained to respond to them. As a First Responder, your primary role in special response emergencies when you are first on the scene is to call for assistance and to provide as much information as possible so that appropriate personnel and equipment are summoned to the scene. When other emergency crews have already responded, assume your role in the Incident Command System as described in the next chapter.

Confined Space Emergencies

 Need to Know

A confined space emergency may occur within a building structure, an underground structure or mine, a well, a storage tank, or another area difficult to access and in which victims are entrapped. Confined spaces include industrial and agricultural storage structures such as silos. Hazards in confined spaces may include low oxygen levels; the presence of toxic or explosive gasses; the risk of collapse, hypothermia or heat stroke; and other hazards.

☑ Confined space rescue teams may be organized by fire departments, industrial organizations, and other agencies.

☑ Special equipment and training are typically needed to eliminate or minimize hazards and access the victim.

☑ Your role is to report the situation if first on the scene, keep bystanders out of the area, and provide support to the rescue team after their arrival.

☑ After the removal of patients, you may assist other EMS personnel in providing care.

Rural and Agricultural Settings

 Need to Know

First Responders serving rural and agricultural areas need to be aware of how emergency response in these areas may differ from that in urban areas. Some key differences are:

Longer response times:

☑ Cellular telephone coverage is still limited in some rural areas, so it may take callers longer to reach a telephone to call in an emergency.

☑ Agricultural and other accidents are often reported some time after the incident occurs, because frequently workers are alone and are not immediately discovered after an accident.

☑ It takes longer for EMS personnel to reach emergency scenes because of greater physical distances. In urban areas, EMTs typically respond within 5 to 10 minutes, but the response time in rural areas can be much longer.

☑ First Responders and other EMS personnel are frequently volunteers who may be some distance away at work or home.

Differences in EMS and healthcare facilities:

☑ EMS professionals responding to emergencies in some rural areas may not have as much sophisticated equipment, or advanced training, as in many urban areas.

☑ Small rural hospitals may not have continuous emergency department coverage and may lack some resources.

☑ Some patients, because of difficulty in receiving routine healthcare at some distance from facilities, may let chronic medical problems become emergencies before seeking help.

Agricultural hazards and injuries:

☑ Work-related deaths among farm workers are higher than almost all other occupations, in part because of the machinery used and the frequent lack of personal protection.

☑ Equipment entanglement may involve lengthy extrication procedures.

☑ The use of hazardous chemicals is common, with exposure risks high.

☑ Temperature extremes frequently contribute stress in an emergency situation.

First Responders in Rural and Agricultural Settings

▶ Need to Do

If you work or volunteer as a First Responder in a rural or agricultural area, take steps to help make your practice more effective:

▶ Be prepared for the needs of patients whose conditions have deteriorated because of a longer response time (e.g., a trauma patient is more likely to already be in shock before your arrival at the scene).

▶ Get to know the area well and the types of hazards most likely to be present at emergency scenes (e.g., agricultural chemicals, dangerous machinery, etc.). In many areas, special training is available for how to manage such hazards **(Figure 18-11)**.

▶ Seek additional training for types of medical care you may need to provide for longer periods while awaiting additional EMS resources.

▶ Be sure to have the right equipment and supplies with you (e.g., you cannot afford to wait for EMTs to arrive with an AED if you do not have one when it is needed). If you are not provided with needed equipment, become an advocate for appropriate funding.

▶ Get advanced training in special skills such as hazardous materials incidents, because special response teams may be some distance away.

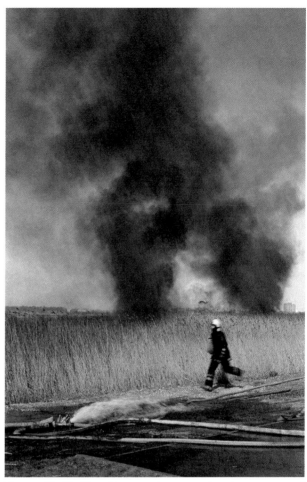

Figure 18-11 First Responders need to be aware of special hazards when responding to emergencies involving agricultural chemicals.

▶ Recognize the need to keep your skills updated because they may not be used frequently; seek out continuing education and refresher courses.

Industrial Settings

✓ Need to Know

Industrial settings are particularly hazardous due to factors such as these **(Figure 18-12)**:

☑ Hazardous machinery and equipment

☑ Presence of hazardous materials

☑ Risks of fire or explosion

☑ Confined spaces

An industrial response team is present in many industries, with specialized training to address hazards specific to the location.

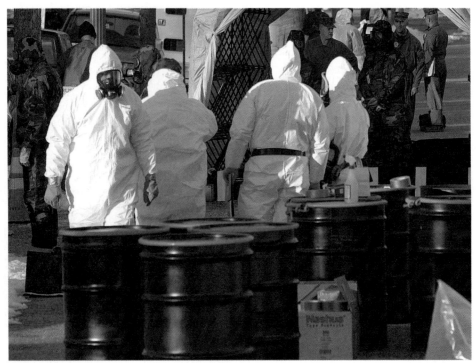

Figure 18-12 Emergencies in industrial settings often involve special hazards.

First Responders in Industrial Settings

▶▶ Need to Do

If you work or volunteer as a First Responder in an industrial area, take steps to help make your practice more effective:

- Know in advance about the availability of special industrial response teams and how to contact them.

- If the industrial site has an emergency plan, ensure it is activated when an emergency occurs. It may be inappropriate for you to enter the scene if such a plan has already been put into effect.

- Remember that your personal safety is your first priority. This is particularly important when unseen hazards may be present.

- Talk to on-site managers or staff to learn about specific hazards before entering the emergency scene.

- Be aware of the potential for multiple patients in an industrial incident, and immediately activate the Incident Command System (see Chapter 19).

Natural Disasters

✓ Need to Know

Natural disasters often cause widespread damage and injury as well as a need to rescue entrapped victims.

- ☑ First Responders reporting to the Incident Command System may have many roles in patient care and cleanup operations **(Figure 18-13)**. Because of the scope of such disasters, responders are often brought in from nearby regions.

- ☑ The National Incident Management System (NIMS), which includes other government agencies such as the Federal Emergency Management Agency (FEMA), directs a coordinated response involving state and local disaster agencies, following a preplanned response (see Chapter 19).

- ☑ Reporting within the command structure and focusing on specific task assignments are important because of the large number of personnel typically involved.

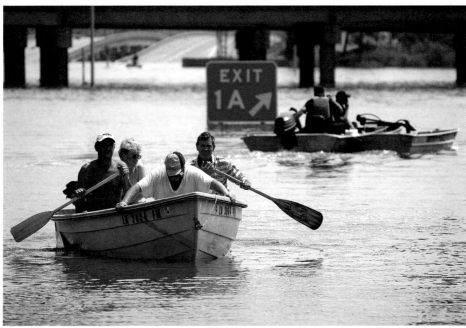

Figure 18-13 First Responders may have many different roles after a natural disaster.

Terrorist Acts

✓ Need to Know

The threat of terrorist acts is omnipresent in our country today. The U.S. Department of Homeland Security created the National Incident Management System (NIMS), which has directed FEMA and other agencies to prepare plans for responding to a wide range of possible attacks, including:

- ☑ Explosions in structures
- ☑ Nuclear explosions
- ☑ Crashes of airliners, surface and subway trains, ferries and other ships, and other vehicles of mass conveyance
- ☑ Release of biological agents such as anthrax
- ☑ Release of chemical agents, such as toxic gases such as ricin, and nerve agents such as sarin
- ☑ Release of radioactive material through a conventional explosive, such as a "dirty bomb"

Preparations for potential terrorist attacks involve every level of government and many separate agencies. First Responders in most jurisdictions receive special training about their role in different types of attacks (see Chapter 19).

All First Responders, however, should maintain an awareness of the possibility of the different types of terrorist attacks and be observant whenever responding to an unusual emergency scene. Should a terrorist incident occur in your area, the number of casualties may depend in part on how quickly an alert is put out and the area evacuated. First Responders should therefore be watchful for unusual activities and suspect a terrorist incident when arriving at an emergency scene involving:

- ☑ A large number of patients
- ☑ Patients with unusual signs and symptoms possibly related to an exposure
- ☑ Any incident at a facility or public place that may be targeted by terrorists
- ☑ Other unusual incidents

Be aware also of the possibility of a secondary device, such as a second explosive at the scene timed to explode after the primary device with the intent of injuring responding emergency personnel.

As always, your responsibilities at the emergency scene include:

- ☑ Maintaining personal safety
- ☑ Evaluating the scene carefully before entering
- ☑ Reporting the emergency as quickly and fully as possible
- ☑ Protecting bystanders and helping maintain scene safety

☑ Following your chain of command for large-scale incidents

☑ Assisting other emergency personnel at the scene, such as with triage and patient care

It is beyond the scope of this text to describe the effects of specific agents that may be used in a terrorist attack. First Responders arriving at an emergency scene where the exposure to any agent may be suspected should treat the scene as a hazardous materials incident and stay at a safe distance to prevent exposure.

Do You Understand?

1. List 3 or 4 hazards that might be present in a confined space emergency.

   _____   _____

   _____   _____

2. In what circumstances should you consider the possibility of a terrorist attack when you arrive at the emergency scene?

   _____

   _____

   _____

Conclusion

In an emergency involving special factors such as hazardous materials or a difficult patient rescue, your role as a First Responder is often to recognize the need for specialized personnel and to manage the scene until they arrive. In the next chapter, which discusses multiple-casualty incidents, you will learn about an additional role—triaging patients—that you may have at the emergency scene.

Key Terms

access (p. 290)

disentanglement (p. 292)

extrication (p. 289)

hazardous materials (haz-mat) (p. 292)

notification (p. 286)

patient packaging (p. 288)

preplanning (p. 286)

removal (p. 292)

Review Questions

1. When you first arrive at any emergency scene, you should
   a. notify dispatch that you have arrived.
   b. get to the patient as quickly as possible.
   c. wait in your vehicle for additional EMS crews to arrive.
   d. survey the area for a potential helicopter landing zone.

2. Preparing the patient for transport is called
   a. accessing.
   b. transferring.
   c. packaging.
   d. disentangling.

3. Which of the following should you *not* do when assisting with a helicopter evacuation?
   a. Shine bright lights on the helicopter as it lands.
   b. Approach from downhill when the helicopter is on a slope.
   c. Approach the helicopter from the front.
   d. Close vehicle doors and windows when the helicopter is landing.

4. What should you do when a vehicle has rolled onto its side?

   a. Attempt to return the vehicle upright.

   b. Stabilize the vehicle with materials at hand.

   c. Climb on top of the vehicle to try that door.

   d. Break the windshield to access the patient.

5. What kind of object or tool is best for breaking a vehicle's side window?

   a. A blunt or rounded object

   b. A flat object, such as a board

   c. A pointed object

   d. Any object is okay

6. What color is an NFPA warning placard that a material in storage is flammable?

   a. White

   b. Blue

   c. Yellow

   d. Red

7. Which of these rescue methods should you try first to help a responsive person in the water not far from a dock?

   a. Throw the victim a life ring with an attached rope.

   b. Reach to the victim with a fishing pole.

   c. Throw the victim a lifejacket.

   d. Paddle a canoe over to the victim.

8. You are in about four feet of water alone with a pulseless patient. What should you do?

   a. Begin CPR immediately while in the water.

   b. Give rescue breaths only while waiting for additional rescuers.

   c. Hold the patient's face out of the water while waiting for a backboard for removing the patient.

   d. Remove the patient from the water as best you can and start CPR.

9. In a confined space emergency, if you are first on the scene, what is your first responsibility?

   a. Call in to report the situation.

   b. Try to open a space for patients to get air.

   c. Cordon off the area to keep bystanders out.

   d. Access the patients by any means possible.

10. If you suspect an emergency scene may have been caused by a terrorist attack, you should

   a. call the special Homeland Security hotline.

   b. tell everyone at the scene to leave as quickly as possible and get away.

   c. treat the scene as a hazardous materials incident.

   d. spray down the entire area with water hoses and fire extinguishers.

The National Incident Management System and Mass-Casualty Incidents

Chapter Preview

- National Incident Management System
- Mass-Casualty Incidents
- Incident Command System for Mass-Casualty Incidents
- Role of First Responders in MCIs
- Triage

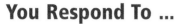

You Respond To …

an emergency scene where a bus tipped on its side after leaving the roadway. Another First Responder arrived just before you and has already called in the emergency as a mass-casualty incident. As you approach, she tells you it looks like there are about a dozen unresponsive patients inside the bus as well as others with injuries.

Introduction

In many cases, you will respond to emergencies with only one patient with a serious injury or medical condition. Other emergencies involve multiple patients or situations in which the patients outnumber the EMS responders. These types of situations require an organized approach for managing the complex scene and treating patients on a priority basis. The National Incident Management System (NIMS), through the Incident Command System (ICS), coordinates and directs the response for mass-casualty incidents as well as other types of large-scale emergencies. Your role within NIMS may be somewhat

different from your everyday role as a First Responder.

The National Incident Management System

✔ Need to Know

EMS systems are local or regional jurisdictions developed to respond to most small-scale emergency situations. A larger-scale emergency, however, such as a mass-casualty incident, natural disaster, or terrorist act, requires the response of emergency personnel and resources from multiple jurisdictions. The **National Incident Management System (NIMS)** was created in 2003 to coordinate and manage the response to such larger incidents. Benefits of NIMS include

- ☑ A unified approach to incident management
- ☑ Standardized command and management structures
- ☑ An emphasis on preparedness, mutual aid, and resource management

NIMS is administered by the U.S. Department of Homeland Security and includes the roles of many other agencies such as the Federal Emergency Management Agency (FEMA). NIMS has developed a National Response Plan (NRP) that coordinates the actions of federal, state, and local governments as well as nongovernment agencies and organizations within a single plan that addresses all large-scale emergencies. The NRP continues to be refined.

Elements of NIMS

NIMS focuses on all the following dimensions of emergency response:

- ☑ Prevention of emergencies and incidents
- ☑ Preparedness
- ☑ Response
- ☑ Recovery
- ☑ Mitigation

The Incident Command System

The **Incident Command System (ICS)** is a part of NIMS that focuses on a coordinated response to emergencies and incidents, including the following:

- ☑ Acts of terrorism
- ☑ Wildfires and urban fires
- ☑ Hazardous materials spills
- ☑ Nuclear accidents
- ☑ Aircraft accidents
- ☑ Earthquakes, hurricanes, tornadoes, floods, and other natural disasters
- ☑ War-related disasters
- ☑ Other mass-casualty incidents

First Responders and other EMS personnel have a crucial role in the ICS, as discussed in the following sections. In addition to preparedness and other elements of NIMS training, most First Responders will receive training related to their role in the ICS.

NIMS and ICS Training

All personnel with a direct role in emergency response and management should receive training in NIMS and ICS. This training is required as a condition for receiving federal preparedness funding assistance.

This requirement includes federal, state, and local government employees within EMS and other disciplines related to emergency services, such as certain hospital, public health, law enforcement, and fire service personnel, as well as some support and volunteer personnel. Different courses are required at different levels. Your instructor will inform you about your training needs related to your First Responder role.

Mass-Casualty Incidents

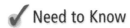 Need to Know

A **mass-casualty incident (MCI)**, also called a multiple-casualty incident, is an emergency in which multiple patients need care. Even when there are only two or three patients with critical injuries, an MCI can be stressful and requires an orderly approach based on setting patient priorities. A large MCI, such as a train wreck, an airline crash, a building collapse, a natural disaster, or a terrorist attack, can strain EMS resources.

Different EMS systems define MCIs in somewhat different ways, sometimes depending on the number of patients involved. A small MCI may be handled within a single EMS system, but larger MCIs require a coordinated response from multiple jurisdictions. Therefore, the ICS, as part of NIMS, is used to direct and manage the emergency response. The ICS, coupled with an effective triage system, is a rapid, logical, and well-organized approach to giving medical care to victims of an MCI.

The Incident Command System for Mass-Casualty Incidents

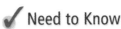 Need to Know

As part of NIMS, the ICS oversees all aspects of response to incidents, including terrorist acts and natural disasters. Many such incidents involve multiple casualties needing medical care. Although this chapter focuses primarily on the medical care aspects of the ICS, First Responders may have additional or other roles as well, as you will learn in your NIMS-ICS training.

The ICS provides an organized approach to a mass-casualty incident:

- ☑ The ICS organizes, coordinates, and controls the resources and personnel necessary to manage the MCI.
- ☑ Similar emergency functions are grouped together for maximum effectiveness, and lines of authority are clearly identified.

In an MCI, the overall supervisory responsibility for workers and resources is assigned to a single person, the **Incident Commander.**

- ☑ The Incident Commander directs the emergency response.
- ☑ Upon determining that the number of critical patients exceeds their capability to manage all of them, the first-responding

unit announces to the dispatcher that an MCI exists and that they are "Command."

☑ As more personnel arrive, command of the incident may be transferred to another person.

☑ The Incident Commander functions from a command post, typically a vehicle near the incident, that provides communications and support personnel for supervising the incident.

Usually, responding rescuers are assigned to a section, or sector, that has specific responsibilities. Each section is supervised by a Section Chief who reports to the Incident Commander. Commonly used medical sections include:

☑ **Triage** — Assesses and categorizes all patients according to the severity of their injuries.

☑ **Treatment** — Treats patients prior to transportation to the hospital. The treatment section may include First Responders, EMTs, Paramedics, nurses, doctors, and other medical personnel.

☑ **Transportation** — Coordinates responding ambulances and helicopters so that patients are expeditiously removed from the scene.

☑ **Staging** — Coordinates all incoming workers and equipment. The staging Section Chief works closely with the Incident Commander and assigns personnel and resources to the other sections as deemed necessary. This section may also coordinate with law enforcement personnel to clear streets and intersections to ensure the uninterrupted arrival of incoming units.

☑ **Supply** — Determines the medical supply needs of other sections.

☑ **Extrication** — Removes any entrapped patients.

Different MCIs require different resources. Smaller MCIs usually do not require all the sections listed.

Role of First Responders in MCIs

▶ Need to Do

If you are the first to respond to an MCI, your first responsibility is to recognize the emergency as an MCI and report it immediately and request assistance. Often the first, knowledgeable EMS provider arriving on the scene becomes the triage officer, until he or she is relieved by a responder with a higher level of training.

ICS TERMINOLOGY

At this time, NIMS continues to evolve and develop to unify the emergency response throughout the country. Previously, different EMS jurisdictions and ICS systems used varying terminology to refer to different sectors used in an MCI and to the different roles and officers within the system. NIMS is in the process of standardizing terminology along with the system, and the terms you learn in your NIMS-ICS training may be slightly different from the terms used here, although the fundamental concepts are the same. When NIMS has fully evolved and is fully implemented throughout the United States, it is expected that a unified system of terminology will be in place.

◆ An initial assessment is first performed on all patients, and a triage category is assigned to each (as described later).

◆ Available personnel and equipment are first directed to patients with the highest priorities for care.

◆ The triage officer usually remains at the scene and is assigned to other responsibilities.

When responding to an MCI where the Incident Command System is in place, First Responders may be assigned to different sections with different responsibilities. Upon arrival, report to the staging section, if one is present, or the command post.

1. Identify yourself and your level of training, and follow directions from the Section Chief or the Incident Commander.

2. Go immediately to your assigned section and report to the Section Chief or the designated individual in charge. Again, give your name and level of training.

3. You may be given a vest to wear that identifies your section. Perform only the task you are assigned.

4. If you complete the assigned task, report to the Section Chief for a new assignment.

5. It is important for all personnel to act only on the direction of supervisory personnel.

MCIs are stressful and may at times seem chaotic. To assist in an orderly, efficient way, accept your assignment without question unless you are inadequately trained for the task. If asked to wait, be patient; your assistance will ultimately be required. Most important, realize that in MCIs some of the usual procedures you are familiar with are likely to be suspended. Accept that in these emergencies, you should perform whatever tasks you are assigned, regardless of your "normal" responsibilities.

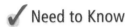 Do You Understand?

1. Who is in charge of resources at a mass-casualty incident?

_____

2. At a large-scale, mass-casualty incident, First Responders may be assigned to
   a. treatment.
   b. triage.
   c. staging.
   d. whatever section the staging Section Chief requests.

Triage

✓ Need to Know

Triage is the process of sorting patients by the severity of their injuries so that those with the highest priority are treated first. Different triage systems have been developed, with varying numbers of triage categories.

The system described in detail here is a three- or four-category system called the **START** system, which stands for Simple Triage and Rapid Treatment.

☑ The START system is useful for rapidly triaging and treating a large number of patients.

☑ It requires only limited medical training, takes less than 60 seconds per patient to complete, and follows a format similar to the initial assessment described in Chapter 6.

In triage, each patient is tagged with a colored tag, indicating his or her triage category **(Figure 19-1)**:

1. Priority 1 — Red — Immediate care needed

☑ Used for patients with airway and breathing difficulties, uncontrolled or severe bleeding, or decreased mental status

2. Priority 2 — Yellow — Urgent care needed

☑ Used for responsive patients with burns without airway problems; major or multiple painful, swollen, deformed extremities; back injuries; and responsive patients with other serious injuries without threats to breathing or circulation

3. Priority 3 — Green — Delayed care

☑ Used for responsive patients with minor painful, swollen, deformed extremities, or minor soft-tissue injuries

4. Priority 4 — Black — No care needed

☑ Used for obviously dead victims or those with a very low likelihood of survival

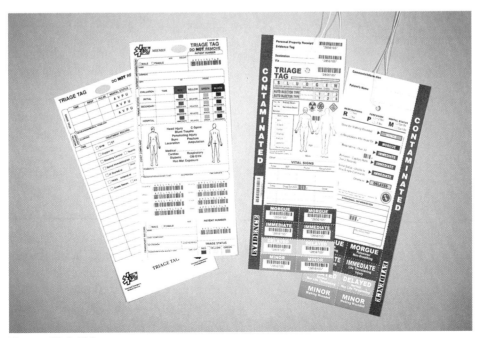

Figure 19-1 Triage tags.

▶ Need to Do

Upon arrival at an MCI, the earliest responders assigned to triage quickly survey the scene. If there are only a few patients, triage can proceed quickly and tags may not be needed. When there are many patients, tags are generally used.

- In a complicated scene with many patients, patients with minor injuries, often called the "walking wounded," are asked to walk aside to a designated area, if they can walk without assistance. They are triaged as Priority 3 to receive care later and may be given a green tag.

- Then emergency personnel can triage the remaining patients. Each triage assessment should take less than 60 seconds to complete.

- The START system evaluates each patient's breathing, circulation, and mental status to assign a triage category, as described in **Box 19-1**.

- As soon as each patient is tagged, move immediately to the next. When all have been triaged, then all personnel begin providing care for Priority 1 patients first.

After the initial START triage, once treatment begins, reevaluation is ongoing. If conditions and numbers of responders allow, observe or check the status of patients originally categorized as Priority 2 or 3 to look for changes in the patient's condition. A Priority 2 patient may become unresponsive, for example, making that patient now a Priority 1 patient.

Pediatric Triage

✓ Need to Know

The START system triage criteria previously described are effective for adults, but less so for infants and children. For example:

- ☑ A respiratory rate faster than 30 breaths/minute indicates a high-priority problem in an adult but may not be a problem in an infant or young child.

- ☑ An adult who is not breathing when the airway is opened is categorized as dead, whereas a child who has just stopped breathing may have a pulse.

- ☑ An adult who cannot follow a simple command is considered unresponsive and tagged Priority 1, but a very young child may not respond for other reasons or be too young to respond as expected.

▶ Need to Do

Pediatric patients are therefore often triaged using an alternate approach called the JumpSTART system.

- In this system, you assess the same characteristics but follow different criteria and take somewhat modified steps, as outlined in **Box 19-2**.

- As with adults, first ask children who can walk to move to one side and tag them as green (Priority 3) to receive care later.

✎ Do You Understand?

1. Match the triage tag colors with the patient's priority status.

   _____ red   a. Immediate care

   _____ black   b. Urgent care

   _____ green   c. Delayed care

   _____ yellow   d. No care

2. An adult breathing slower than _____ or faster than _____ breaths/minute is tagged Priority 1 (red).

3. A child breathing slower than _____ or faster than _____ breaths/minute is tagged Priority 1 (red).

4. How do you triage an adult who is not breathing when the airway is opened?

   _____

5. What do you do next for a child who is not breathing when the airway is opened?

   _____

Conclusion

Mass-casualty incidents can be frightening and stressful, especially with a large number of patients who need care. Using the Incident Command System and following standard triage priorities helps ensure the emergency is managed efficiently and patients are provided care in an organized manner.

BOX 19-1

START TRIAGE ASSESSMENT

1. **Assess Breathing**
   Check whether the patient is breathing. If the patient is breathing at a rate of 8 to 30 breaths/minute, move on to assess circulation. If the patient is breathing at a rate slower than 8 or faster than 30 breaths/minute, tag the patient Priority 1 (red tag). If the patient is not breathing, position the patient's head to open the airway. If still not breathing, tag the patient Priority 4 (black tag). If the patient is breathing when the airway is opened, tag the patient Priority 1 (red tag) because the patient needs airway support.

2. **Assess Circulation**
   For a patient who is breathing without your having to open the airway, next assess circulation by checking the patient's pulse. If the pulse is strong, move on to assess mental status. If the pulse is weak or obviously irregular, tag the patient Priority 1 (red tag). If the patient's pulse is weak and the patient is bleeding severely, quickly apply a pressure dressing to control bleeding, and tag the patient Priority 1 (red tag).

3. **Assess Mental Status**
   For a patient who is breathing and has a pulse, next assess mental status by giving the patient a simple command: "Open your eyes" or "Squeeze my hand." Patients who follow your command are considered alert and responsive and are tagged Priority 2 (yellow tag). Patients who cannot follow a simple command are considered unresponsive and are tagged Priority 1 (red tag).

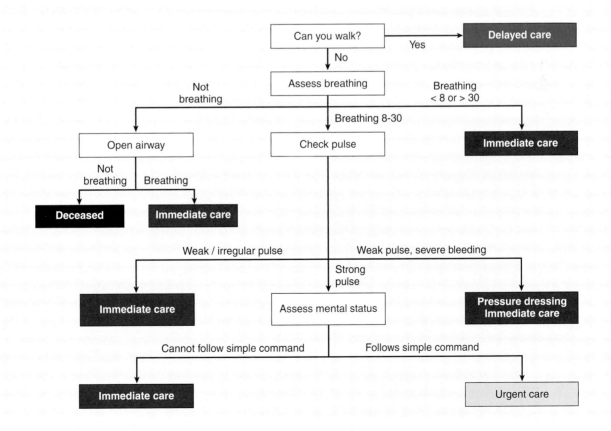

BOX 19-2

JumpSTART PEDIATRIC TRIAGE ASSESSMENT

1. **Assess Breathing**

   Check whether the child is breathing. If the patient is breathing at a rate of 15 to 45 breaths/minute, move on to assess circulation. If the patient is breathing at a rate slower than 15 or faster than 45 breaths/minute, or if breathing is irregular, tag the child Priority 1 (red tag). If the child is not breathing, open the airway. If still not breathing, look in the mouth for a foreign body obstruction and remove one if seen. If the child is now breathing, tag the child Priority 1 (red tag). If not breathing, check for a pulse. If no pulse, tag the patient Priority 4 (black tag). Give a child with a pulse 5 ventilations; if the child begins breathing, tag the child red and move on. If the child does not begin breathing, tag the child black.

2. **Assess Circulation**

   For a child who is breathing 15 to 45 breaths/minute without your having to open the airway, next check the child's pulse in an uninjured extremity. If you feel a pulse, move on to assess mental status. If you do not feel a pulse, tag the patient Priority 1 (red tag).

3. **Assess Mental Status**

   For a child who is breathing and has a pulse, assess mental status with the AVPU assessment. A child who is alert and responds to your voice or pain is tagged Priority 2 (yellow tag). A child who does not respond or who only responds inappropriately to pain is considered unresponsive and tagged Priority 1 (red tag).

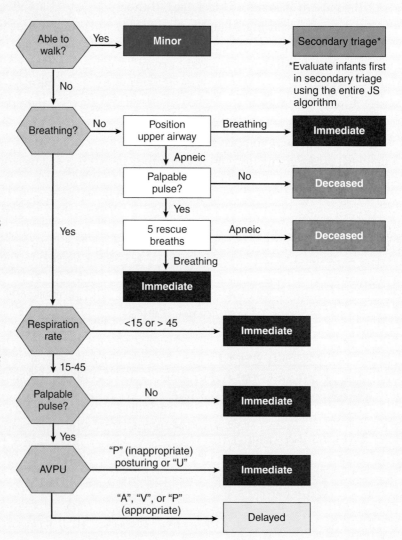

Key Terms

Incident Command System (ICS) (p. 307)

Incident Commander (p. 307)

mass-casualty incident (MCI) (p. 307)

National Incident Management System (NIMS) (p. 306)

START system (p. 309)

triage (p. 309)

Review Questions

1. How many patients must be present before an emergency is considered a mass-casualty incident?
   a. 2
   b. 3
   c. 4
   d. This depends on the specific EMS system.

2. Which Incident Command System section coordinates with law enforcement personnel to clear streets and intersections to ensure the uninterrupted arrival of incoming units?
   a. Transportation
   b. Staging
   c. Supply
   d. Treatment

3. Who usually first acts as the triage officer in a mass-casualty incident?
   a. First EMT or Paramedic on the scene
   b. First arriving provider from the fire department
   c. Responder who most recently took a triage training course
   d. Most knowledgeable EMS provider first on the scene

4. What should you do after completing an assigned task at a mass-casualty incident?
   a. Return to your vehicle and complete your documentation.
   b. Leave the scene to avoid being in the way.
   c. Report to the Section Chief for a new assignment.
   d. Drive to the nearest hospital or receiving facility to assist.

5. Using the START triage system, you should assess and assign each patient to a triage category within
   a. 15 seconds.   c. 60 seconds.
   b. 30 seconds.   d. 2 minutes.

6. A responsive patient with a serious back injury would be given which color triage tag?
   a. Red   c. Green
   b. Yellow   d. Black

7. A responsive patient with a painful, swollen, deformed extremity would be given which color triage tag?
   a. Red   c. Green
   b. Yellow   d. Black

8. An unresponsive, breathing patient with a weak, irregular pulse would be given which color triage tag?
   a. Red   c. Green
   b. Yellow   d. Black

9. A responsive patient who cannot follow your simple command would be given which color triage tag?
   a. Red   c. Green
   b. Yellow   d. Black

10. A responsive child who cannot walk, who is breathing at a rate of 40 breaths/minute, who has a pulse, and who responds to your voice would be given which color triage tag?
    a. Red   c. Green
    b. Yellow   d. Black

A Answers to "Do You Understand?" Exercises and Review Questions

Chapter 1—Introduction to the EMS System

First Responders in Emergencies—"Do You Understand?"

1. The enhanced 911 system automatically provides the dispatcher with the caller's telephone number and location (street address) when using a land telephone line.

2. The First Responder generally assumes patient care and gathers patient information.

3. Transport of the patient is usually performed by the EMTs who assume care from the First Responder.

4. Keep up to date by practicing your skills and taking continuing education or refresher courses.

Roles and Responsibilities of First Responders—"Do You Understand?"

1. True. Unless you maintain your safety, you too may become a patient other EMS personnel will have to treat.

2. Call dispatch (the EMS system) to request additional personnel or equipment.

3. Your first responsibility in patient care is to (d) determine whether there are immediate threats to the patient's life. You must care for any life-threatening conditions before other care or assessments.

Review Questions

1. b
2. c
3. a
4. c
5. d
6. a

Chapter 2—The Well-Being of the First Responder

Emotional Aspects of Emergency Medical Care—"Do You Understand?"

1. Denial. This usually precedes other stages of anger, bargaining, depression, and acceptance.

2. False. Do not offer false reassurances, but let them know that everything that can be done to help will be done.

3. The best answer is (a) Everyone experiences some stress at one time or another.

4. Lifestyle changes that can help you reduce stress include:
   - Stopping smoking
   - Eating a healthy diet
   - Consuming less caffeine and alcohol
   - Controlling body weight
   - Getting regular exercise
   - Learning relaxation techniques

Preventing Disease Transmission—"Do You Understand?"

1. b. Tuberculosis is an airborne disease.

2. The OSHA Bloodborne Pathogens Standard covers anyone who is likely in their work to be exposed to the body fluids of others, including many First Responders.

3. True. To reduce the risk of infectious disease transmission, always wash your hands after giving patient care, even if you wore gloves.

4. If a patient's blood splashes in your eyes, you should flush them out with running water for 20 minutes. Then report the exposure to your supervisor and seek medical care.

Scene Safety—"Do You Understand?"

1. False. Never enter a hazardous scene. Instead, notify EMS and wait for trained personnel with the right equipment.

2. True. A First Responder at a hazardous scene should act to protect himself or herself, the patient, and bystanders.

3. c. Use reflectors, flares, or lights to warn oncoming traffic to help maintain scene safety. Do not try to remove the patient, and stay away from fallen power lines. You cannot disarm the airbag in most vehicles.

Review Questions

1. c
2. a
3. b
4. b
5. d
6. c
7. a
8. d
9. b
10. c

Chapter 3—Legal and Ethical Issues

Scope of Practice & Standard of Care—"Do You Understand?"

1. False. The standard of care for First Responders is to give care as a reasonable, prudent First Responder with similar training would give (not what an EMT would do).

2. True. You should do only what you have been trained to do.

3. Your highest priority (after your personal safety) is meeting your patient's physical and emotional needs.

Legal Principles—"Do You Understand?"

1. You have implied consent when the patient is unresponsive or incompetent or for a minor when a parent or guardian is not present.

2. False. If a competent adult patient refuses consent, you should stay with the patient and wait for additional EMS personnel to arrive.

3. You may be guilty of negligence if you fail to meet the standard of care when treating a patient.

Special Situations—"Do You Understand?"

1. Precautions to take when giving emergency care at a crime scene include:
   - Making sure the scene is safe before entering
   - Ensuring that law enforcement personnel have been notified
   - Not disturbing any item at the scene unless required in order to give care
   - Observing and documenting anything unusual
   - Not cutting through holes in clothing from gunshot or stabbing wounds
   - Following the directions of law enforcement personnel

2. True. Depending on your job description and state laws, you may be obligated to report child abuse to the authorities.

Review Questions

1. b
2. c
3. c
4. d
5. a
6. a
7. c

Chapter 4—The Human Body

Body Regions and Respiratory, Circulatory, and Musculoskeletal Systems—"Do You Understand?"

1. In the anatomical position, the body is facing forward, with arms at sides and palms facing forward.

2. The main function of the respiratory system is to allow oxygen to enter the blood from air breathed in and to remove carbon dioxide.

3. Shock occurs when vital organs are not receiving enough oxygen due to blood loss.

4. Fractures can be life-threatening when nearby organs or larger blood vessels are damaged.

Nervous System, Skin, and Other Body Systems—"Do You Understand?"

1. Changes in a patient's responsiveness, including dizziness and disorientation, are called altered mental status.

2. True. With reduced oxygenation, the skin may be cool, clammy or sweating, and pale or bluish or ashen-colored in a dark-skinned person.

3. a. Prolonged vomiting or diarrhea may result in dehydration as the body loses fluid.

Review Questions

1. b
2. a
3. d
4. b
5. b
6. c
7. a
8. d
9. a
10. c

Chapter 5—Lifting and Moving Patients

Body Mechanics and Patient Positioning—"Do You Understand?"

1. Bend your knees, keep your back straight, and lift with your legs and not with your back.

2. When lifting or carrying a patient, keep the patient close to your body.

3. True. Allow a responsive patient to choose the position that is most comfortable or that makes breathing easiest.

4. The three benefits of the recovery position are:
   - It helps keep the airway open.
   - It allows fluids to drain from the mouth.
   - It prevents the patient from inhaling stomach contents if the patient vomits.

Emergency Moves—"Do You Understand?"

1. Move a patient before assessment and treatment only to escape an immediate danger or because you cannot give lifesaving care in the patient's current position.

2. With the shoulder drag, support the patient's head between your forearms and elbows, or against your chest.

3. c. The two-rescuer extremity carry is best for carrying a patient down stairs because both rescuers face forward and can be at different stair levels.

Nonemergency Moves and EMS Equipment—"Do You Understand?"

1. Before using a nonemergency move, you must:
   - Complete the primary and secondary assessment.
   - Correct any life-threatening problems.
   - Immobilize suspected fractures and dislocations.
   - Ensure there is not a neck or spinal injury.

2. The rescuer at the patient's head usually gives the signal to lift or move with a patient.

3. c. A short backboard is typically used for extricating a patient from inside a vehicle or other confined space.

Review Questions

1. a
2. c
3. d
4. a
5. c
6. b
7. b
8. a
9. d
10. a

Chapter 6—Patient Assessment

Scene Size-Up—"Do You Understand?"

1. In the scene size-up, you look for BSI precautions to take, hazards, the mechanism of injury or nature of the illness, the number of patients, and the need for additional resources.

2. False. Do not delay patient care to thoroughly analyze the mechanism of injury. This is something to observe and consider while approaching the patient.

Initial Assessment—"Do You Understand?"

1. Assess responsiveness in a patient who is not moving or speaking by tapping the person on the shoulder and asking "Are you okay?"

2. Due to a possible spinal injury, open the airway of an unresponsive trauma patient by using the jaw thrust.

3. Look, listen, and feel for breathing.

4. In a responsive adult, check the radial pulse. In an unresponsive adult, check the carotid pulse.

5. False. Control only severe bleeding in the initial assessment. Control minor bleeding after completing the assessment and examination.

Physical Examination—"Do You Understand?"

1. False: A rapid trauma assessment is a complete examination of a trauma patient, looking for any injuries.

2. DOTS stands for Deformities, Open injuries, Tenderness, and Swelling.

3. A clear fluid leaking from the ears is a sign of a skull fracture.

4. In addition to DOTS, assess the extremities for a pulse, movement (motor function), and sensation.

Vital Signs—"Do You Understand?"

1. Signs of respiratory difficulty include gasping or wheezing, very fast or slow respiratory rate, very shallow or deep breathing, shortness of breath, and difficulty speaking.

2. Shock may be indicated by skin that is cool, pale (or ashen), and moist.

3. The pupils are assessed for size, equality, and reactivity.

History—"Do You Understand?"

1. If the patient is unresponsive, talk to family members or others at the scene.

2. False. Ask also about nonprescription medications as well as supplements and other remedies the patient may be taking.

3. Ask about any allergies, including medications, foods, insect stings, and any other substances.

Review Questions

1. a
2. c
3. c
4. c
5. b
6. d
7. a
8. a
9. b
10. c

Chapter 7—The Airway and Breathing Emergencies

Anatomy and Physiology—"Do You Understand?"

1. The epiglottis prevents food from entering the trachea.

2. The large muscle that does most of the work of breathing is the diaphragm.

3. The airway of an infant or young child is more easily obstructed by either the tongue or a foreign body.

The Airway—"Do You Understand?"

1. Use the jaw thrust to open the airway in any trauma patient.

2. False. Sweep the mouth only if you see an obstructing object; never perform a blind sweep.

3. The benefits of using the recovery position for an unresponsive patient who is breathing are:
   - It helps keep the airway open so that you do not need to maintain the head tilt–chin lift or jaw–thrust maneuver.
   - Unrecognized airway obstructions are less likely to occur.
   - It allows fluids to drain from the mouth.
   - It prevents the patient from inhaling stomach contents if the patient vomits.

Breathing—"Do You Understand?"

1. An adult patient breathing fewer than 10 breaths per minute is breathing inadequately.
2. A face mask, also called a pocket mask or resuscitation mask, is preferred for giving a patient ventilations.
3. Each ventilation should take about 1 second.
4. An adult patient who has a pulse but is not breathing should receive 1 ventilation every 5 to 6 seconds.
5. Incorrect actions that may lead to a patient's vomiting during ventilation include:
   - Not opening the airway sufficiently
   - Giving breaths too quickly
   - Continuing to ventilate after the chest has risen
   - Not letting the chest fall between ventilations

Foreign Body Airway Obstructions—"Do You Understand?"

1. The signs of a severe FBAO in a responsive patient include:
   - The patient may look frantic and be clutching at his or her throat.
   - The patient cannot speak.
   - The patient has a pale or bluish coloring around the mouth and nail beds.
   - The patient is coughing very weakly and silently, or not coughing at all.
   - A responsive patient cannot answer the question, "Are you choking?" but indicates that he or she is choking.
2. Give as many abdominal thrusts as are needed to clear the foreign body, or until the patient becomes unresponsive.
3. An unresponsive infant with a severe foreign body airway obstruction should be given CPR.
4. True. Give a pregnant woman chest thrusts instead of abdominal thrusts, and also any patient you cannot get your arms around.

Review Questions

1. a
2. c
3. c
4. b
5. d
6. c
7. c
8. a
9. d
10. b

Chapter 8—Ventilation Devices and Oxygen

Suctioning—"Do You Understand?"

1. True. Never insert the suction tip deeper than the base of the tongue or farther than you can see.
2. In an adult, never suction longer than 15 seconds at a time, or 10 seconds in a child.
3. Always squeeze the bulb before inserting the tip into the mouth and then release the bulb gradually as you withdraw the tip.

Airway Adjuncts—"Do You Understand?"

1. False. An oral airway does not open the patient's airway but helps maintain it open. Therefore, you must position the patient's head to open the airway before inserting the airway.
2. In an adult, an oral airway is inserted with the tip pointing toward the roof of the mouth.
3. Disadvantages of using a nasal airway include that it is difficult to suction a nasal airway and that the patient feels some pain.

Bag Mask—"Do You Understand?"

1. False: Using a BVM, even when it is not connected to supplemental oxygen, provides a higher percentage of oxygen than a pocket mask; the oxygen level in the air is 21%, compared to the 16% in exhaled air blown through a pocket mask.

2. a. Squeeze the bag until the patient's chest rises (usually about 1/2 to 2/3 of the bag's volume). Squeezing further may result in air going into the stomach and causing the patient to vomit.

3. When using a BVM with an adult, give ventilations at the same rate as with a resuscitation mask: one every 5 to 6 seconds.

4. No, do not waste valuable time assembling equipment; use your pocket mask to immediately begin providing ventilations.

Supplemental Oxygen—"Do You Understand?"

1. A full oxygen tank has a pressure of about 2,000 pounds per square inch.

2. Nasal cannulas typically provide the lowest concentration of oxygen: from 24% to 50%, depending on the patient's breathing rate and the oxygen flow rate.

3. False. Do not put oil or grease on any oxygen equipment because these substances are flammable.

4. Always start the flow of oxygen before putting the oxygen delivery device on the patient or else the patient will not be able to breathe when the delivery device is first applied.

Review Questions

1. b
2. d
3. a
4. d
5. c
6. b
7. a
8. a
9. b
10. d

Chapter 9—Cardiac Emergencies and CPR

Circulatory System—"Do You Understand?"

1. The two most important functions of the circulatory system are transporting oxygen and nutrients in the blood to all parts of the body and removing carbon dioxide and other wastes from tissues.

2. Bleeding from arteries is usually the most serious.

3. Irreversible brain damage begins 8-10 minutes after the heart stops beating.

4. True. Different injuries and illnesses may either increase or decrease the heart rate.

Cardiac Arrest and Chain of Survival—"Do You Understand?"

1. Cardiac arrest may be caused by:
   - Heart attack or other heart disease
   - Drowning
   - Suffocation
   - Respiratory arrest from any cause
   - Stroke
   - Poisoning or drug overdose
   - Allergic reaction
   - Diabetic emergency
   - Prolonged seizures
   - Electric shock
   - Trauma
   - Bleeding

2. The cardiac chain of survival consists of 4 links:
   1. Early recognition and access
   2. Early CPR
   3. Early defibrillation
   4. Early advanced care

3. Give an adult 2 minutes of CPR before stopping to call if the patient's cardiac arrest likely resulted from respiratory arrest, as in a drowning patient.

CPR—"Do You Understand?"

1. False. Although in some cases CPR can result in the heart spontaneously restarting, in most cases, defibrillation is needed to return the heart to a normal heart rhythm—and CPR may keep the patient viable until then.

2. The location for chest compressions in a child is the same as in an adult: midway between the nipples on the lower half of the sternum. Use both hands with an adult, and one or both hands with a child.

3. With two-rescuer CPR for an infant or child, use a ratio of 15 compressions and 2 ventilations. A second exception occurs if an advanced airway is in place in the patient: Ventilations are then given without a pause in continuous compressions.

4. CPR problems include compressions that are too shallow and compressions given at too fast a rate.

5. Two rescuers switch positions after 2 minutes (5 cycles) of CPR.

Review Questions

1. a
2. c
3. b
4. d
5. b
6. a
7. d
8. d
9. b
10. d

Chapter 10—Automated External Defibrillation

The Heart's Electrical System—"Do You Understand?"

1. The normal rhythm of the heart is called the sinus rhythm.

2. False. Ventricular fibrillation means the muscle is quivering rather than pumping effec-

tively, and therefore little or no blood is being pumped through the body.

Using an AED—"Do You Understand?"

1. Send for an AED as soon as you encounter an unresponsive patient. Do not delay until you have checked the ABCs.

2. For a child found pulseless (unless seen to have collapsed suddenly), give about 2 minutes of CPR before using the AED.

3. After administering a shock, give CPR for 5 cycles (about 2 minutes).

4. Precautions when using an AED include:

   • Keeping the patient dry

   • Avoiding flammable materials including oxygen

   • Not using the AED when the patient is in motion

   • Not using a cell phone or radio within 6 feet

   • Not touching the patient while the AED is analyzing or giving a shock

Special Considerations—"Do You Understand?"

1. Children at ages 1 to 8 are recommended for AED use with pediatric pads.

2. False. If pediatric pads are unavailable, it is acceptable to use an AED with adult pads on a child.

3. If a patient has a medication patch on the chest where the pad should go, remove the patch and apply the pad.

Review Questions

1. a
2. b
3. d
4. b
5. c
6. c
7. a
8. b

Chapter 11—Medical Emergencies

Heart Attack and Respiratory Emergencies—"Do You Understand?"

1. True. With an unknown sudden illness, the patient should not eat or drink.

2. The common signs and symptoms of a heart attack include shortness of breath, chest pain or pressure, sweating, nausea, pale skin, and dizziness.

3. False. You do not need to know the specific cause of the breathing difficulty to give emergency care. Help the patient rest in the position for easiest breathing, assist with any prescribed medications, give oxygen if allowed, and be prepared to give BLS.

4. The best thing an asthma patient can do during an attack is to use his or her prescribed inhaler; the medication should control the attack.

Altered Mental Status, Stroke, and Seizures—"Do You Understand?"

1. The causes of altered mental status include:
   - Seizures
   - Stroke
   - Head injury
   - Poisoning, drug use or overdose
   - High fever
   - Infection
   - Diabetic emergencies
   - Psychiatric conditions
   - Any condition that causes lowered blood oxygen levels

2. The three assessments of the Cincinnati Prehospital Stroke Scale:

   1. Ask the patient to smile.

   2. Ask the patient, with eyes closed, to raise both arms out in front of the body.

   3. Ask the patient to repeat a sentence.

3. Place something flat and soft under the patient's head. Do not move the patient, do not try to hold the patient still, and do not put anything between the patient's teeth.

Cold, Heat, and Diabetic Emergencies—"Do You Understand?"

1. d. Remove damp clothing and warm a hypothermic patient with a blanket. Do not give him anything to drink, and do not warm him too quickly with a heat source like a fire or a hot shower.

2. Cool down a patient experiencing heatstroke with one of these methods:
   - Wrap the patient in a wet sheet.
   - Sponge the patient with cold water.
   - Spray the skin with water from a spray bottle and fan the area.
   - Put ice bags or cool packs beside the neck, armpits, and groin area.
   - Partly submerge the patient in cool water and splash the skin (do not immerse fully in cold water).

3. If you cannot judge whether the patient has low or high blood sugar, give sugar as for low blood sugar. Ensure EMS has been activated, and provide supportive care. Be prepared to give BLS.

Poisoning, Alcohol and Drug Abuse, Bites and Stings, and Allergic Reactions—"Do You Understand?"

1. The common signs and symptoms of a swallowed poisoning include nausea, dizziness, drowsiness, vomiting, and unresponsiveness.

2. The following actions are appropriate for a patient with a drug or medication overdose:
   - Call the Poison Control Center or medical direction.
   - Check for injuries that may require emergency care.
   - Try to find out what the person took.

   In addition:
   - Position an unresponsive patient in the recovery position because vomiting is likely; do not position the patient on his or her back.
   - Do not allow responsive patients to lie on their back because of the risk of aspiration if they vomit.

- Do not try to induce vomiting with any patient at any time unless so instructed by the Poison Control Center.

- The patient may have altered pain perception, so base emergency care on your assessment of the signs or the injury or illness.

3. d. Breathing problems. These are caused by swelling of the airway and are most serious because they can be life threatening.

Severe Abdominal Pain and Behavioral Emergencies—"Do You Understand?"

1. True. Administer oxygen to a patient experiencing severe abdominal pain, following your local protocol.

2. False. This is a common myth. Talking about suicide is a warning sign that the person is contemplating suicide.

3. Factors that affect whether the force used to restrain a patient is reasonable:

- Using only as much force as is needed to prevent the patient from injuring self or others

- The patient's size, strength, and gender

- The patient's abnormal behavior

- The patient's mental state

- The method of restraint

Review Questions

1. c
2. b
3. a
4. c
5. d
6. b
7. a
8. b
9. c
10. False

Chapter 12—Bleeding and Shock

External Bleeding—"Do You Understand?"

1. False. The first thing to do is control the bleeding. (Also, First Responders do not apply antibiotic ointments.)

2. The steps should be taken in this order:

   1. Put on gloves.
   2. Put direct pressure on the wound.
   3. Apply a pressure dressing.

Internal Bleeding—"Do You Understand?"

1. Pale, cool skin (or ashen colored skin in a dark-skinned person). Skin characteristics are the same as for any patient in shock.

2. The signs and symptoms of internal bleeding include:

- Mental status changes

- Tender, swollen, or rigid abdomen

- Pale, cool, moist clammy skin

Additional signs and symptoms of internal bleeding are:

- Increased respiratory and pulse rates

- Nausea and vomiting

- Thirst

3. Ensure that EMS has been activated (because definitive medical treatment is needed as soon as possible). Then treat for shock.

Shock—"Do You Understand?"

1. False. Never give a patient in shock anything to eat or drink because of the risk of vomiting and because the patient may require surgery.

2. True. Shock may result from many different types of injury and sudden illness.

3. b. Nausea, thirst, and clammy skin are common signs and symptoms of shock.

4. a. Except in cases of minor bleeding, always stop the bleeding first in a patient with shock, because continued bleeding will worsen the shock.

Review Questions

1. b
2. a
3. b
4. c
5. a
6. d
7. a
8. d
9. b

Chapter 13—Soft-Tissue Injuries

Wound Care—"Do You Understand?"

1. A minor wound should be irrigated with running water 5 minutes before dressing and bandaging it.

2. When you must control bleeding, use direct pressure and then a pressure bandage to control the bleeding. Do not try to clean the wound first.

3. False. The bandage should be applied firmly to protect the wound and prevent the dressing from exposure or movement. However, it should not be so tight as to cut off circulation.

4. False. Use roller gauze, not elastic roller bandage, for a pressure bandage to control bleeding.

Specific Injuries 1—"Do You Understand?"

1. c. A puncture wound is most likely to become infected because pathogens are more easily trapped inside the skin and not easily flushed out.

2. Animal bites can be serious for three reasons:
   • Bleeding and tissue damage can be severe.
   • Bacteria are usually present in animals' mouths, increasing the risk for infection.
   • The bite of any animal carries the risk of rabies.

3. True. An amputated part should be kept cold but not put in direct contact with ice; put it inside a sealed bag that is then put in a container with ice and water.

4. Put an occlusive dressing on a sucking chest wound and tape only three sides in place.

5. True. With an open abdominal wound with eviscerated organs, try to prevent the organs from drying out by covering the dressing with a large occlusive bandage.

Specific Injuries 2—"Do You Understand?"

1. A ring bandage is used for a scalp wound when there may be a skull fracture; the ring bandage puts pressure only on the edge of the wound, not in the center where there may be bone fragments.

2. For a chemical splash, flush the eye with running water for at least 20 minutes.

3. Emergency care for ear injuries includes covering the ear with a loose sterile dressing. Do not use tweezers to remove an object, do not flush the ear with water, and do not use direct pressure to try to stop fluid from flowing out.

4. The one exceptional situation in which an impaled object should be removed is an object that has pierced through the cheek; it is removed if it may fall into the mouth and pose a risk to the airway or interfere with ventilation when needed.

Burns—"Do You Understand?"

1. Factors that determine the severity of a burn are:
   • The depth of the burn
   • The size of the burn
   • The specific body areas burned
   • The patient's age and health status

2. False. Never break skin blisters (which may increase the risk for infection), and do not put any substance other than water and a dressing on a burn.

3. Do not use cold water to cool a burn larger than 20% of body surface area because of the risk of hypothermia and shock.

4. Signs and symptoms that may indicate the patient inhaled smoke include:
   • Coughing, wheezing, hoarse voice
   • Possible burned area or blackening on the face or chest
   • Difficulty breathing

5. c. For a chemical splash in the eye, immediately flush the eye with running water and continue for at least 20 minutes.

Review Questions

1. b
2. c
3. b
4. d
5. b
6. c
7. d
8. a
9. a
10. c

Chapter 14—Injuries to Muscles and Bones

Mechanisms of Injury and Types of Musculoskeletal Injuries—"Do You Understand?"

1. Large forces are more likely to result in fractures or dislocations.

2. An elderly patient suffering trauma is more likely than a younger patient to suffer a fracture because of osteoporosis.

3. Severe bleeding from damaged blood vessels may result from a dislocation and cause a serious or even life-threatening condition.

Assessment and Care of Musculoskeletal Injuries—"Do You Understand?"

1. Distal to a musculoskeletal injury, you should assess for circulation, sensation, and movement (CSM).

2. In addition to a weak or absent pulse, impaired circulation may be indicated by a pale or bluish skin color (ashen-colored skin in dark-skinned individuals) and a cool skin temperature.

3. False: The patient's level of pain is not always correlated with the severity of the injury.

4. A cold pack is used on most musculoskeletal injuries to reduce pain and swelling.

Principles of Splinting—"Do You Understand?"

1. Use items such as the following to improvise a rigid splint:
   - A board
   - A cane or walking stick
   - A broom handle
   - A piece of plastic or metal
   - A rolled newspaper or magazine
   - Thick cardboard
   - Other similar items

2. False. Elevate a splinted extremity only if doing so will not cause pain or possibly worsen an injury.

3. Under normal circumstances, always splint an injury in the position found—the one exception is when help will be delayed and circulation is cut off in an extremity distal to the injury.

4. Put the cold pack outside the splint but inside the sling, as close as practical to the injured area.

Splinting Different Areas—"Do You Understand?"

1. An injured elbow, when the arm is straight, should be splinted from the upper arm to the hand.

2. The one injury of the upper extremity in which you do not need to leave the fingers exposed to check CSM is an injury of the hand (or fingers). In this case, you may need to bandage the entire hand.

3. False. Do not use a rigid splint on an injured pelvis. Pad between the legs and gently bandage the legs together unless this causes pain or would require movement.

4. The ribs are supported with a pillow or soft padding, and the arm may be put in a sling to prevent movement and ease pain.

Review Questions

1. b
2. d
3. c
4. a
5. b
6. d
7. a
8. c
9. a
10. b

Chapter 15—Injuries to the Head and Spine

Assessing Head and Spinal Injuries—"Do You Understand?"

1. The following signs and symptoms are common to a head or spinal injury:

   - Changing levels of responsiveness
   - Unequal pupils
   - Headache
   - Clear fluid from the nose or ears
   - Tingling, numbness, or lack of feeling in the feet or hands

   Additional common signs and symptoms include:

   - A lump or deformity in the head, neck, or back
   - A stiff neck
   - Inability to move any body part
   - Pain or tenderness in area of injury or associated with movement
   - Continuous or intermittent pain along the spinal column or extremities independent of movement and palpation

2. The common mechanisms of injury for head and spinal injuries include:

   - Motor vehicle crashes
   - Falls from a height of more than a few feet
   - Diving emergencies involving impact to the head
   - Skiing incidents or other sports injuries
   - Any forceful blunt or penetrating trauma to the head, neck, or torso
   - Hanging incidents

3. False. An unresponsive trauma patient should not be moved unless necessary to provide emergency care (or if necessary to escape a hazard in the scene).

4. False. Even a patient who seems to have only a mild concussion requires medical evaluation because it is difficult to determine the seriousness of such an injury.

Emergency Care for Head and Spinal Injuries—"Do You Understand?"

1. Use the jaw thrust to open the airway of a patient with a suspected spinal injury: Do not tilt the head back but lift the jaw upward using both hands. If you cannot open the airway this way, use the head tilt–chin lift.

2. To control bleeding from a skull fracture, use a ring dressing and apply pressure only around the edges of the wound.

3. Manually stabilize the head and neck of an unresponsive patient with a suspected spinal injury until additional EMS resources have secured the patient to a backboard with the head stabilized.

Review Questions

1. a
2. b
3. c
4. d
5. c
6. c
7. b
8. a
9. b
10. d

Chapter 16—Childbirth

Pregnancy, Labor, and Delivery—"Do You Understand?"

1. The first stage of labor begins with contractions. Rupture of the amniotic sac and the bloody show both may occur before or during labor.

2. The placenta is usually delivered within 30 minutes after childbirth.

Emergency Care in Pregnancy—"Do You Understand?"

1. a. The early signs of a possible miscarriage include vaginal bleeding and abdominal pain or cramping.

2. All six of the signs and symptoms listed could indicate a possible problem with the pregnancy. The woman should see her healthcare provider, or seek emergency care, for any of these.

3. Considering the potential risks of bleeding due to trauma to a pregnant woman is important because:

   • Blood flow is reduced to the fetus, potentially causing unseen fetal problems.

   • Signs of internal blood loss may not be as apparent as in a nonpregnant patient.

Childbirth—"Do You Understand?"

1. Questions to ask the woman when assessing whether delivery is imminent include:

   • Name, age, and due date

   • If she has given birth before

   • If she knows whether she may be having twins or triplets

   • If her water has broken, and if so, to describe it

   • If she has experienced any bleeding

   • Any past or present medical problems

2. The clearest sign that childbirth is imminent is crowning.

3. If there is a delay before the shoulders emerge, you should suction the newborn's mouth and nose.

4. If the mother continues to bleed after childbirth, massage the uterus to stimulate contractions to stop the bleeding.

5. If the newborn has a pulse of 80 and the breathing rate is slow, provide ventilations, following your local protocol to use 100% oxygen, at a rate of 40-60 breaths/minute.

6. When assisting with childbirth follow these guidelines for things not to do:

   • Do not try to delay the birth by having the woman hold her legs together or any other maneuver.

   • Do not place your hands or anything else in the woman's vagina.

   • Do not interfere with the childbirth or touch the infant until the head is completely out.

   • Do not pull on the head or shoulders.

   • Do not try to wash the infant's skin, eyes, or ears.

   • Do not pull on the umbilical cord in an effort to pull out the afterbirth.

Childbirth Problems—"Do You Understand?"

1. In a breech birth, if the head does not deliver soon after the body has emerged, make a breathing space with two fingers alongside the infant's nose.

2. For a prolapsed cord, place the woman in the knee-chest position.

3. If the umbilical cord is tightly wrapped around the infant's neck when the head emerges, and you are unable to free it, you need to clamp or tie the cord and cut it to free it and allow the infant's body to emerge.

Review Questions

1. b
2. a
3. b
4. c
5. c
6. a
7. d
8. d
9. c
10. b

Chapter 17—Infants and Children

Interacting with and Assessing Infants and Children—"Do You Understand?"

1. Things you can do to help calm a young child who is fearful include:
   - Being friendly and calm
   - Talking to the child, not just caretakers, using appropriate language
   - Allowing the child to hold a toy
   - Avoiding separating the child from caretakers unless necessary

2. True. Children can compensate well for both respiratory problems and shock for a time by increasing breathing rate and effort. But decompensation is then often rapid.

3. To assess mental status in a child too young to talk, evaluate how the child interacts with others and the environment:
   - Quality of crying or speaking (energetic or weak)
   - Emotional state (crying, upset, frightened)
   - Behavior (manner appropriate for age, playing, and moving, or listless, motionless)
   - How the child responds to caretakers (comforted, responsive, or combative, irritable, inattentive)
   - How attentive the child is to you (makes eye contact, or disinterested)

4. Start CPR for a child with a pulse less than 60 beats/minute if there are signs of poor perfusion. Follow local protocol to administer oxygen with ventilations.

Airway Management and Breathing Emergences—"Do You Understand?"

1. Do not suction a newborn for longer than 3 to 5 seconds at a time.

2. The signs and symptoms of a mild airway obstruction in a child include:
   - Stridor or crowing
   - Retractions
   - Normal skin color

In addition, the child is usually alert and sitting, has a good pulse, and may be coughing.

3. *Never* perform a blind finger sweep of a child's mouth when you suspect an obstruction. Use the finger sweep only when you see an object; otherwise, you could push an unseen object deeper in the airway.

4. False: When providing blow-by oxygen, the mask can be 2 inches or more from the child's mouth and nose and still increase the child's oxygenation.

5. False: In some cases, a respiratory infection can cause a life-threatening breathing problem. You cannot determine its seriousness in the field. Ensure additional EMS resources arrive to assess and treat the child as needed.

Shock, Seizures, Altered Mental Status, SIDS—"Do You Understand?"

1. In a child, the pulse is usually rapid in early shock, becoming slow in late shock.

2. A febrile seizure in a child is treated the same as any other seizure: Protect the patient, manage the airway, do not attempt to restrain the patient or put anything in the mouth, provide suction if needed, and follow your local protocol to administer oxygen if it is available and you are so trained.

3. Causes of altered mental status in infants and children include:
   - Low blood sugar
   - Poisoning
   - Seizures
   - Infection
   - Head trauma
   - Any condition causing decreased oxygen levels

4. False: When an infant dies of sudden infant death syndrome, ask the parents questions about the circumstances, but do not be judgmental and avoid any comments that might suggest blame.

Trauma, Child Abuse—"Do You Understand?"

1. A motor vehicle crash may cause abdominal and lower spine injuries in an infant or child who was properly restrained.

2. Use the jaw-thrust technique to open a child's airway in all trauma patients.

3. Patterns of injury or marks on the skin of a child that may result from child abuse include:
   - Cigarette burns
   - Whip marks
   - Hand prints
   - Injuries to genitals, inner thighs, or buttocks
   - Rope burns
   - Burns with glove or dip pattern

4. False. Never confront or accuse a caretaker of child abuse. This is not the role of First Responders, and confrontation could delay treatment and transport.

Review Questions

1. a
2. d
3. b
4. c
5. d
6. a
7. b
8. b
9. c
10. a

Chapter 18—EMS Operations

Phases of a Response—"Do You Understand?"

1. Generally the dispatcher will provide you with at least:
   - Nature of the call
   - Name, location, and callback number of the caller
   - Location of patient(s)
   - Number of patients
   - Severity of the problem
   - Other pertinent information, such as help being given to the patient

2. As you approach the emergency scene, consider:
   - The need for body substance isolation precautions
   - Any need to move the patient because of hazards
   - The mechanism of injury or medical emergency
   - The need for additional help
   - The number of patients in a multiple-casualty incident

Helicopter Transport—"Do You Understand?"

1. True. The length of time it may take to extricate a critical patient is a factor when determining whether to ask for air transport. Other factors are how long ground transport would take to reach the appropriate specialty center and whether ground access is impossible or may be delayed.

2. A night landing zone generally should be at least 100 feet square.

3. Approach the helicopter from the front. The rear rotor is dangerous.

Patient Extrication—"Do You Understand?"

1. False. As always, the highest priority when considering patient extrication is your safety. Many types of extrication are too hazardous to attempt without special training and equipment.

2. Generally, it is best to break the side window farthest from the patient.

3. Patient removal comes last in the extrication process, after the patient is accessed, given care and stabilized, and disentangled.

Hazards Materials Incident—"Do You Understand?"

1. The safest area near a hazardous materials incident is generally uphill or upwind of the scene.

2. d. Warning placards identify the type of hazard and use a numerical code to identify the specific substance.

3. Pay special attention to the patient's airway and breathing.

Water and Ice Rescue—"Do You Understand?"

1. Remember the order of safety: reach-throw-go.

2. False. Throw any object that will float. The buoyancy will help the person stay afloat and breathing while you continue the rescue with other means.

3. Splint the patient's head with the patient's arms raised above the head on both sides. Also use this method to hold the head while rolling the patient face up.

4. If you must go on the ice, lie down to distribute your weight over a larger area.

Other Special Response Teams—"Do You Understand?"

1. Hazards that might be present in a confined space emergency include low oxygen levels, the presence of toxic or explosive gases, the risk of collapse, and hypothermia or heat stroke.

2. Consider the possibility of a terrorist attack when there are a large number of patients, when patients have unusual signs and symptoms that possibly relate to an exposure, and when the emergency occurs in a public place that may be targeted by terrorists.

Review Questions

1. a
2. c
3. a
4. b
5. c
6. d
7. b
8. d
9. a
10. c

Chapter 19—The National Incident Management System and Mass-Casualty Incidents

Mass Casualty Incidents—"Do You Understand?"

1. The Incident Commander is in charge of resources at a mass-casualty incident.

2. d. At a large-scale, mass-casualty incident, First Responders may be assigned to any section depending on the needs determined by the staging Section Chief.

Triage—"Do You Understand?"

1. a red   a. Immediate care

   d black   b. Urgent care

   c green   c. Delayed care

   b yellow   d. No care

2. An adult breathing slower than 8 or faster than 30 breaths/minute is tagged Priority 1 (red).

3. A child breathing slower than 15 or faster than 45 breaths/minute is tagged Priority 1 (red).

4. An adult who is not breathing when the airway is opened is tagged black (no care).

5. For a child who is not breathing when the airway is opened, check for a pulse. Give a child with a pulse 5 quick ventilations.

Review Questions

1. d
2. b
3. d
4. c
5. c
6. b
7. c
8. a
9. a
10. b

Glossary

A

abandonment the act of terminating patient care without first ensuring that the care you started is continued by someone with equal or greater training

ABCs an acronym for checking the Airway, Breathing, and Circulation; part of the initial assessment of the patient

abdomen the area below the ribs and above the hips

abdominal cavity the cavity below the diaphragm in which are located the stomach, intestines, and other organs

abdominal quadrants a system by which the abdominal region is divided into four sections by a horizontal line at the umbilicus and a vertical line at the body's midline for the purpose of describing the location of injuries and signs and symptoms

abrasion a wound in which the top layer of skin is scraped off

abuse intentional improper or excessive action that injures or causes harm to someone under the abuser's power, such as a child, elder, or spouse

access to gain entry to a patient entrapped in wreckage or a building in order to provide emergency care

accessory muscles muscles other than the diaphragm used in breathing, especially in respiratory distress

acquired immunodeficiency syndrome (AIDS) a fatal disease caused by the human immunodeficiency virus (HIV)

acute abdomen the medical term for sudden, severe abdominal pain

acute myocardial infarction (AMI) the condition of a sudden reduced blood flow to heart muscle; heart attack

advance directive a legal document in which a person states his or her wishes not to receive specified types of medical care in future situations when the person may be unable to express those wishes

Advanced Cardiac Life Support (ACLS) advanced medical procedures needed to restore a heartbeat; beyond the procedures of Basic Life Support

Advanced Life Support the use of specialized equipment and techniques for patient care, including giving medications, establishing IV lines, and performing endotracheal intubation

agonal respirations reflex gasping that may occur just after cardiac arrest; not true respiration

airborne transmission the process by which a pathogen existing in an infected person is transmitted into a different person through the air, usually via small fluid droplets the infected person coughs or sneezes out

airway the route air moves from the mouth and nose through the pharynx, trachea, and bronchi to the lungs

airway (adjunct) a shaped, tubelike device inserted into the mouth or nose that helps keep a patient's airway open during resuscitation or until the patient receives advanced medical attention

airway obstruction a condition in which the patient's airway is partially or completely obstructed by the tongue, vomit, other body tissue or fluids, or a foreign object, preventing the flow of air to the lungs; choking

altered mental status a phrase used to describe a change from a person's normal responsiveness and awareness, such as confusion, disorientation, dizziness, drowsiness, or partial or complete unresponsiveness

alveoli tiny air sacs in the lungs where oxygen and carbon dioxide pass into and out of small blood vessels

amniotic fluid the fluid surrounding the embryo and fetus within the amniotic sac; in lay language, it is sometimes called "water" (as in "my water broke")

amniotic sac a membrane surrounding the embryo and fetus in the uterus that contains amniotic fluid

amputation the complete cutting or tearing off of all or part of an extremity: a finger or toe, hand or foot, arm or leg

anaphylactic shock a form of shock resulting from an extreme allergic reaction, typically to an insect sting, food, medication, or some other substance; also called anaphylaxis

anaphylaxis another term for anaphylactic shock

anatomical position the position of the body for the purpose of describing location and directions: standing, face forward, with arms at sides and palms facing forward

angina pectoris chest pain caused by heart disease, usually occurring after intense activity or exertion; often called angina

anterior the front of the body

arteries blood vessels that carry oxygenated blood from the heart to all parts of the body

aspiration the movement or breathing in of vomit or other fluids or solids into the lungs

assault the crime of verbally or physically threatening to touch another person without consent

assessment the process of checking the patient for life threats and other medical problems before and during care

asthma a chronic disease in which the airway sometimes becomes narrow and the person has difficulty breathing

atherosclerosis a narrowing and "hardening" of the arteries caused by a buildup of plaque

atria (singular: atrium) the upper two of the heart's four chambers; receive blood back from the body and the lungs

aura a generalized sensation or a hallucinated sensation involving any of the senses that occurs before a seizure

auscultation a general term for listening; specifically, listening to the pulse or breathing using a stethoscope

automated external defibrillator (AED) a device used to detect ventricular fibrillation and deliver a shock to the heart to restore a regular rhythm

AVPU scale a method for evaluating a patient's responsiveness in one of four categories: Alert, responsive to Verbal stimuli, responsive to Pain, or Unresponsive

avulsion an open wound in which an area of skin or other soft tissue is torn partially from the body

B

backboard a device for stabilizing a patient's spine and head before moving; a short backboard is used for patients found in a sitting position, as in a vehicle, and a long backboard is used for patients found lying down

bag-valve-mask (BVM) a resuscitation mask unit with a connected airbag that is squeezed to provide ventilations to a patient; often called a bag mask

barrier device a device like a pocket mask or face shield that provides a barrier between a patient and rescuer when giving rescue breathing, used to reduce the risk of disease transmission

baseline the first measurement taken, such as a patient's initial vital signs

Basic Life Support basic care for the patient's airway, breathing, and circulation provided by First Responders and EMTs

battery the crime of touching another person without consent

behavioral emergency a situation in which the patient's behavior, whether caused by injury or illness or by personality or mental health factors, results in an emergency situation, including the potential for violence or suicide

birth canal the structures from the lower uterus to the vaginal opening through which the infant passes in childbirth

bloodborne transmission the transmission of disease from one person to another through contact with the infected person's blood or certain other body fluids or tissues

blood pressure the force of the blood against the arterial wall as a result of the heart's pumping action; a vital sign revealing information about a patient's condition

bloody show the passing of the mucus plug from the cervix, which had blocked the uterus from possible infection from the vagina, prior to childbirth

blow-by oxygen oxygen administered to a patient from a source placed near the face but not through a mask directly on the face

body mechanics principles for moving and using the body safely to prevent strains and other injuries caused by lifting or other stresses

body substance isolation (BSI) techniques to prevent contact with or exposure to a patient's body fluids and other potentially contaminated materials

body system a group of organs that work together to perform a major body function

brachial pulse the pulse felt over the brachial artery in the inner upper arm, about midway between the shoulder and elbow; typically used for the pulse of an infant

bradycardia a slow heartbeat, usually considered less than 60 beats/minute

breech presentation the position in which the infant's buttocks or feet move first into the birth canal rather than the head; also called breech birth

bronchi (singular: bronchus) the passageways from the trachea to the lungs

bronchodilator a drug that relaxes the muscles of the airway, often administered by an inhaler in a person with asthma

bronchus (plural: bronchi) passageway from the trachea to the lungs

bulb syringe a small bulb made of soft rubber used to suction an infant's mouth and nose

burn damage caused to skin and other tissue by heat, chemicals, or electricity

C

capillaries very small blood vessels between the arteries and veins with thin walls where oxygen and carbon dioxide are exchanged

cardiac arrest the condition in which the heart stops beating or beating effectively enough to circulate blood

cardiac chain of survival a concept emphasizing four steps needed for cardiac arrest patients: (1) early access, (2) early CPR, (3) early defibrillation, and (4) early advanced medical care

cardiopulmonary resuscitation (CPR) a Basic Life Support procedure for a patient who is not breathing and has no heartbeat, consisting of ventilations combined with chest compressions

carotid pulse the pulse felt over the carotid artery in a neck of an adult or child

central nervous system that part of the nervous system formed by the brain and spinal cord

cerebrovascular accident (CVA) the medical terms for a stroke, resulting when blood flow is reduced to a part of the brain

cervix the lower part of the uterus, opening into the vagina

chief complaint the patient's primary problem, as identified by the patient or the person calling EMS for help

choking a physical obstruction of the airway, such as by food or by the tongue in an unresponsive person

chronic a long-term illness or health condition, often incurable; chronic conditions often make the individual more susceptible to the effects of injuries or sudden illnesses

chronic obstructive pulmonary disease (COPD) a group of respiratory diseases, including emphysema and chronic bronchitis, in which breathing can become difficult

Cincinnati Prehospital Stroke Scale (CPSS) a screening process for rapid identification of a stroke outside the hospital

circulatory system the body system that moves the blood to transport oxygen and nutrients throughout the body, to supply cells and remove wastes

citizen responder a lay person, ideally trained in first aid and CPR, who helps an ill or injured person and/or activates the EMS system in an emergency

clavicle the collarbone

closed injury an injury in which the skin is not broken

closed wound another term for a closed injury

clotting the body's process by which blood and other substances thicken to stop bleeding from an injured blood vessel

compensation a mechanism by which the body attempts to make up for decreased blood volume by increasing the heart and breathing rates

competent the victim is able to understand what is happening and the implications of his or her decision about receiving or refusing emergency care

concussion a type of brain injury resulting from a blow to the head, involving a temporary impairment of brain function but usually not permanent damage

consent the act of granting permission for treatment by a conscious, competent adult

contraction the pumping action of the heart

contusion a bruised muscle

cot another term for a stretcher

cramp a tightening of a muscle that usually results from prolonged use

cravat a strip of cloth used to tie a splint in place

crepitus a grating sensation felt or heard when fractured bone ends rub against each other

cricoid pressure a technique of applying pressure to an area of cartilage in the neck to prevent the air given during rescue breathing from moving down the esophagus to the stomach; also called the Sellick maneuver

critical incident an emergency situation particularly stressful to EMS personnel

critical incident stress debriefing (CISD) a program designed to help emergency personnel cope with the severe stress of an emergency situation

critical incident stress management (CISM) programs available in most public safety departments or EMS systems for those who experience uncontrollable stress resulting from a critical incident or from an accumulation of events

croup a viral infection of the upper and lower airway that causes a swelling of the tissues below the voice box

crowning the stage of childbirth when the infant's head is passing into the birth canal and is visible

cyanosis a blue coloring of the nail beds, mucous membranes of the mouth, or skin that results when body tissues do not receive sufficient oxygen

D

debriefing a CISD team meeting generally held within 24 to 72 hours after a major incident to help emergency workers manage their feelings and overcome stress

decompensation the failure of the body's compensating mechanisms for coping with diminished blood volume; shock occurs with decompensation

decontamination the use of physical or chemical means to remove, inactivate, or destroy bloodborne pathogens on a surface or item so that it is no longer infectious

defibrillation the process of administering an electrical shock to a fibrillating heart to restore a normal heart rhythm

defusing a short CISD session, typically less formal and less structured than a debriefing

delirium tremens a condition caused by alcohol withdrawal in a dependent person, causing altered mental status and other signs and symptoms

dependent lividity the settling of blood in the lowest parts of the body after death, causing large areas of a reddish-purple appearance

diabetes a metabolic disorder in which not enough insulin is produced or the body has developed

resistance in the use of insulin, resulting in blood sugar (glucose) levels not being well regulated by the body

diaphragm a muscle between the abdomen and lungs that moves with breathing

diastolic pressure blood pressure when the heart relaxes between beats

direct contact disease transmission that occurs when someone directly contacts an infected person, or fluids or substances from that person

direct medical control the process by which the medical director or designated medical control physician is personally involved in directing patient care provided by EMS personnel through online communications

disentanglement the process of freeing a patient from entrapment in wreckage, a building, or similar situation

disinfectant a substance, such as a bleach solution, that kills most pathogens on contaminated surfaces

dislocation movement of one or more bones out of their normal position in a joint, usually with ligament damage

dispatcher the person within the EMS system who answers 911 or other emergency calls and determines what emergency personnel and equipment to send to the scene; also called an emergency medical dispatcher (EMD)

distal indicates farther away from the trunk of the body

Do Not Resuscitate (DNR) order a type of advance directive in which a person in advance refuses to accept resuscitative efforts in case of cardiac arrest

DOTS an acronym of what to look for in the physical examination of a trauma patient: Deformities, Open injuries, Tenderness (pain), and Swelling

durable power of attorney a type of advance directive by which a person gives another person the legal right and responsibility to make healthcare decisions, including the right to refuse certain types of care

duty to act the legal concept pertaining to people who, by law or job description, have a responsibility to provide medical care

dysrhythmia an irregular heartbeat, also called arrhythmia

E

electrodes the pads of an automated external defibrillator (AED), which detect the patient's heart rhythm for analysis and deliver a shock when appropriate

embryo a developing human from the time of implantation of the fertilized egg in the uterus through the first 8 weeks

Emergency Medical Services (EMS) system a complex healthcare system that provides prehospital care to ill and injured patients, consisting of a tiered approach involving lay persons, First Responders, EMTs, Paramedics, and others

Emergency Medical Technician (EMT) a professional trained in emergency care who has completed an approved Emergency Medical Technician training program at the basic (EMT-B), intermediate (EMT-I), or Paramedic (EMT-P) level

emergency move moving a patient before completing care; this type of move is performed only if the patient and rescuer are in immediate danger or if necessary to provide care

emphysema a respiratory disease that reduces the capacity of the lungs to absorb oxygen

endocrine system the body system that produces hormones that help regulate many body functions

enhanced 911 an EMS communication system in which a call to 911 from a landline telephone provides the dispatcher with the address of the caller

entrance/exit wounds two related wounds such as burned areas on the body where electricity entered and left the body or wounds caused by a bullet entering and exiting the body

epiglottis a tissue flap that prevents solids and liquids from entering the trachea

epiglottitis a rare, life-threatening infection of the epiglottis, which can swell to the point where the airway is completely obstructed

epilepsy a disease affecting the brain that causes seizures

EpiPen® a commercial emergency epinephrine kit used for anaphylactic reactions

esophagus the tube that carries food to the stomach from the throat

evisceration protrusion of abdominal organs through an open wound in the abdominal wall

exposure control plan a plan employers must have in place to prevent exposure to bloodborne pathogens

expressed consent the patient explicitly grants permission for care, usually with verbal agreement or a nod

external respiration the process by which oxygen enters the blood from inhaled air and carbon dioxide exits the blood into exhaled air

extremities the arms and legs

extrication the removal of a patient from an entrapped position such as inside a vehicle or from beneath debris

F

face shield a type of barrier device, shaped from a thin piece of plastic, used when providing ventilations

febrile seizure convulsions caused by a rapidly rising body temperature (fever)

femoral pulse the pulse felt over the femoral artery in the center of the groin crease

femur the long bone of the upper leg

fetus a developing human in the uterus from the age of 8 weeks until birth

fibrillation a serious dysrhythmia, common after a heart attack, in which the heart muscle quivers rather than pumping blood

fibula the smaller of the two bones of the lower leg

first-degree burn an alternate term for a superficial burn

First Responder a person who may be called upon to provide emergency care as a routine part of his or her job and who has a professional duty to respond to medical emergencies

flowmeter a piece of oxygen equipment used to adjust the rate of oxygen delivery to the patient

focused physical exam an incomplete physical exam, used with a responsive medical patient or a trauma patient with only a minor injury, that focuses on the condition

fontanels the "soft spots" of an infant's skull between cranial bones that have not yet fused

foreign body airway obstruction (FBAO) a condition in which the patient's airway is partially or completely obstructed by a foreign object, preventing the flow of air to the lungs; choking

fracture a break in a bone

frostbite a condition in which localized skin and other tissue freezes and dies, caused by exposure to freezing temperatures

full-thickness burn a burn that damages the skin all the way through and may burn muscle or other tissues, causing a medical emergency; a third-degree burn

G

gastrointestinal system the body system that extracts energy and nutrients from food to meet the body's needs

general impression the initial impression a responder forms of the patient's condition based on observations while approaching the patient

glucose blood sugar

Good Samaritan laws laws in most states that protect persons from legal liability who voluntarily render care, in good faith, at the scene of an emergency

H

hand-off report detailed information about the patient given to other responding EMS personnel

hazardous materials (hazmat) substances that can be harmful or toxic to the body or environment, including liquids, solids, and gasses

head tilt–chin lift a maneuver for opening the airway in an unresponsive patient not suspected to have a spinal injury, by tilting the head back and lifting the chin

Health Insurance Portability and Accountability Act (HIPAA) federal legislation concerning how all providers of healthcare must handle patient records and confidentiality

heat exhaustion a condition of dehydration and depletion of salt and electrolytes in the body caused by heavy sweating if the person does not get enough fluids when active in a hot environment

heatstroke a life-threatening condition in which the body's core temperature rises abnormally high when heat loss mechanisms fail to maintain a normal body temperature in a hot environment

hemothorax the accumulation of blood in the thoracic cavity around the lungs caused by internal bleeding

hepatitis the various forms of liver disease caused by the bloodborne hepatitis B virus (HBV), hepatitis C virus (HCV), or other hepatitis viruses

history information gained from the patient and others about the patient's condition and potentially related other factors; see SAMPLE history

HIV the human immunodeficiency virus that causes AIDS

humerus the bone of the upper arm

hyperglycemia high blood sugar, usually in a person with diabetes, which can become a medical emergency

hyperventilation fast, deep breathing usually caused by anxiety or stress

hypoglycemia low blood sugar, usually in a person with diabetes, which can become a medical emergency

hypoperfusion a circulatory system condition resulting from the inadequate delivery of oxygenated blood to body tissues; also called shock

hypothermia a lowering of the body's core temperature; a life-threatening emergency resulting when the body cannot produce enough heat to compensate for heat loss in a cold environment

I

immune system the body system that helps fight disease

immunity the state of being protected against an infectious disease

implied consent the legal concept that assumes that an unresponsive or incompetent adult, or a child without a parent or guardian present, in need of emergency medical care would consent to that care if possible

inadequate breathing a condition in which the patient is not getting enough oxygen because of breathing too slowly (less than 10 breaths/minute) or too weakly

Incident Command System (ICS) an emergency management system that is part of the National Incident Management System (NIMS), designed to control and direct emergency resources at the scene of a large-scale emergency

Incident Commander the person with ultimate responsibility for workers and resources at a mass-casualty incident or a large-scale emergency

indirect contact disease transmission that occurs when someone contacts contaminated objects, food or drink, droplets in the air, or vectors such as insects

indirect medical control the offline or prospective direction provided by the medical director, including protocols (standing orders), standards of training, and quality assurance programs

inferior indicates toward the feet

initial assessment the first patient assessment, performed as soon as the patient is reached, to identify any immediate threats to life

insulin a hormone secreted by the pancreas that helps regulate blood sugar levels

internal bleeding bleeding caused by injury or illness in which the blood remains within the body rather than escaping through an open wound

internal respiration the process of oxygen and carbon dioxide moving into and out of the blood within internal body tissues

irrigate to wash out a wound under running water

J

jaw thrust a maneuver for opening the airway in an unresponsive trauma patient by lifting the jaw upward using both hands

L

laceration a cut in the skin that may penetrate and also damage underlying tissue

lateral indicates away from the midline of the body

ligament a tough, fibrous band that holds bones together in a joint

living will an advance directive specifying the types of healthcare a person does or does not want to receive in future situations when the person may be unable to express those wishes

log roll a technique requiring several responders, this move is used to move a patient from a prone position to a supine position for assessment and treatment or to move a patient onto a backboard or stretcher

lungs the organs in the thoracic cavity where oxygen and carbon dioxide are exchanged in inhaled air

lymphatic system the body system consisting of lymph nodes and lymphatic vessels that helps defend against disease as part of the immune system

M

mass-casualty incident (MCI) an emergency involving multiple patients who require care

mechanism of injury how the patient was injured, including the forces involved

meconium the feces of an infant, which may mix with amniotic fluid prior to childbirth

medial toward the midline of the body

medical director the physician who oversees out-of-hospital emergency medical care

medical oversight the process by which the medical director oversees out-of-hospital emergency medical care

medical patient a patient with signs and symptoms of illness

midline a hypothetical line down the center of the body, dividing the body into left and right halves

miscarriage spontaneous death of the embryo or fetus before the middle of the second trimester; also called spontaneous abortion

musculoskeletal system the body system that gives the body shape and strength and makes movement possible

myocardium heart muscle

N

nasal airway another term for a nasopharyngeal airway

nasal cannula an oxygen delivery device usually used with a breathing patient who does not require a high concentration of oxygen; also called nasal prongs

nasopharyngeal airway (NPA) a nasal airway adjunct inserted through the nose and into the pharynx to help maintain an open airway

nasopharynx the upper section of the airway from the nasal cavity

National Incident Management System (NIMS) a national system directed by the Department of Homeland Security that coordinates and manages preparedness for and response to large-scale emergencies

neglect failing to provide for the basic needs of someone who has a claim to the caretaker's care

negligence the failure to give reasonable care as one has been trained, when such failure results in injury or damage to another

neonate an infant in the first month of life

nervous system the body system that controls all body functions and movement and allows for sensory perception and consciousness

nitroglycerin prescription medication for angina and heart attack, which increases blood flow through partially restricted coronary arteries

nonemergency move moving a patient after emergency care and stabilization have been carried out

nonrebreathing mask an oxygen delivery device composed of a mask and reservoir bag, used with a breathing patient

notification the process of alerting First Responders and other emergency personnel to a medical emergency

O

occlusive dressing an air- and watertight dressing used to seal a wound or burn

Occupational Exposure to Bloodborne Pathogens Standard a set of regulations from the Occupational Safety and Health Administration (OSHA) designed to protect employees from exposure to bloodborne disease pathogens

ongoing assessment reassessment of the patient while awaiting additional EMS resources and giving emergency care

open injury an injury in which the skin is torn or cut open, often causing bleeding

open wound another term for open injury

OPIM acronym for "other potentially infectious materials," a phrase used by OSHA to denote materials other than blood, such as a body tissue or culture, that may transmit a bloodborne pathogen

oral airway another term for an oropharyngeal airway

organ a body part that accomplishes one or more specific functions

oropharyngeal airway (OPA) an oral airway adjunct inserted through the mouth and into the pharynx to help maintain an open airway

oropharynx the lower section of the airway (throat) from the oral cavity

orthopedic stretcher a type of portable stretcher that splits apart lengthwise for positioning under a patient from both sides; also called a scoop stretcher

osteoporosis a bone condition involving a loss of calcium; more common in old age

oxygen delivery device a piece of equipment, such as a resuscitation mask, that provides oxygen to the patient

oxygen reservoir a bag attached to a mask that temporarily holds supplemental oxygen from the tank for the patient to inhale

P

pacemaker a small, electronic device implanted under the skin in some patients with heart disease, which helps the heart maintain a regular rhythm

palpate to feel a body area to identify signs and symptoms of injury or illness

Paramedic an EMT who has completed an approved Paramedic training program involving many advanced emergency procedures including the administration of intravenous fluids and drugs

partial-thickness burn a burn that damages the skin's deeper layers but does not penetrate to tissues beneath the skin; a second-degree burn

patella the bone of the kneecap

patent a condition of being open and clear, as in a patent airway

pathogen infectious substance, such as bacteria or a virus, capable of inducing disease

patient packaging the process of completely stabilizing and preparing a patient for transport, including treatment for life-threatening problems, bandaging, splinting, and spinal stabilization

pelvic cavity the cavity within the pelvic structures in which the bladder and other organs are located

pelvis generally the area below the abdomen and specifically the pelvic bones between the hip and the lower spine

perfusion the flow of blood through a body area

personal protective equipment (PPE) barriers, such as gloves and resuscitation masks, that prevent being exposed to blood and other body fluids when caring for a patient in an emergency or working around potentially infected materials

pharynx the section of the airway at the back of the oral and nasal cavities; the throat

physical examination the process of examining an injured or ill patient head to toe to find conditions requiring treatment

placenta an organ that develops in pregnancy to supply the embryo and fetus with oxygen and nutrients from the mother by means of the umbilical cord

pneumothorax accumulation of air in the thoracic cavity around the lungs, caused by escape of air from the lung due to an injury or a puncture of the chest wall

Poison Control Center (PCC) one of a national network of centers designed to provide information about specific poisons in an emergency

posterior the back of the body

prehospital care the phase of emergency medical care provided before a patient is delivered to a hospital

pre-planning a process of developing an organized plan in anticipation of an emergency likely in a given location; the pre-plan should identify responding personnel, possible scene hazards, routes of evacuation, and other action guidelines

pressure dressing a dressing that maintains pressure on an open wound to control bleeding

pressure regulator a piece of oxygen equipment that connects to the oxygen tank to reduce the pressure of oxygen leaving the tank to a safe level

prolapsed cord a situation in which a segment of the umbilical cord protrudes through the birth canal before childbirth

prone lying facedown

proximal closer toward the trunk of the body

pulmonary refers to the lungs; for example, the pulmonary artery carries blood to the lungs to be oxygenated, and the pulmonary vein carries oxygenated blood from the lungs to the heart to be pumped throughout the body

pulse rhythmic changes in the blood pressure in arteries caused by the heartbeat, which can be felt in certain body locations

puncture an injury into the skin caused by a sharp, penetrating object that may also damage deeper tissues

R

rabies a viral disease, fatal if not treated in time, usually transmitted by the bite of an infected animal

radial pulse the pulse felt over the radial artery in the wrist at the base of the thumb

radius one of the two bones of the lower arm

rapid trauma assessment the complete physical exam of an unresponsive patient or a patient with a significant mechanism of injury

recovery position a position used for nontrauma, unresponsive, breathing patients; the patient is positioned on the side to keep the airway open and allow fluids to drain from the mouth

removal the act of removing a patient from wreckage or a building after providing emergency care and disentangling the patient

reproductive system the body system that makes human reproduction possible

respiratory arrest a condition in which breathing has completely stopped

responsiveness a patient's mental status, ranging from being conscious and alert to being completely unresponsive to all stimuli

restraint a device used to restrain a violent or potentially violent patient, such as plastic or leather loops used to cuff the hands

resuscitation mask a barrier device used to give ventilations; also called a pocket face mask or a face mask

retractions areas between bones of the thorax and neck that move inward with the work of breathing in a patient in respiratory distress

rule of nines a method calculating the percentage of body surface area of a burn

S

SAMPLE history an acronym for information gathered in a patient history: Signs and symptoms, Allergies, Medications, Pertinent previous problems, Last food or drink, and Events

scapula the bone of the shoulder blade

scene size-up the process of checking the emergency scene on arrival for safety and other factors, including taking BSI precautions, looking for hazards, and checking for clues about what happened

scoop stretcher another term for an orthopedic stretcher

scope of practice the level of care that can be provided by a healthcare professional with a specified level of training

second-degree burn an alternate term for a partial-thickness burn

shaken baby syndrome a pattern of internal injuries that typically result when a caretaker becomes frustrated with a crying infant and shakes the infant

shock a life-threatening condition that occurs when vital body organs are not receiving enough oxygen; hypoperfusion

sign an objective observation or measurement such as warm skin or a deformed extremity

sinus rhythm the heart's normal rhythm

sling a device used to support and immobilize the arm, made of a wide bandage or cloth tied around the neck

spinal column refers generally to the vertebrae that extend from the base of the brain to the "tailbone," as well as to the nerves, or spinal cord, running through the vertebrae

spinal cord the bundle of nerves running through the vertebrae

splint a device for immobilizing a part of the body

spontaneous abortion the medical term for a miscarriage

sprain damage to ligaments and other structures in a joint

stair chair a device for carrying a patient in a seated position down stairs or through a confined space where a stretcher cannot be used

standard of care the minimal standard and quality of care expected of First Responders; the care that a reasonable, prudent First Responder with similar training would give a patient in similar circumstances

standard precautions a set of safety guidelines for treating all blood and other potentially infectious materials as if they are contaminated; also called universal precautions

START system "Simple Triage And Rapid Treatment" triage system for evaluating and treating multiple patients when resources and personnel are limited

sterilize to use a chemical or physical procedure to destroy all microbial life on an item

sternum breastbone

stoma a hole in the neck, used for breathing, surgically created as a result of an injury or illness

strain a tearing of muscle or tendon tissue

stress a mental and emotional state that also has many physical effects, resulting from any negative experience that causes psychological strain or disequilibrium

stretcher a device for moving or transporting a patient; a standard stretcher has wheels, rails, and legs that fold as the stretcher is slid into an ambulance; also called a cot or gurney

stridor a high-pitched whistling sound on inhaling, such as may be caused by an obstruction

sucking chest wound an open wound in the chest caused by a penetrating injury that lets air move in and out of the chest during breathing

suction negative relative pressure produced by a device, used to clear the airway of liquid or semi-liquid material

sudden illness a medical crisis that occurs with no or little warning and requires emergency care until the patient can be seen by a medical professional

sudden infant death syndrome (SIDS) the unexpected and sudden death of a seemingly normal and healthy infant that occurs during sleep

superficial burn a usually minor burn that damages only the skin's outer layer

superior toward the head

supine lying face up

supplemental oxygen oxygen in a tank administered to ill or injured patients

symptom a subjective observation reported by the patient, such as pain or nausea

systolic pressure blood pressure when the heart contracts

T

tendon a fibrous band of tissue that attaches muscle to bone

tetanus a serious infection caused by common bacteria, also called lockjaw

third-degree burn an alternate term for a full-thickness burn

thoracic cavity the area inside the chest where the heart and lungs are located

thorax the chest area enclosed by the ribs (including the back of the body)

tibia the larger of the two bones of the lower leg

tourniquet a band rarely applied around an extremity above a wound as an extreme last resort to control bleeding by cutting off circulation to the extremity

trachea the tube carrying air from the larynx to the bronchi

trauma dressing thick, bulky dressings used with large or irregular wounds, or dressings used to stabilize an impaled object

trauma patient a patient with an injury

triage the process of sorting patients by the severity of their injuries so that those with the highest priority are treated first

triage category classification that describes the severity of a patient's injuries: immediate, urgent, delayed, or no care

tripod position the position often taken by a person in respiratory distress: sitting and leaning forward, with hands on knees

tuberculosis (TB) a highly contagious airborne disease caused by bacteria

U

ulna one of the two bones of the lower arm

umbilical cord an organ containing an artery and vein that connects the embryo and fetus to the mother

urinary system the body system that removes liquid wastes from the body and helps maintain the body's water balance

uterus the muscular, hollow female organ in which an embryo and fetus develops and to which the placenta is attached

V

vaccine a drug that stimulates the immune system to produce antibodies to a specific disease, thereby making a person immune to the disease

vagina the hollow tubelike female organ opening outside the body, through which an infant passes in childbirth

vasoconstriction the contraction of blood vessels

vasodilation the dilation of blood vessels

veins blood vessels that return deoxygenated blood from the body to the heart

ventilation the process of moving air or oxygen into the lungs of a patient who is not breathing or is breathing inadequately; also refers to each breath given

ventricles the lower two of the heart's four chambers, which pump blood to the body and lungs

ventricular fibrillation (V-fib) an abnormal heart rhythm, which commonly occurs with heart attacks, in which the ventricles of the heart are quivering instead of beating rhythmically

vernix a protective, white, cheesy-looking coating found on a newborn's skin

vertebrae the bones in the back and neck

vest extrication device a device that helps stabilize the head and spine when extricating a patient from a vehicle or other sitting position

vital signs observable characteristics of a patient's status, generally including assessments of respirations, pulse, skin characteristics, pupils, and blood pressure

Index

A